The ABSITE Review

Third Edition

The ABSITE Review

Third Edition

Steven M. Fiser, MD

Cardiac Surgery Specialists
Bon Secours Heart and Vascular Institute
Richmond, Virginia

. Wolters Kluwer | Lippincott Williams & Wilkins
Health
Philadelphia • Baltimore • New York • London
Buenos Aires • Hong Kong • Sydney • Tokyo

Acquisitions Editor: Brian Brown
Managing Editor: Jamie Elfrank
Production Manager: Bridgett Dougherty
Marketing Manager: Lisa Lawrence
Manufacturing Manager: Kathleen Brown
Design Coordinator: Stephen Druding
Compositor: Aptara, Inc.

Library of Congress Cataloging-in-Publication Data

Fiser, Steven M., 1971-
 The ABSITE review / Steven M. Fiser.—3rd ed.
   p. ; cm.
 Other title: American Board of Surgery In-Training Examination review
 Includes bibliographical references and index.
 Summary: "The ABSITE Review was developed to serve as a quick and thorough study guide for the ABSITE, such that it could be used independently of other material and would cover nearly all topics found on the exam. The outline format makes it easy to hit the essential points on each topic quickly and succinctly, without having to wade through the extraneous material found in most textbooks. As opposed to question-and-answer reviews, the format also promotes rapid memorization. Although specifically designed for general surgery residents taking the ABSITE, the information contained in The ABSITE Review is also especially useful for certain other groups"—Provided by publisher.
  ISBN 978-1-60831-607-6 (pbk. : alk. paper)
  1. Surgery—Examinations, questions, etc. 2. Surgery, Operative—Examinations, questions, etc.
I. Title. II. Title: American Board of Surgery In-Training Examination review.
  [DNLM: 1. Surgical Procedures, Operative—Outlines. 2. Clinical Medicine—Outlines.
WO 18.2 F531a 2010]
  RD37.2.F58 2010
  617.0076—dc22

                                                                              2010020006

                                                              10 9 8 7 6 5 4 3 2 1

CCS0810

CONTENTS

CREDITS

FIGURE CREDITS

Figures on the page numbers listed are reprinted with permission from: *Greenfield's Surgery: Scientific Principles & Practice, 4e,* Mulholland MW, Lillemoe KD, Doherty GM, Maier RV, Upchurch GR, eds. Philadelphia, PA: Lippincott Williams & Wilkins; 2006.
1, 2, 3, 16, 17, 18, 42, 46, 56, 58, 62, 63, 64, 66, 70, 73, 76, 81, 82, 83, 84, 90, 92, 99, 100, 104, 110, 114, 122, 126, 128, 129, 141, 143, 148, 149, 151, 152, 153, 156, 160, 161, 169, 171, 176, 177, 178, 179, 181, 183, 186, 187, 189, 190, 193, 194, 205, 207, 209, 211, 212, 214, 215, 217, 218, 219, 221, 223, 224, 231, 234, 235, 236, 240, 247, 250, 252, 255, 257, 258, 259, 260, 261, 262, 265, 267, 269, 271, 276, 279, 280, 281, 283, 286, 287, 288, 289, 292, 293, 294, 295, 297, 298, 302, 303, 304, 307, 308, 309, 310, 311, 313, 314, 331, 333, 335, 336, 337, 345, 349, 350, 351, 352, 354, 355, 357, 358, 360

TABLE CREDITS

Tables on the page numbers listed are reprinted with permission from the following chapters in *Greenfield's Surgery: Principles and Practice, 4e.* Mulholland MW, Lillemoe KD, Doherty GM, Maier RV, Upchurch GR, eds. Philadelphia, PA: Lippincott Williams & Wilkins; 2006.

Dellinger EP. Surgical Infections.
21, 23

Gibran NS. Burns.
103, 104, 105

Rutter TW, Tremper KK.
Anesthesiology and Pain Management.
35, 36 (top), 37 (bottom)

Smith JS Jr, Frankenfield DC,
Souba WW. Nutrition and Metabolism.
43, 44

Libutti SK. Cancer.
50, 53 (top)

Merion RM. Organ Preservation.
59

Cuschieri J. Shock.
72 (top)

Chesnut RM. Head Trauma.
72

Wisner DH, Hoyt DB. Abdominal Trauma.
90

Nathens AB, Maier RV. Critical Care.
100 (bottom)

Chang AE, Johnson TM, Gira AK.
Cutaneous Neoplasms.
111, 112

Sabel MS. Sarcomas of Bone and Soft
Tissue.
115

Moyer JS, Teknos TN. Head and Neck.
119, 121

Morrow M, Khan S. Breast Disease.
149, 151, 152, 154, 155, 157, 158

Lane JS, Messina LM. Cerebrovascular
Occlusive Disease.
180 (top)

Mulholland MW. Gastroduodenal
Ulceration.
222, 224

Turner DJ, Bass BL. Small Intestinal
Neoplasms.
229

PREFACE TO THE FIRST EDITION

Each year, thousands of general surgery residents across the country express anxiety over preparation for the American Board of Surgery In-Training Examination (ABSITE), an exam designed to test residents on their knowledge of the many topics related to general surgery.

This exam is important to the future career of general surgery residents for several reasons. Academic centers and private practices searching for new general surgeons use ABSITE scores as part of the evaluation process. Fellowships in fields such as surgical oncology, trauma, and cardiothoracic surgery use these scores when evaluating potential fellows. Residents with high ABSITE results are looked upon favorably by general surgery program directors, as high scorers enhance program reputation, helping garner applications from the best medical students interested in surgery.

General surgery programs also use the ABSITE scores, with consideration of feedback on clinical performance, when evaluating residents for promotion through residency. Clearly, this examination is important to general surgery residents.

Much of the anxiety over the ABSITE stems from the issue that there are no dedicated outline-format review manuals available to assist in preparation. *The ABSITE Review* was developed to serve as a quick and thorough study guide for the ABSITE, such that it could be used independently of other material and would cover nearly all topics found on the exam. The outline format makes it easy to hit the essential points on each topic quickly and succinctly, without having to wade through the extraneous material found in most textbooks. As opposed to question-and-answer reviews, the format also promotes rapid memorization.

Although specifically designed for general surgery residents taking the ABSITE, the information contained in *The ABSITE Review* is also especially useful for certain other groups:

- General surgery residents preparing for their written American Board of Surgery certification examination
- Surgical residents going into another specialty who want a broad perspective of general surgery and surgical subspecialties (and who may also be required to take the ABSITE)
- Practicing surgeons preparing for their American Board of Surgery recertification examination

PREFACE TO THE THIRD EDITION

I do *not* want to waste your time. I do want to provide you with the most comprehensive, accurate, and efficient books available for the ABSITE. Residency is time consuming, with the average resident working 80 hours per week. It is hard to squeeze in sufficient time to study for the ABSITE. In addition, these scores matter for fellowships and appointments. The books I write distill the essential information required for the ABSITE down into usable blocks, making your study time much more efficient and powerful.

This book has been updated to reflect information from recent examinations. Additional diagrams and algorithms have been added as well. This book is also in color, which adds further depth to the illustrations.

Again, I thank all of the residents who gave me feedback on the books or came up to me at meetings saying "Hey, I used your books in residency and they really saved me." I am glad to have helped out.

Thank you again and good luck on the ABSITE.

CHAPTER 1. CELL BIOLOGY

CELL MEMBRANE

- **A lipid bilayer** that contains protein channels, enzymes, and receptors
- **Cholesterol** increases membrane fluidity
- Cells are negative inside compared with outside, based on Na/K ATPase (3 Na^+ out/2 K^+ in)
- The Na^+ gradient that is created is used for cotransport of glucose, proteins, and other molecules

Electrolyte Concentrations of Intracellular and Extracellular Fluid Compartments

	Extracellular Fluid (mEq/L) Plasma	Intracellular Fluid (mEq/L)
CATIONS		
Na^+	140	12
K^+	4	150
Ca^{2+}	5	10^{-7}
Mg^{2+}	2	7
ANIONS		
Cl^-	103	3
HCO_3^-	24	10
SO_4^{2-}	1	—
HPO_4^{3-}	2	116
Protein	16	40
Organic anions	5	—

Adapted from Wait RB, et al. Fluids and electrolytes and acid–base balance. In: Greenfield LJ, et al., eds. *Surgery: Scientific Principles and Practice*. 3rd ed. Philadelphia: Lippincott Williams & Wilkins; 2001:245)

- **Desmosomes/hemidesmosomes** – these are adhesion molecules (cell–cell and cell–extracellular matrix), which anchor cells
- **Tight junctions** – these are cell–cell occluding junctions and form an impermeable barrier (i.e., epithelium)
- **Gap junctions** – these allow communication between cells (connexin subunits)
- **G proteins** – intramembrane protein, transduce signal from receptor to response enzyme
- **Ligand-triggered protein kinase** – receptor and response enzyme are a single transmembrane protein

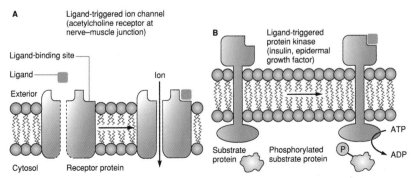

Types of cell surface receptors. *(A)* Ligand-activated ion channel; binding results in a conformational change, opening or activating the channel. *(B)* Ligand-activated protein kinase; binding activates the kinase domain, which phosphorylates substrate proteins. *(continued)*

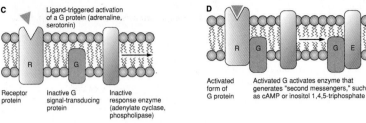

Types of cell surface receptors. (*Continued*) (*C* and *D*) Ligand activation of a G protein, which then activates an enzyme that generates second, or intracellular, messengers.

- **ABO blood-type antigens** – glycolipids on cell membrane
- **HLA-type antigens** – glycoproteins (Gp) on cell membrane

- **Osmotic equilibrium** – water will move from an area of low solute concentration to an area of high solute concentration and approach osmotic equilibrium

CELL CYCLE
- G1, S (protein synthesis, chromosomal duplication), G2, M (mitosis, nucleus divides)
- G1 most variable, determines <u>cell cycle length</u>
- Growth factors affect cell during G1
- Cells can also go to G0 (quiescent) from G1

Mitosis
- **Prophase** – centromere attachment, spindle formation, nucleus disappears
- **Metaphase** – chromosome alignment
- **Anaphase** – chromosomes pulled apart
- **Telophase** – separate nucleus reforms around each set of chromosomes

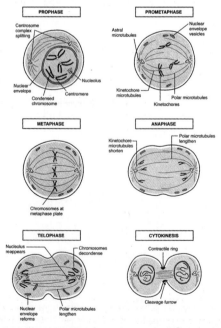

Diagram of the stages of the M (mitosis) phase. (From Dudek RW. *High-Yield Cell and Molecular Biology*. 2nd ed. Philadelphia: Lippincott Williams & Wilkins; 2007, with permission.)

- vWF links **GpIb receptor on platelets to collagen**
- PT normal; PTT can be normal or abnormal
- Have long **bleeding time** (ristocetin test)
- **Type I is most common** (70% of cases) and often has only mild symptoms
- **Type III causes the most severe bleeding**

- **Type I and III** – reduced quantity of circulating vWF
  - Tx: recombinant VIII:vWF, DDAVP, cryoprecipitate, conjugated estrogens
- **Type II** – defect in vWF molecule itself, have enough vWF but does not work well
  - Tx: recombinant VIII:vWF, cryoprecipitate

- ■ **Hemophilia A (VIII deficiency)**
  - Sex-linked recessive
  - Need levels 100% preoperatively; keep 30% after surgery
  - Prolonged PTT and normal PT
  - **Factor VIII crosses placenta** → newborns may not bleed at circumcision

  - **Hemophiliac joint – no aspiration**
    - Tx: ice, keep joint mobile with range of motion exercises, factor VIII concentrate or cryoprecipitate

  - Epistaxis, intracerebral hemorrhage, and hematuria may occur
    - Tx: recombinant VIII:vWF or cryoprecipitate; possibly DDAVP

- ■ **Hemophilia B (IX deficiency)** – Christmas disease
  - Sex-linked recessive
  - Need level 100% preoperatively
  - Prolonged PTT and normal PT
  - Tx: recombinant factor IX concentrate or FFP

- ■ **Factor VII deficiency** – prolonged PT and normal PTT, bleeding tendency. Tx: recombinant factor VII concentrate, **FFP**

Clinical Manifestations of Hemophilia A

Clinical Severity	Amount of Factor VIII Present (%)	Manifestations
Mild hemophilia	>5	May bleed after trauma or surgery
Moderate hemophilia	2–5	Usually only bleed after trauma or surgery
Severe hemophilia	<2	Spontaneous bleeds into muscles and joints

From O'Connell C, Dickey VL. *Blueprints Hematology and Oncology*. Philadelphia: Lippincott Williams & Wilkins; 2005, with permission.

Classification of von Willebrand Disease

Type I	Partial deficit of vWF	Autosomal dominant inheritance
Type II	Qualitative defect of vWF	Autosomal dominant inheritance
Type III	Complete deficiency (rare)	Autosomal recessive inheritance

From O'Connell C, Dickey VL. *Blueprints Hematology and Oncology*. Philadelphia: Lippincott Williams & Wilkins; 2005, with permission.

Perioperative Treatment of Bleeding Disorders

Hemophilia A (factor VIII)
Goal: Raise FVIII to 80%–100%
Approach: FVIII concentrate[a]. No. of units = (% × kg BW)/2
If inhibitors present:
  (1) 70–150 U/kg bolus, then 5–15 U/kg qh or 40 U/kg plus 20 U/kg for each Bethesda unit qh human FVIII
  (2) Plasmapheresis to remove inhibitor; replace FVIII with porcine or recombinant FVIII
  (3) Recombinant FIX or VII

Goal: Maintain FVIII at 80%–100% for 10–14 days
Approach: Same as for preop; reinfuse every 8–12 hours (or longer if surgery extensive)
Monitor FVIII levels as guide to therapy

Hemophilia B (factor IX)
Goals: (1) Factor IX levels to 80%–100%
Approach: (1) FIX concentrate[b]. No. of units = % × kg BW
                        (2) Use FFP if deficit and surgery minimal
N.B. FIX concentrate may cause thrombosis. Consider adding heparin 5,000 units SQ every 8 hours

Goal: Maintain FIX levels at 40%–50% for 2–3 days, then 20% for 7–10 days or longer, depending on the response
Approach: Same as preop
Monitor FIX levels as guide to therapy

von Willebrand's (vW factor)
Goals: (1) Raise vWf to 80–100 U/dL
                        (2) Replace abnormal vWf
                        (3) Raise FVIII as needed
Approach: (1) DDAVP – 0.3 pg/kg IV in 20 mL saline over 30 minutes; repeat q12–24h
                        (2) If DDAVP failure, use FVIII concentrate using same approach as above
                        (3) Replace FVIII as needed
Goals: (1) Maintain vWf at 40 U/dL for 2–3 days or longer as needed
                        (2) Maintain FVIII at 80%–100% levels for 4–5 days or longer
                        (3) Monitor vWf:R:Co and FVIII as guide to therapy

In hemophilia B, when the dose of factor IX for replacement therapy is calculated as described above and given as purified factor IX, the plasma factor IX level rises to only half of that expected from the units of factor IX listed on the bottle. This may reflect binding of infused factor IX to vascular endothelium.

An antifibrinolytic (ε-aminocaproic acid 2.5–4 g po qid for 1 week or tranexamic acid 1.0–1.5 g po tid or qid for 1 week) should be given to prevent late bleeding after dental extraction or other causes of oropharyngeal mucosal trauma (e.g., tongue laceration).

[a]Viral inactivated or recombinant factor VIII concentrate.
[b]Highly purified viral inactivated factor IX concentrate.
From Spence RK, Green A. Surgery in patients with congenital clotting deficiencies. In: Spiess BD, et al., eds. *Perioperative Transfusion Medicine.* 2nd ed. Philadelphia: Lippincott Williams & Wilkins; 2006, with permission.

- ■ **Platelet disorders** – cause bruising, epistaxis, mucosal bleeding, petechiae, purpura
  - **Acquired thrombocytopenia** – can be caused by H_2 blockers, heparin
  - **Glanzmann's thrombocytopenia** – GpIIb/IIIa receptor deficiency on platelets (cannot bind to each other)
    - Fibrin normally links the GpIIb/IIIa receptors together
    - Tx: <u>platelets</u>
    - **Bernard Soulier** – GpIb receptor deficiency on platelets (cannot bind to collagen)
    - vWF normally links GpIb to collagen
    - Tx: <u>platelets</u>
  - **Uremia** – inhibits platelet function
    - Tx: <u>hemodialysis</u> (1st), DDAVP, platelets

- **Ticlopidine** – decreases ADP in platelets, prevents exposure of GpIIb/IIIa. Tx: <u>platelets</u>
- **Dipyridamole** – inhibits cAMP phosphodiesterase, increases cAMP, decreases ADP-induced platelet aggregation. Tx: <u>platelets</u>
- **Pentoxifylline** – inhibits platelet aggregation. Tx: <u>platelets</u>
- **Clopidogrel (Plavix)** – ADP receptor antagonist. Tx: <u>platelets</u>
- **PCN/cephalosporins** – bind platelets, can **increase bleeding time**

Heparin-induced thrombocytopenia (HIT)
- Thrombocytopenia due to antiplatelet antibodies (IgG PF4 antibody) results in platelet destruction
- Can also cause platelet aggregation and thrombosis (HIT**T**; **T** = thrombosis)
- Forms a **white clot**
- Can occur with low doses of heparin
- Low-molecular-weight heparin may have a decreased risk of causing HIT
- Tx: stop heparin; argatroban, hirudin, ancrod, or dextran to anticoagulate

Disseminated intravascular coagulation (DIC)
- Decreased platelets, prolonged PT, prolonged PTT
- Low fibrinogen, high fibrin split products, high D-dimer
- Often initiated by tissue factor
- Need to treat underlying cause

ASA – stop 7 days before surgery; patients will have prolonged bleeding time
- <u>Inhibits cyclooxygenase in platelets, ↓ TXA_2</u>

Coumadin – stop 7 days before surgery, consider starting heparin while Coumadin wears off

Platelets – keep >50,000 before surgery, >20,000 after surgery

Prostate surgery – can release urokinase, activates plasminogen → thrombolysis
- Tx: ε-Aminocaproic acid (Amicar)

H and P – best way to predict the bleeding risk

Normal circumcision – does not rule out bleeding disorders; can still have clotting factors from mother

Abnormal bleeding with tooth extraction or tonsillectomy – picks up 99% patients with bleeding disorder

Epistaxis – common with vWF deficiency and platelet disorders

Menorrhagia – common with bleeding disorders

CONDITIONS CAUSING ABNORMAL HYPERCOAGULABILITY
Leiden factor – 30% of spontaneous venous thromboses
- **Most common congenital hypercoagulability disorder**
- Resistance to activated protein C, **defect on factor V**
- Tx: heparin, warfarin

Hyperhomocysteinemia – 10% of spontaneous venous thromboses
- **Tx: folic acid and B_{12}**

Prothrombin gene defect G20210 A – 5% of spontaneous venous thromboses
- **Tx**: heparin, warfarin

Protein C or S deficiency – 5% of spontaneous venous thromboses
- **Tx**: heparin, warfarin

◼ **Antithrombin III deficiency** – 2%–3% of spontaneous venous thromboses
  • **Heparin does not work in these patients**
  • Can develop after previous heparin exposure
  • Tx: recombinant AT-III concentrate or FFP (highest concentration of AT-III) followed by heparin or hirudin or ancrod; warfarin

◼ **Polycythemia vera** – defect in platelet function; usually have thrombosis, can have bleeding
  • Keep Hct < 48 and platelets < 400 before surgery
  • Tx: ASA

◼ **Lupus anticoagulant** – antiphospholipid antibodies
  • Not all of these patients have SLE
  • Procoagulant (get prolonged PTT but are hypercoagulable)
  • Dx: prolonged PTT (not corrected with FFP), positive Russell viper venom time, false-positive RPR test for syphilis
  • Tx: heparin, warfarin

◼ **Acquired hypercoagulability – tobacco** (most common factor causing acquired hypercoagulability), malignancy, inflammatory states, inflammatory bowel disease, infections, oral contraceptives, pregnancy, rheumatoid arthritis, postop patients, myeloproliferative disorders

Venous Thrombotic Workup

  ◼ Rule out obvious causes
  ◼ Activated protein C resistance[a]
  ◼ Lupus anticoagulant[a]
  ◼ Anticardiolipin antibodies by enzyme-linked immunosorbent assay
  ◼ Prothrombin 20210 mutation testing by polymerase chain reaction
  ◼ Antithrombin activity (functional)[a]
  ◼ Protein C and S activity (functional)[a]
  ◼ Factor VIII level with sedimentation rate or C-reactive protein
  ◼ Fasting total plasma homocysteine level
  ◼ Factor V Leiden mutation
  ◼ ᴅ-Dimer
  ◼ Complete blood cell count

  Older than 55 years, no other cause found, computed tomography scan of chest/abdomen/pelvis screen for cancer.

  [a]Preferable to n test in the setting of acute clot or heparin or Coumadin treatment.
  From O'Connell C, Dickey VL. *Blueprints Hematology and Oncology*. Philadelphia: Lippincott Williams & Wilkins; 2005, with permission.

Arterial Thrombotic Workup

  Venus workup
  Transthoracic echocardiogram with bubble study looking for patent shunt, foramen ovale
  Lipid panel and lipoprotein(a)

  From O'Connell C, Dickey VL. *Blueprints Hematology and Oncology*. Philadelphia: Lippincott Williams & Wilkins; 2005, with permission.

◼ **Cardiopulmonary bypass** – factor XII (Hageman factor) activated; results in hypercoagulable state
  • Tx: heparin

◼ **Warfarin-induced skin necrosis**
  • Occurs when placed on Coumadin without being heparinized first
  • Due to short half-life of proteins C and S, which are first to decrease in levels compared with the procoagulation factors; results in relative hyperthrombotic state

- **Patients with relative protein C deficiency are especially susceptible**
- Tx: heparin if it occurs; prevent by placing patient on heparin before starting warfarin

■ **Key elements in the development of venous thromboses (Virchow's triad)** – stasis, endothelial injury, and hypercoagulability
■ **Key element in the development of arterial thrombosis** – endothelial injury

DEEP VENOUS THROMBOSIS
■ Stasis, venous injury, and hypercoagulability risk factors
■ Treatment
  - **1st** – warfarin for 6 months
  - **2nd** – warfarin for 1 year
  - **3rd** or significant PE – warfarin for lifetime
■ **Greenfield filters** – for patients with contraindications to anticoagulation; with documented PE while on anticoagulation; with free-floating iliofemoral, IVC, or femoral deep venous thrombosis (DVT); who have undergone pulmonary embolectomy
  - temporary filters can be inserted in patients at high risk for DVT (i.e., head injury patients on prolonged bed rest)

General Guidelines for Duration of Treatment Time for Anticoagulation

Condition	Duration
Provoked DVT	3–6 mo
Idiopathic DVT	6 mo
Idiopathic DVT, recurrent	Indefinite
Cancer	Until cancer is no longer active
Idiopathic PE	Indefinite
ITD and no history of clotting	No treatment
DVT and antiphospholipid syndrome	Indefinite
Recurrent DVT and ITD	Indefinite

DVT, deep venous thrombosis; ITD, inherited thrombotic disorder; PE, pulmonary embolism.
From O'Connell C, Dickey VL. *Blueprints Hematology & Oncology*. Philadelphia: Lippincott Williams & Wilkins; 2005, with permission.

Patients Who Are at *High* Risk for Thrombosis Recurrence After the Standard 6 Months of Anticoagulation

■ Active cancer of receiving chemotherapy
■ Hyperhomocysteinemia
■ Antiphospholipid antibodies
■ Antithrombin, protein C or S deficiency
■ Homozygous factor V Leiden mutation, not heterozygous
■ Inflammatory bowel disease
■ Multiple minor risk factors
■ Recurrent idiopathic thrombosis

Current recommendation is to continue anticoagulants indefinitely, unless the risk of bleeding is high in a specific individual situation.

From O'Connell C, Dickey VL. *Blueprints Hematology and Oncology*. Philadelphia: Lippincott Williams & Wilkins; 2005, with permission.

PULMONARY EMBOLISM
■ If patient has coded and is in shock despite massive inotropes, go to OR; otherwise give heparin (thrombolytics have not shown an improvement in survival) or suction catheter–based intervention
■ ⅓ of positive V/Q scans have negative duplexes
■ Most common from the **iliofemoral region**

HEMATOLOGIC DRUGS

■ **Anticoagulation agents**
• **Warfarin** – <u>prevents vitamin K–dependent decarboxylation of glutamic residues</u> on vitamin K–dependent factors

• **Dextran** – inhibits platelets and coagulation factors

• **Sequential compression devices** – improve venous return but also induce fibrinolysis with compression (release of tPA [tissue plasminogen activator])

• **Heparin**
  • Activates <u>antithrombin III</u>
  • Reversed with **protamine** (1–1.5 protamine/100 U heparin (or 1 mg heparin) follow PTT
  • Half-life of heparin is 60–90 minutes; **cleared by reticuloendothelial system**
  • **Long-term heparin** – osteoporosis, alopecia; <u>does not cross placental barrier</u> → <u>warfarin does</u>
  • **Protamine** – cross-reacts with NPH insulin or previous protamine exposure;
    • 4%–5% of all patients (regardless of previous exposure) get protamine reaction – hypotension, bradycardia, and decreased heart function

• **Hirudin (Hirulog)** – leeches, <u>irreversible</u> direct thrombin inhibitor; also the most potent direct inhibitor of thrombin; at increased risk for bleeding complications want PTT 60–90

• **Argatroban** – direct thrombin inhibitor; metabolized in the liver, half-life is 50 minutes, often used in patients w/HITT

• **Bivalirudin (Angiomax)** – reversible direct thrombin inhibitor, metabolized by proteinase enzymes in the blood; half-life is 25–30 minutes

• **Ancrod** – Malayan pit viper venom; stimulates tPA release

■ **Procoagulant agents (antifibrinolytics)**
• **ε-Aminocaproic acid (Amicar)**
  • Inhibits fibrinolysis by inhibiting **plasmin**
  • Used in DIC, persistent bleeding following cardiopulmonary bypass, thrombolytic overdoses

■ **Thrombolytics**
• **Streptokinase** – has high antigenicity; **urokinase, tPA**
• For thrombolytics to work, a **guidewire** must get past the obstruction
• **Need to follow fibrinogen levels** – fibrinogen < 100 associated with increased risk and severity of bleeding

Contraindications to Thrombolytic Use (Urokinase, Streptokinase, TPA)	
Degree	**Contraindications**
Absolute	Active internal bleeding; recent CVA (<2 mo); intracranial pathology
Major	Recent (<10 d) surgery, organ biopsy, or obstetric delivery; left heart thrombus; active peptic ulcer or gastrointestinal abnormality; recent major trauma; uncontrolled hypertension
Minor	Minor surgery; recent CPR; atrial fibrillation with mitral valve disease; bacterial endocarditis; hemostatic defects (i.e., renal or liver disease); diabetic hemorrhagic retinopathy; pregnancy

Data from NIH Consensus Development Conference. Thrombolytic therapy in treatment. *Ann Intern Med* 1980;93:141.

All blood products carry the risk of HIV and hepatitis, except **albumin and serum globulins** (these are heat treated)

CMV-negative blood – use in low-birth-weight infants, bone marrow transplant patients, and other transplant patients

Clerical error leading to ABO incompatibility is #1 cause of death from transfusion reaction

Stored blood is low in 2,3-DPG $\rightarrow$ causes left shift (increased affinity for oxygen)

HEMOLYSIS REACTIONS
- **Acute hemolysis** – ABO incompatibility; antibody mediated
  - Back pain, chills, tachycardia, fever, hemoglobinuria
  - Can lead to ATN, DIC, shock
  - Haptoglobin <50 mg/dL (binds Hgb, then gets degraded), free hemoglobin > 5 g/dL, increase in unconjugated bilirubin
  - Tx: fluids, diuretics, HCO_3^-, pressors, histamine blockers (Benadryl)
  - In anesthetized patients, transfusion reactions may present as **diffuse bleeding**
- **Delayed hemolysis** – antibody-mediated against minor antigens
  - Tx: observe if stable
- **Nonimmune hemolysis** – from squeezed blood
  - Tx: fluids and diuretics

OTHER REACTIONS
- **Febrile nonhemolytic transfusion reaction** – <u>most common transfusion reaction</u>
  - Usually recipient antibody reaction against **WBCs** in donor blood
  - Tx: discontinue transfusion if patient had previous transfusions or if it occurs soon after transfusion has begun
  - Use WBC filters for subsequent transfusions
- **Anaphylaxis** – bronchospasm, hypotension, urticaria
  - **Usually IgG against IgA in IgA-deficient recipient**
  - Tx: fluids, Lasix, pressors, steroids, epinephrine, histamine blockers (Benadryl)
- **Urticaria** – usually nonhemolytic
  - **Usually a reaction against plasma proteins or IgA in the transfused blood**
  - Tx: histamine blockers (Benadryl), supportive
- **Transfusion-related acute lung injury (TRALI) – rare**
  - Caused by antibodies to recipient's WBCs, clot in pulmonary capillaries

OTHER TRANSFUSION PROBLEMS
- **Cold** – **poor clotting** can be caused by cold products or cold body temperature; patient needs to be warm to clot correctly
- **Dilutional thrombocytopenia** – occurs after 10 units of PRBCs
- **Hypocalcemia** – occurs with massive transfusion; Ca is required for the clotting cascade
- **Antiplatelet antibodies** – develop in 20% of patients after 10–20 platelet transfusions
- **Hetastarch (Hespan)** – can use up to 1 L without the risk of bleeding complications

- Most common bacterial contaminate – **GNRs (usually *E. coli*)**
- Most common blood product source of contamination – **platelets (not refrigerated)**
- **Chagas' disease** – can be transmitted with blood transfusion

Risk of Transfer of Infectious Diseases

Disease	Approximate Risk per Unit of Blood
HIV	1:1,000,000–2,000,000
Hepatitis B or C	1:250,000–500,000

Frequency of Blood Types in the United States

Type	Frequency (%)
O+	38.0
A+	36.0
B+	8.0
O−	7.0
A−	6.0
AB+	3.4
B−	1.5
AB−	0.6

From O'Connell C, Dickey VL. *Blueprints: Hematology and Oncology*. Philadelphia: Lippincott Wilkins & Williams; 2005, with permission.

Blood Product Compatibility

Type of Blood	Required Component Type
Whole blood	Must be identical to recipient's blood
RBCs	Must be compatible with recipient's plasma
WBCs	Must be compatible with recipient's plasma
FFP	Should be compatible with recipient's RBCs
Cryoprecipitate	All ABO groups compatible
Platelets	All ABO groups acceptable; components compatible with recipient's RBCs are preferred

FFP, fresh frozen plasma; RBC, red blood cell; WBC, white blood cell.
From O'Connell C, Dickey VL. *Blueprints: Hematology and Oncology*. Philadelphia: Lippincott Williams & Wilkins; 2005, with permission.

Routinely Performed Infectious Disease Screening Tests on U.S. Blood Donations in 2005

Pathogen	Screening Test
Treponema pallidum	Standard Serological Test (STS) for syphilis
Hepatitis B virus (HBV)	HBV surface antigen (HBsAg) antibody to HBV core antigen (anti-HBc)
Hepatitis C virus (HCV)	Antibody to HCV (anti-HCV) nucleic acid test (NAT) for HCV RNA
Human immunodeficiency virus (HIV)	Antibody to HIV-1/2 (anti-HIV-1/2) NAT for HIV-1 RNA
Human T cell lymphotropic virus (HTLV)	Antibody to HTLV-1/11 (anti-HTLV-1/11)
West Nile Virus (WNV)	NAT for WNV RNA

From Fiebig EW, Busch MP. Infectious risks of transfusion. In: Spiess BD, et al., eds. *Perioperative Transfusion Medicine*. 2nd ed. Philadelphia: Lippincott Williams & Wilkins; 2006, with permission.

Blood Component Characteristics

	Dose	Volume per Dose	Shelf Life	Storage Conditions	Expected Response
PRBC	1 unit	250–325 mL	21–42 d	1°C–6°C	1 g/dL increase in Hgb
FFP	Factor replacement 10–15 mL/kg	200 mL	Frozen: 1 yr; Thawed: 24 h	Frozen: ≤−18°C Thawed: 1°C–10°C	Correct PT/aPTT/ INR by replacement of coagulation factors
Platelets	4–6 pooled whole blood–derived platelets or 1 unit pheresis platelet	200–250 mL	5 d	20°C–24°C with continuous and gentle agitation	30–60 × 109/L/dose
Cryoprecipitate	10 pooled units	100 mL	Frozen: 1 yr Thawed/ pooled: 4 h	Frozen: ≤−18°C Thawed: 1°C–10°C	Increases fibrinogen von Willebrand factor, factor VIII, factor XIII

From Sanford KW, Roseff SD. A surgeon's guide to blood banking and transfusion medicine. In: Spiess BD, et al., eds. *Perioperative Transfusion Medicine*. 2nd ed. Philadelphia: Lippincott Williams & Wilkins; 2006, with permission.

T CELLS (THYMUS) – CELL-MEDIATED IMMUNITY

■ **Helper T cells (CD4)**
- Release **IL-4 (most potent)**, which causes **B-cell** maturation into **plasma cells**
- Release **IL-2 (most potent),** which causes maturation of **cytotoxic T cells**
- Involved in **delayed-type hypersensitivity** (brings in inflammatory cells by chemokine secretion)

- **Th1 helper T cells**
  - Predominant release of proinflammatory cytokines (IL-2, INF-γ)
  - Involved in cell-mediated responses
- **Th2 helper T cells**
  - Predominant release of anti-inflammatory cytokines (IL-4 → inhibits macrophages)
  - Involved in atopy and allergic responses

■ **Suppressor T cells (CD8)** – regulate CD4 and CD8 cells
■ **Cytotoxic T cells (CD8)** – recognize and attack non–self-antigens attached to <u>MHC class I receptors (e.g., viral gene products)</u>

■ **Intradermal skin test (i.e., TB skin test)** – used to test cell-mediated immunity
■ **Infections associated with defects in cell-mediated immunity** – intracellular pathogens (TB, viruses)
■ **Nucleotides** – can ↑ T-cell–mediated immunity

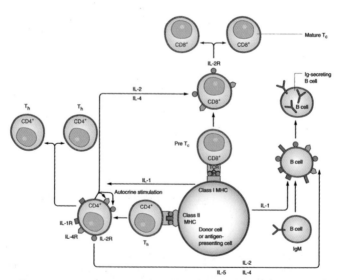

T- and B-Cell Activation. Two signals are required. First, alloantigen binds to antigen-specific receptors—the TCR (T cells) or surface IgM (B cells). The second, or costimulatory, signal is provided by IL-1 released by the antigen-presenting cell. CD41 helper T cells (T$_h$) release IL-2, IL-4, and IL-5, which provide help for CD81 T cells (T$_c$) and for B-cell activation.

B CELLS (BONE) – ANTIBODY-MEDIATED (HUMORAL) IMMUNITY
▓ IL-4 from helper T cells stimulates B cells to become plasma cells (antibody secreting)

MHC CLASSES
▓ **MHC class I (A, B, and C)**
  • CD8 cell activation
  • Present on all nucleated cells
  • Single chain with 5 domains
  • Target for cytotoxic T cells

▓ **MHC class II (DR, DP, and DQ)**
  • CD4-cell activation
  • Present on B cells, dendrites, monocytes, and antigen-presenting cells
  • 2 chains with 4 domains each
  • Activator for helper T cells
  • Stimulate antibody formation

Viral infection – endogenous viral proteins produced, are bound to class I MHC, go to cell surface, and are recognized by CD8 cytotoxic T cells

Bacterial infection – endocytosis, proteins get bound to class II MHC molecules, go to cell surface, recognized by CD4 helper T cells → B cells which have already bound to the antigen are then activated by the CD4 helper T cells; they then produce the antibody to that antigen and are transformed to plasma cells and memory B cells

These pathways are the general mechanisms by which viral and bacterial infections are handled. There are some examples of crossover between MHC class I and class II immunity, meaning viruses get presented through MHC II pathway and bacteria through MHC I pathway

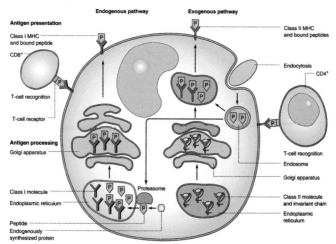

Antigen processing and presentation. Endogenously synthesized or intracellular proteins are degraded into peptides that are transported to the ER. These peptides bind to class I MHC molecules and are transported to the surface of the antigen-presenting cell. CD8$^+$ cells recognize the foreign peptide bound to class I MHC by way of the TCR complex. Exogenous antigen is endocytosed and broken down into peptide fragments in endosomes. Class II molecules are transported to the endosome in association with the invariant chain, bind the peptide, and are delivered to the surface of the antigen-presenting cell, where they are recognized by CD4$^+$ cells.

NATURAL KILLER CELLS
- Not restricted by MHC, do not require previous exposure, do not require antigen presentation
- Not considered T or B cells
- <u>Recognize cells that **lack self-MHC**</u>
- Part of the body's natural immunosurveillance for cancer

ANTIBODIES
- **IgM** – initial antibody made after exposure to antigen. Is the largest antibody, having 5 domains (10 binding sites)
- **IgG** – most abundant antibody in body. Responsible for secondary immune response. Can cross the placenta and provides protection in newborn period
- **IgA** – found in secretions, in Peyer's patches in gut, and in breast milk (additional source of immunity in newborn); helps prevent microbial adherence and invasion in gut
- **IgD** – membrane-bound receptor on B cells (serves as an antigen receptor)
- **IgE** – allergic reactions, parasite infections (see table on hypersensitivity reactions, below)
- **IgM and IgG are opsonins**
- **IgM and IgG fix complement** (requires 2 IgGs or 1 IgM)
- **Variable region** – antigen recognition
- **Constant region** – recognized by PMNs and macrophages
  - Fc fragment does <u>not</u> carry variable region
- **Polyclonal antibodies** have multiple binding sites to the antigen at multiple epitopes
- **Monoclonal antibodies** have only 1 binding site to 1 epitope

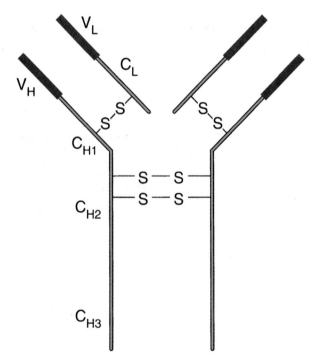

Structure of immunoglobulin (IgG). Variable (V) and constant (C) regions of heavy (H) and light (L) chains are joined by disulfide bonds.

Hypersensitivity Reactions

Type	Description	Examples
I	Immediate hypersensitivity reaction (allergic reaction) IgE mediated: mast and basophils release histamine, serotonin, and bradykinin in response to release of major basic protein from eosinophils, which have IgE receptors for the antigen	Bee stings, peanuts, hay fever
II	IgG or IgM reacts with cell-bound antigen	ABO blood type incompatibility, Rh incompatibility, Graves disease, myasthenia gravis, ITP
III	Immune complex deposition	Serum sickness, rheumatoid arthritis, SLE
IV	Delayed-type hypersensitivity Antigen stimulation of previously sensitized T cells	TB skin test, contact dermatitis

- **Basophils** – major source of histamine in blood
- **Mast cells** – major source of histamine in tissue (other than stomach)
- **Primary lymphoid organs** – liver, bone, thymus
- **Secondary lymphoid organs** – spleen and lymph nodes
- **Immunologic chimera** – 2 different cell lines in one individual (bone marrow transplant patients)

IL-2
- **Converts lymphocytes to lymphokine-activated killer (LAK)** cells by enhancing their immune response to tumor
- Also converts lymphocytes into tumor-infiltrating lymphocytes (TILs)
- Has been shown to be successful for melanoma

TETANUS
- **Non–tetanus-prone wounds** – give tetanus toxoid only if patient has received <3 doses or tetanus status unknown
- **Tetanus-prone wounds** (>6 hours old; obvious contamination and devitalized tissue; crush, burn, frostbite, or missile injuries) – always give tetanus toxoid unless patient has had ≥3 doses and it has been <5 years since last booster
- **Tetanus immune globulin** – give only to patient with tetanus-prone wounds who have not been immunized or if immunization status unknown

Malnutrition – most common immune deficiency

MICROFLORA
- Stomach – virtually sterile; some GPCs, some yeast
- Proximal small bowel – 10^5 bacteria, mostly GPCs
- Distal small bowel – 10^7 bacteria, GPCs, GPRs, GNRs
- Colon – 10^{11} bacteria, almost all anaerobes, some GNRs, GPCs

- **Anaerobes**
  - Most common organisms in the GI tract
  - More common than bacteria in the colon (1,000:1)
  - ***Bacteroides fragilis*** – most common anaerobe in the colon
- ***Escherichia coli*** – most common aerobic bacteria in the colon

GRAM-NEGATIVE SEPSIS
- *E. coli* most common
- **Endotoxin** (lipopolysaccharide lipid A) is released
- Triggers the release of TNF-α (from macrophages), activates complement and coagulation cascade
- Early gram-negative sepsis – $\downarrow$ insulin, $\uparrow$ glucose (impaired utilization)
- Late gram-negative sepsis – $\uparrow$ insulin, $\uparrow$ glucose secondary to insulin resistance
- **Hyperglycemia** – often occurs just before the patient becomes clinically septic
- **Optimal glucose level in a septic patient** – 100–120 mg/dL

CLOSTRIDIUM DIFFICILE COLITIS
- Dx: fecal leukocytes in stool, *C. difficile* toxin
- Tx: oral – vancomycin or Flagyl; IV – Flagyl; lactobacillus can also help
- Stop other antibiotics or change them

ABSCESSES
- 90% of abdominal abscesses have anaerobes
- 80% of abdominal abscesses have both anaerobic and aerobic bacteria
- Abscesses are treated by **drainage**
- Usually occur 7–10 days after operation
- Antibiotics need to be started in patients w/ diabetes, cellulitis, clinical signs of sepsis, fever, elevated WBC, or who have bioprosthetic hardware (e.g., mechanical valves, hip replacements)

WOUND INFECTION
- **Clean** (hernia): 2%
- **Clean contaminated** (elective colon resection with prepped bowel): 3%–5%
- **Contaminated** (gunshot wound to colon with repair): 5%–10%
- **Gross contamination** (abscess): 30%

- ***Staphylococcus aureus*** – coagulase-positive
  - **Most common organism overall** in surgical wound infections
- ***Staphylococcus epidermidis*** – coagulase-negative

- **Exoslime** released by staph species is an **exopolysaccharide matrix**
- *E. coli* – **most common GNR** in surgical wound infections
- *B. fragilis* – **most common anaerobe in surgical wound infections**
  - Recovery from tissue indicates necrosis or abscess (only grows in low redox state)
  - Also implies translocation from the gut

- $\geq 10^5$ **bacteria** needed for wound infection; less bacteria needed if foreign body present
- **Risk factors for wound infection**: long operations, hematoma or seroma formation, advanced age, chronic disease (COPD, renal failure, liver failure, diabetes mellitus), malnutrition, immunosuppressive drugs

- **Surgical infections within 48 hours of procedure**
  - Injury to bowel with leak

Category 1 Recommendations From the Hospital Infection Control Practices Advisory Committee for the Prevention of Surgical Site Infections

Do not operate on patients with active infections	Avoid flash sterilization
Do not shave patient in advance	Wear a mask[a]
Control glucose in diabetic patients	Cover all hair[a]
Stop tobacco use in patient	Wear sterile gloves[a]
Have patient shower with antiseptic soap	Use gowns and drapes that resist fluid penetration
Prepare skin with appropriate agent	Gentle tissue handling
Surgeon's nails should be short	Closed suction drains (when used)
Surgeons scrub hands	Delayed primary closure for heavily contaminated wound
Exclude infected surgeons	Sterile dressing for 24–48 h
Give prophylactic antibiotics when indicated	Use CDC definitions for SSI
Maintain prophylactic antibiotic levels during operation	SSI surveillance with feedback to surgeons
Keep O.R. doors closed	
Use sterile instruments	

[a]These items are required by OSHA regulations and are not actually supported by class 1 data. From Mangram AJ, et al. Guideline for prevention of surgical site infection, 1999. Hospital Infection Control Practices Advisory Committee. *Control Hosp Epidemiol.* 1999;20:250–278.

  - Invasive soft tissue infection – *Clostridium perfringens* and beta-hemolytic strep can present within hours postoperatively (produce exotoxins)

- Most common nonsurgical infection – **urinary tract infection (most commonly *E. coli*)**
  - Biggest risk factor – urinary catheters

- Leading cause of infectious death after surgery – **nosocomial pneumonia**
  - Related to the length of ventilation; aspiration from duodenum thought to have a role
  - Most common organisms in ICU pneumonia – **#1 *S. aureus***, #2 *Pseudomonas*
  - GNRs #1 class of organisms in ICU pneumonia

LINE INFECTIONS
- **#1 *S. epidermidis***, #2 *S. aureus*, #3 yeast
- **Femoral lines** at higher risk for infection compared with subclavian and intrajugular lines
- 50% line salvage rate with antibiotics; much less likely with yeast line infections

- **Central line cultures** – >15 colony forming units = line infection → need new site
- **Site shows signs of infection** → move to new site
- If worried about line infection, best to pull out the central line and place peripheral IVs if central line not needed

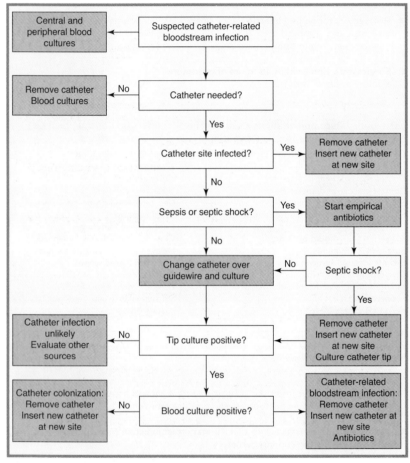

Algorithm for catheter infection. (From Soeters PB, Dejong CHC, Olde Damink SWM, et al. Operative risk, nutritional assessment and intravenous support. In: Fischer JE, et al., eds. *Mastery of Surgery*. 5th ed. Philadelphia: Lippincott Wilkins & Williams; 2007, with permission.)

NECROTIZING SOFT TISSUE INFECTIONS
- Beta-hemolytic *Streptococcus* (group A), *C. perfringens*, and mixed organism
- Usually occur in patients who are immunocompromised (diabetes mellitus) or who have poor blood supply
- Can present very quickly after surgical procedures (within hours)

Signs and Symptoms of Necrotizing Soft Tissue Infection

White blood cell count $20,000/mm^3$
Thin, gray drainage
Marked induration
Edema of entire limb
Hyponatremia (Na $<$ 135 mEq/L)
Skin blistering/sloughing
Skin necrosis
Crepitus/soft tissue gas on x-ray
Pain out of proportion to skin findings
Sepsis (tachycardia, hypotension, high fluid requirements)

■ **Necrotizing fasciitis** – beta-hemolytic group A strep; can be polyorganismal
  • Overlying skin may be pale red and progress to purple with blister or bullae development
  • Overlying skin can look normal in the early stages
  • Thin, gray, foul-smelling drainage; crepitus
  • Tx: early debridement, high-dose penicillin; may want broad spectrum if thought to be-polyorganismal

■ *C. perfringens* **infections**
  • <u>Necrotic tissue</u> decreases oxidation-redux potential, setting up environment for *C. perfringens*
  • *C. perfringens* has alpha toxin
  • Pain out of proportion to exam
  • May not show skin signs with deep infection
  • Gram stain shows GPRs without WBCs
  • **Myonecrosis and gas gangrene** – common presentations
  • Can occur with farming injuries
  • Tx: early debridement, high-dose penicillin

■ **Fournier's gangrene**
  • Severe infection in perineal and scrotal region
  • Risk factors – diabetes mellitus and immunocompromised state
  • Caused by mixed organisms (GPCs, GNRs, anaerobes) Hyponatremia,
  • Tx: early debridement; try to preserve testicles if possible; antibiotics

■ **Mixed organism infection** can also cause necrotizing soft tissue infections

FUNGAL INFECTION
■ Need fungal coverage for positive blood culture, 2 sites other than blood, 1 site with severe symptoms, endophthalmitis, patients on prolonged bacterial antibiotics with failure to improve
■ *Actinomyces* **(not a true fungus)** – pulmonary symptoms most common; can cause tortuous abscesses in cervical, thoracic, and abdominal areas   Sulfur granules/crystals
  • Tx: drainage and penicillin G
■ *Nocardia* **(not a true fungus)** – pulmonary and CNS symptoms most common
  • Tx: drainage and sulfonamides (Bactrim)
■ **Histoplasmosis** – pulmonary symptoms most common; Mississippi and Ohio River valleys
  • Tx: amphotericin for severe infections

- ■ **Cryptococcus** – CNS symptoms most common
  - Tx: amphotericin for severe infections
- ■ **Coccidioidomycosis** – pulmonary symptoms; Southwest
  - Tx: amphotericin for severe infections
- ■ **Candida** – common inhabitant of the respiratory tract
  - Tx: fluconazole (some *Candida* resistant), amphotericin for severe infections

SPONTANEOUS (PRIMARY) BACTERIAL PERITONITIS
- ■ Protein < 1 g/dL in peritoneal fluid – risk factor
- ■ Monobacterial (50% *E. coli*, 30% *Streptococcus*, 10% *Klebsiella*)
- ■ Secondary to decreased host defenses (intrahepatic shunting, impaired bactericidal activity in ascites); <u>not</u> due to transmucosal migration
- ■ Fluid cultures negative in many cases
- ■ PMNs > 500 cells/cc diagnostic
- ■ Tx: ceftriaxone or other 3rd-generation cephalosporin
- ■ Need to rule out intra-abdominal source (diverticular abscess, perforation) if not getting better on antibiotics or if cultures are polymicrobial
- ■ Liver transplantation not an option with active infection
- ■ Fluoroquinolones good for short-term prophylaxis

SECONDARY BACTERIAL PERITONITIS
- ■ Intra-abdominal source (transmucosal migration, perforated viscus)
- ■ Polymicrobial – *B. fragilis*, *E. coli*, *Enterococcus* most common organisms
- ■ Tx: usually need laparotomy to find source

HIV
- ■ **Exposure risk** – HIV blood transfusion 70%
  - Infant from positive mother 30%
  - Needle stick from positive patient 0.3%
  - Mucous membrane exposure (1%)[1]
  - Seroconversion occurs in 6–12 weeks
  - AZT and lamivudine can help ↓ seroconversion after exposure
  - Should be given within 1–2 hours of exposure

- ■ **Opportunistic infections** – most common cause for laparotomy in HIV patients (CMV infection most common)
  - Neoplastic disease – 2nd most common reason for laparotomy
- ■ **CMV colitis** – most common intestinal manifestation of AIDS (can present with pain, bleeding, or perforation)
- ■ **Lymphoma in HIV patients** – <u>stomach</u> most common followed by rectum
  - Mostly non-Hodgkin's, 70% B cell
  - Tx: chemotherapy
- ■ **GI bleeds** – lower GI bleeds are more common than upper GI bleeds in HIV patients
  - **Upper GI bleeds** – <u>Kaposi's sarcoma</u>, lymphoma
  - **Lower GI bleeds** – <u>CMV</u>, bacterial, HSV
- ■ **CD4 counts**: 800–1,200 normal; 300–400 symptomatic disease; 200 opportunistic infections

---

[1]Deziel DJ, et al. *Rush University Review of Surgery*. 3rd ed. Philadelphia: WB Saunders; 2000:149.

HEPATITIS C
- Now rarely transmitted with blood transfusion (0.0001%/unit)
- 1%–2% of population infected
- Fulminant hepatic failure rare
- <u>Chronic infection</u> occurs in 60%
- <u>Cirrhosis</u> in 15% over 20 years
- <u>Hepatocellular carcinoma</u> in 1%–5%
- Interferon may help prevent development of cirrhosis

OTHER INFECTIONS
- **Brown recluse spider bites** – Tx: dapsone initially; may need resection of area and skin graft for large ulcers later
- **Acute septic arthritis** – *Gonococcus*, staph, *H. influenzae*, strep
  - Tx: drainage, 3rd-generation cephalosporin and vancomycin until cultures show organism
- **Diabetic foot infections** – mixed staph, strep, GNRs, and anaerobes
  - Tx: broad-spectrum antibiotics (Unasyn, Zosyn)
- **Cat/dog/human bites** – polymicrobial
  - *Eikenella* found only in human bites; can cause permanent joint injury
  - *Pasteurella multocida* found in cat and dog bites
  - Tx: broad-spectrum antibiotics (Augmentin)

- **Impetigo, erysipelas, cellulitis, and folliculitis** – staph and strep most common organisms
- **Furuncle** – boil; usually *S. epidermidis* or *S. aureus*. Tx: drainage +/− antibiotics
- **Carbuncle** – a multiloculated furuncle

- **Peritoneal dialysis catheter infections**
  - *S. aureus* and *S. epidermidis* most common
  - Fungal infections hard to treat
  - Tx: intraperitoneal vancomycin and gentamicin; increased dwell time and intraperitoneal heparin may help
  - Removal of catheter for peritonitis that lasts for 4–5 days
  - Fecal peritonitis requires laparotomy to find perforation
  - Some say need removal of peritoneal dialysis catheter for all fungal, tuberculous, and *Pseudomonas* infections

- **Sinusitis**
  - **Risk factors** – nasoenteric tubes, intubation, patients with severe facial fractures
  - Usually polymicrobial
  - CT head shows air–fluid levels in the sinus ; Dx : tap
  - Tx: broad-spectrum antibiotics; rare to have to tap sinus percutaneously for systemic illness

- Use **clippers** preoperatively instead of razors to decrease chance of wound infection

CHAPTER 6. ANTIBIOTICS

Antiseptic – kills and inhibits organisms on body
Disinfectant – kills and inhibits organisms on inanimate objects
Sterilization – all organisms killed
Common antiseptics in surgery
>   **Iodophors (Betadine)** – good for GPCs, GNRs, and poor fungi
>   **Chlorhexidine gluconate (Hibiclens)** – good for GPCs, GNRs, and fungi

MECHANISM OF ACTION
- **Inhibitors of cell wall synthesis** – penicillins, cephalosporins, carbapenems, monobactams, vancomycin
- **Inhibitors of the 30s ribosome and protein synthesis** – tetracycline, aminoglycosides (tobramycin, gentamicin), linezolid
- **Inhibitors of the 50s ribosome and protein synthesis** – erythromycin, clindamycin, chloramphenicol, Synercid
- **Inhibitor of DNA helicase (DNA gyrase)** – quinolones (bid dosing)
- **Inhibitor of RNA polymerase** – rifampin
- **Produces oxygen radicals that breakup DNA** – metronidazole (Flagyl)

- **Sulfonamides** – PABA analogue, inhibit purine synthesis
- **Trimethoprim** – inhibits dihydrofolate reductase, inhibits purine synthesis
- **Bacteriostatic antibiotics** – chloramphenicol, tetracycline, clindamycin, erythromycin (all have reversible ribosomal binding), Bactrim
- **Aminoglycosides** – have irreversible binding to ribosome and are considered **bactericidal**

MECHANISM OF ANTIBIOTIC RESISTANCE
- **PCN resistance** – plasmids for beta-lactamase
- **Transfer of plasmids** – most common method of antibiotic resistance
- **Methicillin-resistant *S. aureus* (MRSA)** – resistance to methicillin caused by **mutation of cell wall–binding protein**
- **Vancomycin-resistant *Enterococcus*** – resistance develops from **mutation in cell wall–binding protein**
- **Gentamicin resistance** – resistance due to modifying enzymes leading to decrease in active transport

APPROPRIATE DRUG LEVELS
- **Vancomycin** – peak 20–40 μg/mL; trough 5–10 μg/mL
- **Gentamicin** – peak 6–10 μg/mL; trough <1 μg/mL
- **Peak too high** $\rightarrow$ decrease amount of each dose
- **Trough too high** $\rightarrow$ decrease frequency of doses (increase time interval between doses)

SPECIFIC ANTIBIOTICS
- **Penicillin**
  - GPCs – streptococci, syphilis, *Neisseria meningitides* (GPR), *Clostridium perfringens* (GPR), beta-hemolytic *Streptococcus*, anthrax
  - Not effective against *Staphylococcus* or *Enterococcus*

- **Oxacillin/nafcillin**
  - Anti-staph penicillins (staph only)

■ **Ampicillin/amoxicillin**
  - Same as penicillin but also picks up <u>enterococci</u>

■ **Unasyn (ampicillin/sulbactam) and Augmentin (amoxicillin/clavulanic acid)**
  - Broad spectrum – pick up GPCs (staph and strep), GNRs, $+/-$ anaerobic coverage
  - Effective for enterococci; <u>not</u> effective for *Pseudomonas, Acinetobacter,* or *Serratia*
  - **Sulbactam and clavulanic acid** are beta-lactamase inhibitors

■ **Ticarcillin/piperacillin** (antipseudomonal penicillins)
  - **GNRs** – enterics, *Pseudomonas, Acinetobacter,* and *Serratia*
  - Side effects: inhibits platelets; high salt load

■ **Timentin (ticarcillin/clavulanic acid) and Zosyn (piperacillin/sulbactam)**
  - Broad spectrum – pick up **GPCs** (staph and strep), **GNRs, anaerobes**
  - Effective for enterococci; effective for *Pseudomonas, Acinetobacter,* and *Serratia*
  - Side effects: inhibits platelets; high salt load

■ **First-generation cephalosporins** (cefazolin, cephalexin)
  - **GPCs** – staph and strep
  - <u>Not</u> effective for *Enterococcus*; does not penetrate CNS
  - Ancef (cefazolin) has the longest half-life → best for prophylaxis
  - Side effects: can produce positive Coombs test

■ **Second-generation cephalosporins** (cefoxitin, cefotetan, cefuroxime)
  - **GPCs, GNRs,** $+/-$ anaerobic coverage; lose some staph activity
  - <u>Not</u> effective for *Enterococcus, Pseudomonas, Acinetobacter,* or *Serratia*
  - Effective only for community-acquired GNRs
  - Cefotetan has longest half-life → best for prophylaxis
  - Side effects: prolonged PT

■ **Third-generation cephalosporins** (ceftriaxone, ceftazidime, cefepime, cefotaxime)
  - **GNRs mostly,** $+/-$ **anaerobic coverage**
  - <u>Not</u> effective for *Enterococcus*; effective for *Pseudomonas, Acinetobacter,* and *Serratia*
  - Side effects: cholestatic jaundice (ceftriaxone), sludging in gallbladder (ceftriaxone)

■ **Monobactam (aztreonam)**
  - GNRs; picks up *Pseudomonas, Acinetobacter,* and *Serratia*

■ **Carbapenems (meropenem/imipenem)**
  - Broad spectrum – GPCs, GNRs, and anaerobes
  - <u>Not</u> effective for **MEPP:** **M**RSA, **E**nterococcus, **P**roteus, and **P**seudomonas (which can develop resistance)
  - **Cilastatin** – prevents renal hydrolysis of the drug and increases half-life
  - Side effects: carbapenems can cause seizures

■ **Bactrim**
  - GNRs, $+/-$ GPCs
  - <u>Not</u> effective for *Enterococcus, Pseudomonas, Acinetobacter,* and *Serratia*
  - Side effects (numerous): teratogenic, allergic reactions, renal damage, Stevens–Johnson syndrome (erythema multiforme), hemolysis in G6PD-deficient patients

■ **Quinolones (ciprofloxacin, levofloxacin, trovafloxacin)** → bactericidal
  - GPCs, mostly GNRs

- <u>Not</u> effective for *Enterococcus*; picks up *Pseudomonas*, *Acinetobacter*, and *Serratia*
- 40% of MRSA sensitive; same efficacy PO and IV

Aminoglycosides (gentamicin, tobramycin, amikacin)
- GNRs
- Good for *Pseudomonas*, *Acinetobacter*, and *Serratia*; not effective for anaerobes (need O_2)
- **Resistance due to modifying enzymes leading to decreased active transport**
- Synergistic with ampicillin for *Enterococcus* – beta-lactams (ampicillin/amoxicillin)
  - Facilitate aminoglycoside penetration
  - Side effects: reversible nephrotoxicity, irreversible ototoxicity

Erythromycin (macrolides)
- GPCs; best for community-acquired pneumonia and atypical pneumonias
- Side effects: nausea (PO), cholestasis (IV)
- Also binds motilin receptor and is prokinetic for bowel

Vancomycin (glycopeptides)
- GPCs, *Enterococcus*, *Clostridium difficile* (with PO intake), MRSA
- Binds cell wall proteins
- **Resistance develops from change in cell wall–binding sites**
- Side effects: HTN, Redman syndrome (histamine release), nephrotoxicity, ototoxicity

Synercid (streptogramin – quinupristin-dalfopristin)
- GPCs; includes MRSA, VRE

Linezolid (oxazolidinones)
- GPCs; includes MRSA, VRE

Tetracycline
- GPCs, GNRs, syphilis
- Side effects: tooth discoloration in children

Clindamycin
- Anaerobes, some GPCs
- Good for aspiration pneumonia
- Can be used to treat *C. perfringens*
- Side effects: pseudomembranous colitis

Metronidazole
- Anaerobes
- Side effects: disulfiram-like reaction, peripheral neuropathy

Carbenicillin and ticarcillin can interfere with aminoglycosides
Tetracyclines can interfere with beta-lactams
Broad-spectrum antibiotics can lead to **superinfection**

Antifungal drugs
- **Amphotericin** – binds sterols in wall and alters membrane permeability
  - Side effects: nephrotoxic, fever, decreased potassium, hypotension, anemia
- **Fluconazole** – <u>not</u> all *Candida* spp. are sensitive
- **Ketoconazole** – <u>not</u> all *Candida* spp. are sensitive
- Prolonged broad-spectrum antibiotics $+/-$ fever $\rightarrow$ **fluconazole**
- Possible fungal sepsis $\rightarrow$ **amphotericin**

- **Antituberculosis drugs**
  - **Isoniazid** – inhibits mycolic acids
    - Side effects: hepatotoxicity, B_6 deficiency
  - **Rifampin** – inhibits RNA polymerase
    - Side effects: hepatotoxicity; GI symptoms; high rate of resistance
  - **Pyrazinamide**
    - Side effect: hepatotoxicity
  - **Ethambutol**
    - Side effect: retrobulbar neuritis

- **Antiviral drugs**
  - **Acyclovir** – inhibits DNA polymerase, usually used for HSV infections; can be used for EBV
  - **Ganciclovir** – used for CMV infections
    - Side effects: decreased bone marrow, CNS toxicity

Effective for *Enterococcus* – vancomycin, Timentin/Zosyn, ampicillin/amoxicillin, or gentamicin with ampicillin

Effective for *Pseudomonas*, *Acinetobacter*, and *Serratia* – ticarcillin/piperacillin, Timentin/Zosyn third-generation cephalosporins, aminoglycosides (gentamicin and tobramycin), meropenem/imipenem (resistance can develop in *Pseudomonas*), or fluoroquinolones
Double cover *Pseudomonas*

Perioperative antibiotics
Used to prevent incisional wound infections
Need to be given within 1 hours before incision

Extended Prophylactic Antibiotic Complications

Complication	<24 h Antibiotics ($n = 92$)	>48 h Antibiotics ($n = 59$)
Clostridium difficile colitis	10	31[a]
Candida infections	9	17
Central line infections	19	34[a]

[a]$P < 0.005$.
From Cheadle WG, Branson R, Franklin GA. Pulmonary risk and ventilatory support. In: Fischer JE, Bland KI, et al., eds. *Mastery of Surgery.* 5th ed. Philadelphia: Lippincott Wilkins & Williams; 2005, with permission.

Sublingual and rectal drugs – do not pass through the liver first
Skin absorption – based on lipid solubility through the epidermis
CSF absorption – restricted to nonionized, lipid-soluble drugs

Albumin – largely responsible for binding drugs (PCNs and warfarin 90% bound)
Sulfonamides – will displace unconjugated bilirubin in newborns
Tetracycline and heavy metals – stored in bone

0 order kinetics – constant amount of drug is eliminated regardless of dose
1st order kinetics – drug eliminated proportional to dose
Takes 5 half-lives for a drug to reach steady state
Volume of distribution = amount of drug in the body divided by amount of drug in plasma or blood
  • Drugs with a high volume of distribution have higher concentrations in the **extravascular compartment** (e.g., fat tissue) compared with **intravascular concentrations**
Bioavailability – fraction of unchanged drug reaching the systemic circulation
Assumed to be 100% for intravenous drugs, less for other routes (i.e., oral)

ED_{50} – drug level at which <u>desired effect</u> occurs in 50% of patients
LD_{50} – drug level at which <u>death</u> occurs in 50% of patients

Hyperactive – effect at an unusually low dose
Tachyphylaxis – tolerance after only a few doses
Potency – dose required for effect
Efficacy – ability to achieve result without untoward effect

Microsomal drug metabolism (hepatic cell endoplasmic reticulum, P-450 system)
  • **Phase I** – demethylation, oxidation, reduction, hydrolysis reactions (mixed function oxidases, requires NADPH/oxygen)
  • **Phase II** – glucuronic acid (#1) and sulfates attached (forms **water-soluble metabolite**); often inactive and ready for excretion. Biliary excreted drugs may become deconjugated in intestines with reabsorption, some in active form

  • **Inhibitors of P-450** – cimetidine, isoniazid, ketoconazole, erythromycin, Cipro, Flagyl, allopurinol, verapamil, amiodarone, MAOIs, disulfiram
  • **Inducers of P-450** – cruciform vegetables, ETOH, insecticides, cigarette smoke, phenobarbital (barbiturates), Dilantin, theophylline, warfarin

  • **P-450 system** transforms aromatic hydrocarbons into carcinogens

Kidney – most important organ for eliminating most drugs (glomerular filtration and tubular secretion)

Polar drugs (ionized) – more <u>water soluble</u> and more likely to be eliminated in unaltered form
Nonpolar drugs (nonionized) – more <u>fat soluble</u> and more likely to be metabolized before excretion

Gout – caused by uric acid buildup; end product of purine metabolism
  • **Colchicine** – anti-inflammatory; binds tubulin and inhibits migration
  • **Indomethacin** – anti-inflammatory

- **Allopurinol** – xanthine oxidase inhibitor, blocks uric acid formation from xanthine
- **Probenecid** – ↑ renal secretion of uric acid

Lipid-lowering agents
- **Cholestyramine** – can bind vitamin K and cause bleeding tendency
- **HMG-CoA reductase inhibitors (statin drugs)** – can cause liver dysfunction, rhabdomyolysis
- **Niacin (inhibits cholesterol synthesis)** – can cause flushing. Tx: ASA

GI drugs
- **Promethazine** (Phenergan, antiemetic) – **causes** tardive dyskinesia (inhibits dopamine receptors)
  - Tx: diphenhydramine (Benadryl)
- **Metoclopramide** (Reglan, prokinetic) – dopamine receptor blocker that can be used to increase gastric motility and gut motility in general
- **Ondansetron (Zofran)** – serotonin receptor inhibitor; antiemetic
- **Omeprazole** – proton pump inhibitor; blocks H/K ATPase in stomach
- **Cimetidine/ranitidine** – histamine H_2 receptor blockers; decrease acid in stomach
- **Octreotide** – somatostatin analogue that is longer acting

Cardiac drugs
- **Digoxin**
  - **Inhibits Na/K ATPase and increases myocardial calcium**
  - ↑ atrial contraction rate but **slows AV conduction**
  - Also acts as an **inotrope**
  - ↓ **blood flow** to intestines – has been implicated in causing **mesenteric ischemia**
  - **Hypokalemia** – ↑ sensitivity of heart to digitalis; can precipitate arrhythmias or AV block
  - **Is not cleared with dialysis**
  - Other side effects: visual changes (yellow hue), fatigue, arrhythmias

- **Procainamide** – can cause lupus-like syndrome, pulmonary fibrosis, and torsades
  - **Magnesium** – used to treat torsades
  - Follow drug levels and QT intervals: >400 milliseconds is concerning
  - Normal procainamide level: 4–12 μg/mL
  - Normal NAPA level: <30 μg/mL

- **Adenosine** – causes transient interruption of the AV node

- **ACE (angiotensin-converting enzyme) inhibitors** – captopril
  - Best single agent shown to reduce mortality in patients with CHF
  - Can prevent CHF post-MI
  - Can prevent progression of renal dysfunction in patients with hypertension and DM
  - Can precipitate renal failure in patients with renal artery stenosis

- **Beta-blockers** – may prolong life in patients with severe LV failure
  - **Reduce risk of MI and atrial fibrillation postoperatively**

- **Atropine** – acetylcholine antagonist; increases heart rate
Metyrapone and aminoglutethimide – inhibit adrenal steroid synthesis
Used in patients with adrenocortical CA

Leuprolide – analogue of GnRH and LHRH
Inhibits release of LH and FSH from pituitary when given continuously (paradoxic effect)

Vasopressin (ADH) – acts on V-1 receptors found on vascular smooth muscle (constriction)
- Can be used in patients with <u>gastrointestinal bleeding</u> by reducing intestinal blood flow

Indomethacin – inhibits prostaglandin production
- Used to close patent ductus arteriosus (PDA) in children and used in patients with gout

Misoprostol – PGE_1 derivative; a protective prostaglandin used to prevent peptic ulcer disease
- Consider use in patients on chronic NSAIDs

NSAIDs – inhibit prostaglandin synthesis and lead to $\downarrow$ mucus and HCO_3^- secretion and $\uparrow$ acid production (mechanism of ulcer formation in patients on NSAIDs)

Haldol – can cause extrapyramidal manifestations; inhibits dopamine receptors

ASA poisoning – tinnitus, headaches, nausea, and vomiting
    1st – respiratory alkalosis
    2nd – metabolic acidosis

Gadolinium – side effect: nausea

Tylenol overdose – Tx: *N*-acetylcysteine

Activated protein C (Xigris) – used for sepsis
    Mechanism is **fibrinolysis**
    Drug inactivates the inhibitor of protein C, creating activated protein C

CHAPTER 8. ANESTHESIA

INHALATIONAL AGENTS
- **MAC** – minimum alveolar concentration = smallest concentration of inhalational agent at which 50% of patients will not move with incision
  - Small MAC → more lipid soluble = more potent
  - Speed of induction is inversely proportional to solubility
  - Nitrous is fastest but has high MAC (low potency)

- Inhalational agents cause unconsciousness, amnesia, and some degree of analgesia
- Blunt hypoxic drive
- Most are associated with some degree of **myocardial depression,** ↑ cerebral blood flow, and ↓ renal blood flow

- **NO$_2$ (nitrous oxide)** – fast, minimal myocardial depression
- **Halothane** – slow, highest degree of cardiac depression and arrhythmias; least pungent, which is good for children
  - Halothane hepatitis – fever, eosinophilia, jaundice, ↑ LFTs
- **Enflurane** – can cause seizures
- **Isoflurane** – good for neurosurgery; higher cost
- **Sevoflurane** – less myocardial depression, fast onset/offset, less laryngospasm; higher cost

INDUCTION AGENTS
- **Sodium thiopental (barbiturate)** – fast acting
  - Side effects: ↓ cerebral blood flow and metabolic rate, ↓ blood pressure

- **Propofol** – very rapid distribution and on/off; amnesia; sedative
  - Side effects: hypotension, respiratory depression
  - **Not an analgesic**
  - Do not use in patients with egg allergy
  - Metabolized in liver and by plasma cholinesterases

- **Ketamine** – dissociation of thalamic/limbic systems; places patient in a cataleptic state (amnesia, analgesia)
  - No respiratory depression
  - Side effects: hallucinations, catecholamine release (↑ carbon monoxide, tachycardia), ↑ airway secretions, and ↑ cerebral blood flow
  - **Contraindicated in patients with head injury**
  - Good for **children**

- **Etomidate** – fewer hemodynamic changes; fast acting
  - Continuous infusions can lead to adrenocortical suppression

- **Rapid sequence intubation** – can be indicated for recent oral intake, GERD, delayed gastric emptying, pregnancy, bowel obstruction

MUSCLE RELAXANTS (PARALYTICS)
- **Diaphragm** – last muscle to go down and 1st muscle to recover from paralytics
- **Neck muscles and face** – 1st to go down and last to recover from paralytics

- ■ **Depolarizing agent – the only one is succinylcholine**
  - **Succinylcholine** – fast, short acting; causes fasciculations at first, ↑ ICP; many side effects
    - **Malignant hyperthermia**
    - Defect in calcium metabolism
    - Calcium released from sarcoplasmic reticulum causes muscle excitation – contraction syndrome
    - Side effects: 1st sign is ↑ **end-tidal CO_2,** then fever, tachycardia, rigidity, acidosis, hyperkalemia
    - Tx: **dantrolene** (10 mg/kg) inhibits Ca release and decouples excitation complex, cooling blankets, HCO_3, glucose, supportive care
    - **Hyperkalemia** – depolarization releases K (see also Chap. 9)
    - **Do not use** in burn patients, neurologic injury, neuromuscular disorders, spinal cord injury, massive trauma, acute renal failure
    - **Open-angle glaucoma** can become closed-angle glaucoma
    - **Atypical pseudocholinesterases** – cause prolonged paralysis (Asians)

- ■ **Nondepolarizing agents**
  - Inhibit neuromuscular junction by competing with acetylcholine
  - Can get prolongation of these agents with hypothermia, hypercarbia, certain antibiotics, electrolyte abnormalities, myasthenia gravis

  - **Cis-atracurium** – undergoes **Hoffman degradation**
    - **Can be used in liver and renal failure**
    - Histamine release
  - **Mivacurium** – fast, short acting; degradation by **plasma cholinesterases**
    - Histamine release
  - **Rocuronium** – fast, intermediate duration; hepatic metabolism
  - **Pancuronium** – slow acting, long-lasting; renal metabolism
    - Most common side effect – **tachycardia**

  - **Reversing drugs for nondepolarizing agents**
    - **Neostigmine** – counters nondepolarizing agents, blocks **acetylcholinesterase,** increasing acetylcholine
    - **Edrophonium** – counters nondepolarizing agents, blocks **acetylcholinesterase,** increasing acetylcholine
    - **Atropine or glycopyrrolate** should be given with <u>neostigmine or edrophonium</u> to counteract effects of generalized acetylcholine overdose

LOCAL ANESTHETICS
- ■ Work by increasing **action** potential threshold, preventing Na influx
- ■ Can use 0.5 cc/kg of 1% lidocaine
- ■ Infected tissues hard to anesthetize secondary to **acidosis**
- ■ Length of action – bupivacaine > lidocaine > procaine
- ■ Epinephrine allows higher doses to be used, stays locally
  - **No epinephrine** with arrhythmias, unstable angina, uncontrolled hypertension, poor collaterals (penis and ear), uteroplacental insufficiency
- ■ Side effects: tremors, seizures, tinnitus, arrhythmias (CNS symptoms occur before cardiac)

- ■ **Amides** (all have an "i" in first part of the name) – lidocaine, bupivacaine, mepivacaine; rarely allergic reactions
- ■ **Esters** – tetracaine, procaine, cocaine; ↑ allergic reactions secondary to PABA analogue

Analgesics

	Potency	Sedation Dose	Duration	Infusion Dose
OPIOIDS				
Morphine	1	0.02–0.1 mg/kg IV	2–7 h	—
Meperidine	0.1	0.2–1 mg/kg IV	2–4 h	—
Fentanyl	100	0.5–1 mg/kg IV	30–60 min	—
Sufentanil	1,000	Not recommended		
Alfentanil	25	10–20 mg/kg IV	10–15 min	
Remifentanil[a]	—	Not recommended	10 min	0.1–0.2 mg/kg/min
OTHER ANALGESICS AND ANESTHETICS				
Propofol		0.1–0.5 mg/kg IV[b,c]		25–50 mg/kg/min
Ketamine		0.1–0.5 mg/kg IV[b]		—
		1.0–2.0 mg/kg IM		

IM, intramuscular; IV, intravenous.
[a]Will produce apnea.
[b]May produce apnea.
[c]Produces pain on injection that can be reduced by treatment with 20 mg of lidocaine IV.

NARCOTICS (OPIOIDS)
- Morphine, fentanyl, Demerol, codeine
- Act on mu receptors
- Profound analgesia, respiratory depression (↓ CO_2 drive), no cardiac effects, blunt sympathetic response
- Metabolized by the liver and excreted via kidney
- Overdose of narcotic drugs – Tx: **Narcan**
- Avoid use of narcotics in patients on **MAOIs** → can cause **hyperpyrexic coma**

- **Morphine** – analgesia, euphoria, respiratory depression, miosis, ↓ cough, constipation, histamine release
  - **Active metabolites** can build up in patients with renal failure
- **Demerol** – analgesia, euphoria, respiratory depression, miosis, tremors, fasciculations, convulsions
  - **No histamine release**
  - Avoid in patients with renal failure → can get buildup of **normeperidine analogue and result in seizures** (also need to be careful with the amount given)
- **Methadone** – simulates morphine, less euphoria
- **Fentanyl** – 80× strength of **morphine** (does not cross-react in patients with morphine allergy)
  - No histamine release
- **Sufentanil, alfentanil, remifentanil** – very fast-acting narcotics with short half-lives

BENZODIAZEPINES
- Hepatically metabolized; anticonvulsant, amnesic, anxiolytic, respiratory depression; not analgesic
- **Versed (midazolam)** – short acting; contraindicated in pregnancy, crosses placenta
- **Ativan (lorazepam)** – long acting
- **Valium (diazepam)** – long acting
- Overdose of these drugs – Tx: flumazenil (competitive inhibitor; may cause seizures and arrhythmias; contraindicated in patients with elevated ICP or status epilepticus)

Anxiolytics and Amnesics (Benzodiazepines)

Name	Dose (mg/kg)	Duration (h)	Strengths	Weaknesses
Midazolam (Versed)	0.05 (infusion dose 0.25 mg/kg/min)	0.5	Water soluble Short duration Good for sedation for short procedures	Acute respiratory depression
Diazepam (Valium)	0.1	1	Intermediate duration	Irritation on IV injection Phlebitis Acute respiratory depression after IV overdose
Lorazepam (Ativan)	0.02–0.08	6–8	Long duration	—
BENZODIAZEPINE REVERSAL				
Flumazenil (Romazicon)	4–20 mg/kg (0.2 mg repeated every 2–10 min until reversal is achieved) Maximum dose 1 mg	45–90 min	—	May produce seizures, panic, arrhythmias

IV, intravenous.

EPIDURAL AND SPINAL ANESTHESIA
■ **Epidural** – causes sympathetic denervation, vasodilation
  • **Morphine** in epidural can cause **respiratory depression**
  • **Lidocaine** in epidural can cause **decreased heart rate and blood pressure**
  • Dilute concentrations allow sparing of motor function
  • **Tx for acute hypotension and bradycardia:** turn epidural down; fluids, phenylephrine, atropine

Opioid Protocols in Epidural Opiate Analgesia

	Morphine[a]	Fentanyl[b]
Length of onset	Longer (30–60 min)	Shorter (15–30 min)
Duration	Longer (6–24 h for single bolus)	Shorter (1–2 h for single bolus)
Cephalad spread and side effects	More prone	Less prone
Indication	Favored for lumbar administration after abdominal surgery	Favored for thoracic administration after chest surgery
Dose	Typically 3–5 mg, q6–8h	Typically 50–75 mg/h ($\pm$dilute bupivacaine)

[a] Hydrophilic: slow in, slow out.
[b] Lipophilic: fast in, fast out.

  • T-5 epidural can affect cardiac accelerator nerves
  • Epidural contraindicated with hypertrophic cardiomyopathy, cyanotic heart disease → can get inadvertent spinal anesthesia

■ **Spinal anesthesia** – injection into subarachnoid space, spread determined by baricity and patient position
  • Neurologic blockade is above motor blockade
  • Spinal contraindicated with hypertrophic cardiomyopathy, cyanotic heart disease

■ **Caudal block** – through sacrum, good for pediatric hernias and perianal surgery

■ **Epidural and spinal complications** – hypotension, headache, urinary retention, abscess/hematoma formation, neurologic impairment
  • High spinal – respiratory depression

■ **Spinal headaches** – Tx: rest, increased fluids, caffeine, analgesics; blood patch to site if persists >24 hours. Headache gets worse sitting up

PERIOPERATIVE COMPLICATIONS
■ **CHF and renal failure** – associated with most postoperative hospital mortality

■ **Postop MI** – may have no pain or EKG changes; can have hypotension, arrhythmias, ↑ filling pressures, oliguria, bradycardia

■ **Patients who need cardiology workup** – angina, previous MI, shortness of breath, CHF, walks <2 blocks due to shortness of breath or chest pain, FEV_1 < 70%, aortic stenosis murmur, PVCs > 5/min, age > 70, patients undergoing major vascular surgery

ASA Classes

Class	Description
I	Healthy
II	Mild disease without limitation (controlled hypertension, obesity, diabetes mellitus, significant smoking history, older age)
III	Severe disease (angina, previous MI, poorly controlled hypertension, diabetes mellitus with complications, moderate COPD)
IV	Severe constant threat to life (unstable angina, CHF, renal failure, liver failure, severe COPD)
V	Moribund (ruptured AAA, saddle pulmonary embolus, ascending aortic dissection resulting in heart failure)
VI	Donor
E	Emergency

■ Most **vascular procedures** are considered moderate- to high-risk surgery

■ **Biggest risk factors for postop MI**: age > 70, DM, previous MI, CHF, and unstable angina

Cardiac Risk[a] Stratification for Noncardiac Surgical Procedures

High (reported cardiac risk often >5%)
• Emergent major operations, particularly in the elderly
• Aortic and other major vascular surgery
• Peripheral vascular surgery
• Anticipated prolonged surgical procedures associated with large fluid shifts and/or blood loss

Intermediate (reported cardiac risk generally <5%)
• Carotid endarterectomy
• Head and neck surgery
• Intraperitoneal and intrathoracic surgery
• Orthopedic surgery
• Prostate surgery

Low[b] (reported cardiac risk generally <1%)
• Endoscopic procedures
• Superficial procedures
• Cataract surgery
• Breast surgery

[a]Combined incidence of cardiac death and nonfatal myocardial infarction.
[b]Do not generally require further preoperative cardiac testing.

Best determinant of esophageal vs. tracheal intubation – **end-tidal CO_2**
Intubated patient undergoing surgery with sudden transient rise in $ETCO_2$
    Dx: most likely alveolar hypoventilation
    Tx: ↑ tidal volume (most likely do to atelectasis) or ↑ respiratory rate

Intubated patient with sudden drop in $ETCO_2$ – likely became disconnected from the
    vent; could also be due to pulmonary embolism or significant hypotension

Endotracheal tube – should be placed 2 cm above the carina

MC PACU complication – nausea and vomiting

CHAPTER 9. FLUIDS AND ELECTROLYTES

TOTAL BODY WATER
- Roughly ⅔ of the total body weight is water (men); **infants** have a little more body water, **women** have a little less
- ⅔ of water weight is intracellular (mostly muscle)
- ⅓ of water weight is extracellular
  - ⅔ of extracellular water is interstitial
  - ⅓ of extracellular water is in plasma

- **Proteins** – determine <u>plasma/interstitial</u> compartment osmotic pressures
- **Na** – determines <u>intracellular/extracellular</u> osmotic pressure

- **Volume overload** – most common cause is iatrogenic; first sign is **weight gain**
- **Cellular catabolism** – can release a significant amount of H_2O

- **0.9% normal saline**: Na 154 and Cl 154
- **Lactated Ringer's solution (LR; ionic composition of plasma)**: Na 130, K 4, Ca 2.7, Cl 109, bicarb 28

- **Plasma osmolarity**: $(2 \times Na) + (glucose/18) + (BUN/2.8)$
  - Normal: 280–295

ESTIMATES OF VOLUME REPLACEMENT
- 4 cc/kg/h for 1st 10 kg
- 2 cc/kg/h for 2nd 10 kg
- 1 cc/kg/h for each kg after that
- Best indicator of adequate volume replacement is **urine output**

- During open abdominal operations, fluid loss is **0.5–1.0 L/h** unless there are measurable blood losses
- Usually do not have to replace blood lost unless it is **>500 cc**
- **Insensible fluid losses** – 10 cc/kg/day, 75% skin, 25% respiratory, pure water

- **IV replacement after major adult gastrointestinal surgery**
  - During operation and 1st 24 hours, use **LR**
  - After 24 hours, switch to **D5 ½ NS with 20 mEq K^+**
    - 5% dextrose will stimulate **insulin release,** resulting in amino acid uptake and protein synthesis (also prevents protein catabolism)
    - D5 ½ NS @ 125/h provides 150 g glucose per day (525 kcal/day)

GI FLUID SECRETION
- Stomach   1–2 L/day
- Biliary system   500–1,000 mL/day
- Pancreas   500–1,000 mL/day
- Duodenum   500–1,000 mL/day

- **Normal K^+ requirement:** 0.5–1.0 mEq/kg/day
- **Normal Na^+ requirement:** 1–2 mEq/kg/day

GI ELECTROLYTE LOSSES
- Sweat – hypotonic
- Saliva – K^+ (highest concentration of K^+ in body)

- Stomach – H^+ and Cl^-
- Pancreas – HCO_3^-
- Bile – HCO_3^-
- Small intestine – HCO_3^-, K^+
- Large intestine – K^+

- **Gastric losses** – replacement is D5 ½ NS with 20 mg K^+
- **Pancreatic/biliary/small intestine losses** – replacement is LR with HCO_3^-
- **Large intestine (diarrhea) losses** – replacement is LR with K^+
- **GI losses** – should generally be replaced **cc/cc**
- **Urine output** – should be kept at least 0.5 cc/kg/h; should not be replaced, usually a sign of normal postoperative diuresis

POTASSIUM (NORMAL 3.5–5.0)
- **Hyperkalemia** – peaked T waves initial finding on EKG
  - **Calcium gluconate** (membrane stabilizer for heart)
  - **Sodium bicarbonate** (causes alkalosis, K enters cell in exchange for H)
  - **10 U insulin and 1 ampule of 50% dextrose** (K driven into cells along with glucose)
  - **Kayexalate**
  - **Dialysis** if refractory
- **Hypokalemia** – T waves disappear ; ↓ DTRs.
  - May need to replace Mg^+ before you can correct K^+

SODIUM (NORMAL 135–145)
- **Hypernatremia** – restlessness, irritability, ataxia, seizures

  - Correct with D5 water slowly to avoid brain swelling

  - Total free water deficit = 0.6 × patient's weight (kg) × $[(Na^+/140) - 1]$

  - Water requirement = $\dfrac{\text{desired change in } Na^+ \text{ over 1 day} \times \text{TBW}}{\text{desired } Na^+ \text{ after giving the water requirement}}$

    - TBW (total body water) = 0.6 × patient's weight (kg)

    - Change Na more than 0.7 mEq/h (16 mEq/day for below)

    - For the equation above, if the Na was 165 for a 70-kg man:

    - (16 × 42)/149 = 4.5 L

- **Hyponatremia** – headaches, delirium, seizures, nausea, vomiting

  - Na deficit = 0.6 × (weight in kg) × (140 − Na)

  - **Water restriction** is the first treatment for hyponatremia, then **diuresis,** then NaCl replacement
  - Correct Na slowly to avoid **central pontine myelinosis (no more than 1 mEq/h)**
  - **Hyperglycemia can cause pseudohyponatremia** – for each 100 increment of glucose over normal, add 2 points to the Na value
  - SIADH results in hyponatremia

CALCIUM (NORMAL 8.5–10.0; NORMAL IONIZED Ca 4.4–5.5)
- **Hypercalcemia** (Ca usually > 13 or ionized > 6–7) – causes lethargic state
  - Breast cancer most common malignant cause

- No lactated Ringer's (contains Ca^{2+})
- No thiazide diuretics (these retain Ca^{2+})
- Tx: NS at 200–300 cc/h, Lasix
  - For **malignant disease** → mithramycin, calcitonin, alendronic acid, dialysis
- **Hypocalcemia** (Ca usually < 8 or ionized Ca < 4) – hyperreflexia, Chvostek's sign (tapping on face produces twitching), perioral tingling and numbness, Trousseau's sign (carpopedal spasm), prolonged QT interval
  - May need to **correct Mg** before being able to correct Ca
  - **Protein adjustment for calcium** – for every 1-g decrease in protein, add 0.8 to Ca

MAGNESIUM (NORMAL 2.0–2.7)
- **Hypermagnesemia** – causes lethargic state; burn, trauma, and renal dialysis patients
  - Tx: calcium
- **Hypomagnesemia** – signs similar to hypocalcemia

METABOLIC ACIDOSIS
- **Anion gap = Na − (HCO₃ + Cl)**
  - Normal: <10–15

- **Anion gap acidosis** – "MUDPILES" = **m**ethanol, **u**remia, **d**iabetic ketoacidosis, **p**araldehydes, **i**soniazid, **l**actic acidosis, **e**thylene glycol, **s**alicylates

- **Normal gap acidosis** usually due to loss of Na/HCO_3^- (ileostomies, small bowel fistulas)

- Tx: underlying cause; keep pH > 7.20 with bicarbonate; severely ↓ pH can affect myocardial contractility

METABOLIC ALKALOSIS
- Usually a contraction alkalosis
- **Nasogastric suction** – results in **hypochloremic, hypokalemic, metabolic alkalosis, and** paradoxical **aciduria**
- Loss of Cl^- and H ion from stomach secondary to nasogastric tube (hypochloremia and alkalosis)
- Loss of water causes kidney to reabsorb Na in exchange for K^+ (Na/K ATPase), thus losing K^+ (hypokalemia)
- Na^+/H^- exchanger activated in an effort to reabsorb water along with K^+/H^- exchanger in an effort to reabsorb K^+ → results in paradoxical aciduria

Acid–Base Balance			
Condition	pH	CO_2	HCO_3
Respiratory acidosis	↓	↑	↑
Respiratory alkalosis	↑	↓	↓
Metabolic acidosis	↓	↓	↓
Metabolic alkalosis	↑	↑	↑

- **Henderson–Hesselbach equation**
  - $pH = pK + \log [HCO_3^-]/[CO_2]$
  - Ratio of base to acid (HCO_3^- to CO_2) of 20:1 = pH of 7.4

ACUTE RENAL FAILURE
- **FeNa** = (urine Na/Cr)/(plasma Na/Cr) – <u>best test for azotemia</u>

- **Prerenal** – FeNa < 1%, urine Na < 20, BUN/Cr ratio > 20, urine osmolality > 500 mOsm
  - 70% of renal mass must be damaged before ↑ Cr and BUN

- **Contrast dyes** – <u>volume expansion</u> best prevents renal damage: HCO_3^- and *N*-acetylcysteine gtt
- **Myoglobin** – converted to <u>ferrihemate</u> in acidic environment, which is toxic to renal cells
  - Tx: <u>alkalinize urine</u>

TUMOR LYSIS SYNDROME
- Release of purines and pyrimidines leads to ↑ **PO_4 and uric acid,** ↓ Ca
- Can result in ↑ BUN and Cr, EKG changes
- Tx: hydration, allopurinol (↓ uric acid production), diuretics, alkalinization of urine

VITAMIN D (CHOLECALCIFEROL)
- Made in skin (UV sunlight) from 7-dehydrocholesterol
- **Goes to liver for (25-OH),** then **kidney for (1-OH).** This creates the active form of vitamin D
- **Active form of vitamin D** – ↑ **calcium-binding protein,** leading to ↑ intestinal Ca absorption

CHRONIC RENAL FAILURE
- ↓ **Active vitamin D** (↓ 1-OH hydroxylation) → ↓ Ca reabsorption from gut (↓ Ca-binding protein)
- **Anemia** – from low erythropoietin

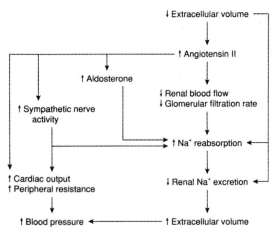

Multiple effects of increased angiotensin II release in response to the stimulus of decreased extracellular volume.

Transferrin – transporter of iron
Ferritin – storage form of iron

Hypophosphatemia : ↓ cell membrane integrity poor wound healing, hemolysis, rhabdomyolysis, muscle weakness

Caloric Need – approximately 25 kcal/kg/day

Composition of a Standard Central Venous Solution

Volume	10% Amino acid solution	500 mL
	50% Dextrose solution	500 mL
	Fat emulsion	—
	Electrolytes + vitamins + minerals	~50 mL
	Total volume	~1,050 mL
Composition	Amino acids	50 g
	Dextrose	250 g
	Total N	50/6.25 = 8 g
	Dextrose kcal	250 g × 3.4 kcal/g = 840 kcal
	MOsms/L	~2,000

Electrolytes Added to Total Parenteral Nutrition Solutions

Electrolyte	Usual Concentration (mEq/L)	Range of Concentrations (mEq/L)
Sodium	60	0–150
Potassium	40	0–80
Acetate	50	50–150
Chloride	50	0–150
Phosphate	15	0–30
Calcium[a]	4.5	0–20
Magnesium	5	5–15

[a]Generally added as calcium gluconate or calcium chloride 1 ampule of calcium gluconate = 1 g of calcium = 4.5 mEq.

Fat	9 kcal/g
Protein	4 kcal/g
Oral carbohydrates	4 kcal/g
Dextrose	3.4 kcal/g

10% lipid solution contains 1.1 kcal/cc; 20% lipid solution contains 2 kcal/cc

Nutritional requirements for average healthy adult male
1 g protein/kg/day is needed, of which 20% should be essential amino acids
30% fat calories – important for essential fatty acids
Rest of calories should be as **carbohydrates**

Trauma, surgery, or sepsis stress can increase kcal requirement 20%–40%
Pregnancy increases kcal requirement 300 kcal/day
Lactation increases kcal requirement 500 kcal/day
Protein requirement also increases with these

Burns
Calories: 25 kcal/kg/day + (30 kcal/day × % burn)
Protein: 1–1.5 g/kg/day + (3 g × % burn)

Much of the energy expenditure is used for **heat production**
Basal metabolic rate **increases 10%** for each degree above 38.0°C

If overweight, use equation: weight = [(actual weight − ideal body weight) × 0.25] + IBW
Harris–Benedict equation calculates basal energy expenditure based on **weight, height, age, and gender**

Central line TPN – glucose based; **maximum glucose administration** – 3 g/kg/h
Peripheral line parenteral nutrition (PPN) – fat based

Metabolic Differences Between the Responses to Simple Starvation and to Injury		
	Simple Starvation	**Severe Starvation**
Basal metabolic rate	−	+ +
Presence of mediators	−	+ + +
Major fuel oxidized	Fat	Mixed
Ketone body production	+ + +	±
Hepatic ureagenesis	+	+ + +
Negative nitrogen balance	+	+ + +
Gluconeogenesis	+	+ + +
Muscle proteolysis	+	+ + +
Hepatic protein synthesis	+	+ + +

Short-chain fatty acids – fuel for **colonocytes**
Glutamine – fuel for **small bowel enterocytes**
 Most common amino acid in **bloodstream and tissue**
 Releases NH_4 in kidney, thus helping with **nitrogen excretion**
 Can be used for gluconeogenesis

Primary fuel for neoplastic cell – glutamine

PREOPERATIVE NUTRITIONAL ASSESSMENT
■ **Approximate half-lives**
 • Albumin – 20 days
 • Transferrin – 10 days
 • Prealbumin – 2 days

■ Normal **protein** level: 6.0–8.5
■ Normal **albumin** level: 3.5–5.5

■ **Acute indicators of nutritional status** – retinal binding protein, prealbumin, transferrin, total lymphocyte count

■ **Ideal body weight (IBW)**
 • Men = 106 lb + 6 lb for each inch over 5 ft
 • Women = 100 lb + 5 lb for each inch over 5 ft

■ **Preoperative signs of poor nutritional status**
 • Acute weight loss >10% in 6 months
 • Weight <85% of IBW
 • Albumin <3.0
 • Low albumin (<3.0) – **strong risk factor for morbidity and mortality after surgery**

RESPIRATORY QUOTIENT (RQ)
■ Ratio of CO_2 produced to O_2 consumed – measurement of energy expenditure

■ **RQ > 1** = lipogenesis (overfeeding)
 • Tx: ↓ carbohydrates and caloric intake
 • High carbohydrate intake can lead to CO_2 buildup and ventilator problems

▓ **RQ < 0.7** = ketosis and fat oxidation (starving)
  • Tx: ↑ carbohydrates and caloric intake

▓ **Pure fat metabolism** – RQ = 0.7
▓ **Pure protein metabolism** – RQ = 0.8
▓ **Pure carbohydrate metabolism** – RQ = 1.0

POSTOPERATIVE PHASES
▓ **Diuresis phase** – postoperative days 2–5
▓ **Catabolic phase** – postoperative days 0–3 (negative nitrogen balance)
▓ **Anabolic phase** – postoperative days 3–6 (positive nitrogen balance)

STARVATION OR MAJOR STRESS (SURGERY, TRAUMA, SYSTEMIC ILLNESS)
▓ **Glycogen stores**
  • Depleted after 24–36 hours of starvation (⅔ in skeletal muscle, ⅓ in liver) → **body then switches to fat**
  • Skeletal muscle lacks **glucose-6-phosphatase** (found only in **liver**)
  • Glucose-6-phosphate stays in muscle after breakdown from glycogen and is utilized

▓ **Gluconeogenesis precursors** – amino **acids** (especially alanine), lactate, pyruvate, glycerol
  • **Alanine** is the simplest amino acid precursor for gluconeogenesis
    ◦ Primary substrate for gluconeogenesis
  • **Alanine and phenylalanine** – only amino acids to increase during times of stress
  • **Late starvation** – gluconeogenesis occurs in <u>kidney</u>

▓ **Starvation**
  • Protein-conserving mechanisms **do not occur after trauma** (or surgery) secondary to catecholamines and cortisol
  • Protein-conserving mechanisms do occur with **starvation**
  • **Fat** (ketones) is the main source of energy in trauma and starvation

  • Most patients can tolerate a 15% weight loss without major complications
  • Patients can tolerate about **7 days** without eating; if longer than that, place a **Dobbhoff tube or start TPN**
  • Try to feed gut to avoid **bacterial translocation** (bacterial overgrowth, increased permeability due to starved enterocytes)
  • **Elemental formula** – all protein given in the form of amino acids (given IV, expensive)
  • **PEG** – consider when regular feeding not possible (e.g., CVA) or predicted to not occur for >4 weeks

  • **Brain** – utilizes <u>ketones</u> with progressive starvation (normally uses glucose)
  • **Peripheral nerves, adrenal medulla, red blood cells, and white blood cells** – obligate glucose users

  • **Refeeding syndrome**
    ◦ Occurs when feeding after prolonged starvation/malnutrition
    ◦ Results in ↓ **K, Mg, and PO$_4$;** causes cardiac dysfunction and fluid shifts
    ◦ Prevent this by starting at a **low rate** (10–15 kcal/kg/day)
  • **Cachexia** – anorexia, weight loss, wasting
    ◦ Thought to be mediated by TNF-α
    ◦ Glycogen breakdown, lipolysis, protein catabolism
  • **Kwashiorkor** – protein deficiency
  • **Marasmus** – starvation

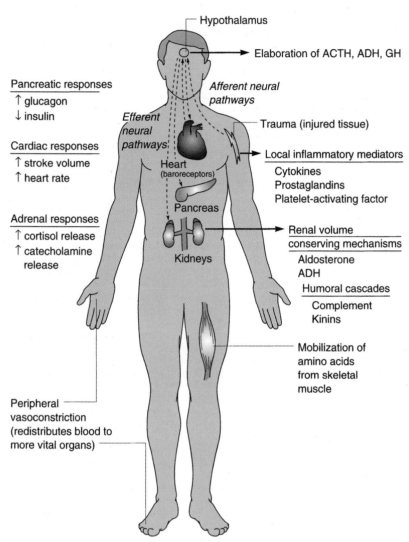

Homeostatic adjustments initiated after injury.

Hypothalamus
Elaboration of ACTH, ADH, GH

Pancreatic responses
↑ glucagon
↓ insulin

Afferent neural pathways

Efferent neural pathways

Trauma (injured tissue)

Cardiac responses
↑ stroke volume
↑ heart rate

Heart (baroreceptors)

Local inflammatory mediators
Cytokines
Prostaglandins
Platelet-activating factor

Pancreas

Adrenal responses
↑ cortisol release
↑ catecholamine release

Kidneys

Renal volume conserving mechanisms
Aldosterone
ADH
Humoral cascades
Complement
Kinins

Mobilization of amino acids from skeletal muscle

Peripheral vasoconstriction (redistributes blood to more vital organs)

NITROGEN BALANCE
- **6.25 g of protein contains 1 g of nitrogen**
- **N balance** = (N in − N out) = ([protein/6.25] − [24-hour urine N + 4 g])
  - Positive N balance – more protein ingested than excreted (anabolism)
  - Negative N balance – more protein excreted than taken in (catabolism)
- Total protein synthesis for a healthy, normal 70-kg male is **250 g/day**

- **Liver**
  - Responsible for amino acid production and breakdown
  - **Urea production** to get rid of ammonia from amino acid breakdown
  - Majority of protein breakdown from skeletal muscle is **glutamine and alanine**

FAT DIGESTION

■ **Triacylglycerides (TAGs), cholesterol, and lipids**
  • Broken down by pancreatic lipase, cholesterol esterase, and phospholipase to micelles and free fatty acids
  • **Micelles** – aggregates of bile salts, long-chain free fatty acids, and monoacylglycerides
    • Enter enterocyte by fusing with membrane
    • **Bile salts** – increase absorption area for fats, helping form **micelles**
    • **Cholesterol** – used to synthesize bile salts
    • **Fat-soluble vitamins (A, D, E, K)** – absorbed in micelles
  • **Medium- and short-chain fatty acids** – enter enterocyte by simple diffusion

■ **Micelles and other fatty acids enter enterocytes** → **chylomicrons** are formed, which enter **lymphatics** (thoracic duct)
■ **Chylomicrons** – 90% TAGs, 10% phospholipids/proteins/cholesterol
  • **Medium- and short-chain fatty acids** – enter **portal system** (same as amino acids and carbohydrates)
  • **Long-chain fatty acids** – enter **lymphatics** along with chylomicrons

■ **Lipoprotein lipase** – on liver endothelium; clears <u>chylomicrons and TAGs</u> from the blood, breaking them down <u>to fatty acids and glycerol</u>, which are then taken up by hepatocyte
■ **Free fatty acid–binding protein** – on liver endothelium; binds short- and medium-chain fatty acids

■ **VLDL** – most important route of entry for dietary cholesterol; synthesized in the liver

■ **Saturated fatty acids** – used for fuel by cardiac and skeletal muscles
  • **Fatty acids** (ketones – acetoacetate, beta-hydroxybutyrate) – preferred source of energy for the <u>liver, heart, and skeletal muscle</u>
■ **Unsaturated fatty acids** – used as structural components for cells

■ **Hormone-sensitive lipase** – in fat cells; breaks down **TAGs** (storage form of fats) **to fatty acids and glycerol;** released into blood (sensitive to growth hormone, catecholamines, glucocorticoids)

■ **Essential <u>fatty acids</u> – linolenic, linoleic**
  • Needed for prostaglandin synthesis (long-chain fatty acids)
  • Important for immune cells
■ **Omega-3 fatty acids** – PGI_3, TXA_3, LTB_5 (all odd) – thought to have antioxidant properties
■ **Omega-6 fatty acids** – PGE_2, TXA_2, LTB_4 (all even)

CARBOHYDRATE DIGESTION

■ Begins with **salivary amylase,** then pancreatic amylase and disaccharidases
■ **Glucose and galactose** – absorbed by secondary active transport; released into portal vein
■ **Fructose** – facilitated diffusion; released into portal vein
■ **Sucrose** = fructose + glucose
■ **Lactose** = galactose + glucose
■ **Maltose** = glucose + glucose

PROTEIN DIGESTION

■ Begins with **stomach pepsin,** then trypsin, chymotrypsin, and carboxypeptidase

- Trypsinogen released from pancreas and activated by enterokinase released from duodenum
  - Other pancreatic protein enzymes are then activated by trypsin
  - Trypsin can then also autoactivate other trypsinogen molecules
- **Protein** broken down to amino acids, dipeptides, and tripeptides by proteases
- Absorbed by secondary active transport; released as free amino acids into portal vein
- May want to limit protein intake in patients with **liver failure and renal failure to avoid ammonia buildup** and possible worsening encephalopathy

- **Branched-chain** <u>amino acids</u> – **leucine, isoleucine, valine** ("LIV")
  - Metabolized in **muscle**
  - Possibly important in patients with liver failure
  - Are **essential amino acids**

Deficiencies	
Deficiency	Effect
Chromium	Hyperglycemia, encephalopathy, neuropathy
Selenium	Cardiomyopathy, weakness, hair loss
Copper	Pancytopenia
Zinc	Hair loss, poor healing, rash
Trace elements	Poor wound healing
Phosphate	Weakness (failure to wean off ventilator), encephalopathy, decreased phagocytosis
Thiamine (B_1)	Wernicke's encephalopathy, cardiomyopathy, peripheral neuropathy
Pyridoxine (B_6)	Sideroblastic anemia, glossitis, peripheral neuropathy
Cobalamin (B_{12})	Megaloblastic anemia, peripheral neuropathy, beefy tongue
Folate	Megaloblastic anemia, glossitis
Niacin	Pellagra (diarrhea, dermatitis, dementia)
Essential fatty acids	Dermatitis, hair loss, thrombocytopenia
Vitamin A	Night blindness
Vitamin K	Coagulopathy
Vitamin D	Rickets, osteomalacia
Vitamin E	Neuropathy

CORI CYCLE
- Glucose is utilized and converted to **lactate** in muscle
- Lactate then goes to the liver and is converted back to **pyruvate** and eventually **glucose** via <u>gluconeogenesis</u>
- Glucose is then transported back to muscle

Cancer #2 cause of death in the United States

MC CA in women – breast CA
MC cause of CA-related death in women – lung CA
MC CA in men – prostate CA
MC cause of CA-related death in men – lung CA

PET (positron emission tomography) scan – used to identify metastases → **detects fluorodeoxyglucose molecules**

T cells need MHC complex to attack tumor
Natural killer cells can independently attack tumor cells
Tumor antigens are random unless viral-induced tumor

Hyperplasia – increased number of cells
Metaplasia – replacement of one tissue with another (GERD squamous epithelium in esophagus changed to columnar gastric tissue)
Dysplasia – altered size, shape, and organization (Barrett's esophagus)

TUMOR MARKERS
- CEA – colon CA
- AFP – liver CA
- CA 19-9 – pancreatic CA
- CA 125 – ovarian CA
- Beta-HCG – testicular CA, choriocarcinoma
- PSA – prostate CA (thought to be the tumor marker with the **highest sensitivity**)
- NSE – small cell lung CA, neuroblastoma
- BRCA I and II – breast CA
- **Half-lives** – CEA: 18 days; PSA: 18 days; AFP: 5 days

ONCOGENESIS
- **Cancer transformation**
  - Heritable alteration in genome
  - Loss of growth regulation
- **Latency period** – time between exposure and formation of clinically detectable tumor
- **Initiation** – carcinogen acts with DNA
- **Promotion** of cancer cells
- **Progression** of cancer cells to clinically detectable tumor

- Neoplasms can arise from **carcinogenesis** (e.g., smoking), **viruses** (e.g., EBV), or **immunodeficiency** (e.g., HIV)
- **Retroviruses contain oncogenes**
  - Epstein-Barr virus – associated with Burkitt's lymphoma (8:14 translocation) and nasopharyngeal CA (c-myc)

Malignancies Associated With Infectious Agents

Malignancy	Associated Infectious Agent
Cervical cancer	Human papillomavirus
Gastric cancer	*Helicobacter pylori*
Hepatocellular carcinoma	Hepatitis B and hepatitis C viruses
Kaposi's sarcoma	HHV-8
Primary effusion lymphoma	HHV-8
Splenic lymphoma	Hepatitis C virus
Nasopharyngeal carcinoma	EBV
Burkitt's lymphoma	EBV
Adult T-cell leukemia/lymphoma	Human T-cell leukemia virus-1
Various lymphomas	HIV

EBV, Epstein-Barr virus; HHV-8, human herpesvirus-8; HIV, human immunodeficiency virus
From O'Connell C, Dickey VL. *Blueprints: Hematology and Oncology.* Philadelphia: Lippincott Williams & Wilkins; 2005, with permission.

■ **Proto-oncogenes are human genes with malignant potential**

RADIATION THERAPY (XRT)
■ **M phase** – most vulnerable stage of cell cycle for XRT
■ Most damage done by formation of **oxygen radicals** → maximal effect with **high oxygen levels**
■ Main target is **DNA** – oxygen radicals cause damage of DNA and other molecules
■ XRT itself can also cause some damage by causing small breaks in DNA

■ **Higher-energy radiation has skin-preserving effect** (maximal ionizing potential not reached until deeper structures)
■ **Fractionate doses**
   • Allows **repair** of normal cells
   • Allows **reoxygenation** of tumor
   • Allows **redistribution** of tumor cells in cell cycle
■ Very radiosensitive tumors – **seminomas, lymphomas**
■ Very radioresistant tumors – **epithelial, sarcomas**
■ Kidneys, lungs, liver, and lymphocytes have increased sensitivity to XRT
■ **Large tumors** – less responsive to XRT due to <u>lack of oxygen in the tumor</u>
■ **Brachytherapy** – source of radiation in or next to tumor (Au-198, I-128); delivers high, concentrated doses of radiation

CHEMOTHERAPY AGENTS
■ **Cell cycle–specific agents** (5FU, methotrexate) – exhibit plateau in cell-killing ability
■ **Cell cycle–nonspecific agents** – linear response to cell killing

■ **Tamoxifen (blocks estrogen receptor)** – decreases short-term (5 year) risk of breast CA 45%
   • 1% risk of blood clots
   • 0.1% risk of endometrial CA
■ **Taxol** promotes microtubule formation and stabilization that cannot be broken down; cells are ruptured
■ **Bleomycin and busulfan** – can cause pulmonary fibrosis

■ **Cisplatin** (platinum alkylating agent) – nephrotoxic, neurotoxic, ototoxic

▩ **Carboplatin** (platinum alkylating agent) – **bone** (myelo) suppression

▩ **Vincristine** (microtubule inhibitor) – peripheral neuropathy, neurotoxic
▩ **Vinblastine** (microtubule inhibitor) – **bone** (myelo) suppression

▩ **Alkylating agents** – transfer alkyl groups; form covalent bonds
   • **Cyclophosphamide – acrolein** is the active metabolite
      ◦ Side effects: gonadal dysfunction, SIADH, hemorrhagic cystitis
      ◦ **Mesna** can help with hemorrhagic cystitis
   • **Isofosfamide**
▩ **Levamisole – anthelminthic drug** thought to stimulate immune system against cancer
▩ **Methotrexate** – inhibits <u>dihydrofolate reductase (DHFR)</u>, which inhibits purine and DNA synthesis
   • Side effects: renal toxicity, radiation recall
   • **Leucovorin rescue** – ↓ folate (tetrahydrofolic acid); reverses effects of methotrexate
▩ **5-Fluorouracil (5FU)** – inhibits <u>thymidylate synthesis</u>, which inhibits purine and DNA synthesis
   • **Leucovorin** – ↑ toxicity of 5FU
▩ **Doxorubicin** – DNA intercalator, O_2 radical formation
   • Heart toxicity secondary to O_2 radicals at >500 mg/m^2
▩ **Etoposide** (VP-16) – inhibits topoisomerase (which normally unwinds DNA)

▩ **Least myelosuppression** – bleomycin, vincristine, busulfan, cisplatin
▩ **GCSF** (granulocyte colony-stimulating factor) – used for neutrophil recovery after chemo
   • Side effects: Sweet's syndrome (acute febrile neutropenic dermatitis)

Resection of a normal organ to prevent cancer
   Colon – FAP
   Breast – BRCA I or II with strong family history
   Thyroid – RET proto-oncogene or MENIN gene with family history of MEN or thyroid CA

Tumor suppressor genes
   Retinoblastoma (Rb1) – chromosome 13; involved in **cell cycle**
   p53 – chromosome 17; involved in **cell cycle** (normal gene induces cell cycle arrest and apoptosis; abnormal gene allows unrestrained cell growth)
   APC – chromosome 5; involved with **cell adhesion and cytoskeleton function**
   DCC – chromosome 18; involved in **cell adhesion**
   bcl – involved in **apoptosis** (programmed cell death)
   BRCA

Proto-oncogenes
   ras proto-oncogene – G protein defect
   src proto-oncogene – tyrosine kinase defect
   sis proto-oncogene – platelet-derived growth factor receptor defect
   erb B proto-oncogene – epidermal growth factor receptor defect
   myc (c-myc, n-myc, l-myc) proto-oncogenes – transcription factors

Li–Fraumeni syndrome – defect in p53 gene → patients get childhood sarcomas, breast CA, brain tumors, leukemia, adrenal CA

Medullary CA of the thyroid (see also Chap. 22)
   Associated with Ret proto-oncogene (chromosome 10)
   Patients with Ret gene defect plus family history →90% get medullary CA of thyroid; need prophylactic total thyroidectomy

Colon CA
Genes involved in development include **APC, p53, DCC, and K-ras**
APC involved in cell adhesion and cytoskeleton function – thought to be the initial mutation in the development of colon CA
Colon CA usually does not go to bone

Carcinogens
Coal tar – larynx, skin, bronchial CA
Beta-naphthylamine – urinary tract CA (bladder CA)
Benzene – leukemia
Asbestos – mesothelioma

Cancer spread
Suspicious supraclavicular nodes – neck, breast, lung, stomach (Virchow's node), pancreas
Suspicious axillary node – lymphoma (#1), breast, melanoma
Suspicious periumbilical node – pancreas (Sister Mary Joseph's node)
Ovarian metastases – stomach (Krukenberg tumor), colon
Bone metastases – breast (#1), prostate
Skin metastases – breast, melanoma
Small bowel metastases – melanoma (#1)

Clinical trials
Phase I – is it safe and at what dose?
Phase II – is it effective?
Phase III – is it better than existing therapy?
Phase IV – implementation and marketing

Types of therapy
Induction – sole treatment; often used for advanced disease or when no other treatment exists
Primary (neoadjuvant) – chemotherapy given 1st, followed by another (secondary) therapy
Adjuvant – combined with another modality; given after other therapy is used
Salvage – for tumors that fail to respond to initial chemotherapy

Lymph nodes have poor barrier function → better to view them as signs of **probable metastasis**

En bloc multiorgan resection can be attempted for some tumors (colon into uterus, adrenal into liver, gastric into diaphragm)
Aggressive local invasiveness is different from metastatic disease

Palliative surgery – tumors of hollow viscus causing obstruction or bleeding (colon CA), pancreatic CA with biliary obstruction, breast CA with skin or chest wall involvement

Sentinel lymph node biopsy – no role in patients with clinically palpable nodes; you need to go after and sample these nodes

Colon metastases to the liver – 25% 5-year survival rate if successfully resected

Most successfully cured metastases with surgery – colon CA in liver, sarcoma to the lung, but survival still low overall for these

Predictors of Mortality and Survival Following Resection of Hepatic Colorectal Metastases

Prognostic Factor	P Value	RR Death
Disease-free interval < 12 mo	0.002	1.56
Tumor number > 3	0.01	1.56
CEA > 200 mg/L	0.05	1.45
Size > 5 cm	0.01	1.46
Node positive primary	0.05	1.34

Survival Based on Number of Factors

Number of Factors	5-yr Survival (%)	Median OS
0	57	74
1	57	73
2	47	50
3	16	30
4	8	15

CEA, carcinoembryonic antigen; OS, overall survival; RR, relative risk.
Adapted from Fong Y, Fortner J, Sun RL, et al. Clinical score for predicting recurrence after hepatic resection for metastatic colorectal cancer: analysis of 1001 consecutive cases. *Ann Surg.* 1999;230:309.

Ovarian CA – one of the few tumors for which **surgical debulking** improves chemotherapy (not seen in other tumors)
Curable solid tumors with chemotherapy only – Hodgkin's disease, non-Hodgkin's lymphoma
   Most lymphomas are **B cell**
T-cell lymphomas – HTLV-1 (skin lesions), mycosis fungoides (Sézary cells)
HIV-related malignancies – Kaposi's sarcoma, non-Hodgkin's lymphoma

CHAPTER 12. TRANSPLANTATION

TRANSPLANT IMMUNOLOGY
- **HLA-A, -B, and -DR** – most important in recipient/donor matching
- **HLA-DR** – most important overall
- **ABO blood compatibility** – generally required for all transplants (except liver)

- **Crossmatch**
  - Detects preformed recipient antibodies by mixing recipient serum with donor lymphocytes → would generally cause **hyperacute rejection (except liver)**

- **Panel reactive antibody (PRA)**
  - Technique identical to crossmatch; detects preformed recipient antibodies using a panel of typing cells
  - Get a percentage of cells that the serum reacts with
  - Transfusions, pregnancy, previous transplant, and autoimmune diseases can all increase PRA

- **Mild rejection** – pulse steroids
- **Severe or secondary rejection** – OKT3 or other drugs

- **Skin cancer** – #1 malignancy following any transplant (squamous cell CA #1)

- **Posttransplant lymphoproliferative disorder (PTLD)** – next most common malignancy following transplant – **Epstein-Barr virus related**
  - **Tx**: withdrawal of immunosuppression; may need chemotherapy and XRT for aggressive tumor

DRUGS
- **Azathioprine (Imuran)**
  - Inhibits de novo purine synthesis, which inhibits T cells
  - **6-Mercaptopurine** is the active metabolite (formed in the liver)
  - Side effects: myelosuppression
  - Keeps WBCs > 3

- **Mycophenolate** – similar action to azathioprine

- **Steroids** – inhibit genes for cytokine synthesis (IL-1, IL-6) and macrophages

- **Cyclosporin (CSA)**
  - Binds **cyclophilin protein** and inhibits genes for cytokine synthesis (IL-2, IL-3, IL-4, INF-γ)
  - Side effects: nephrotoxicity, hepatotoxicity, HUS, tremors, seizures
  - Keeps trough 200–300
  - Undergoes **hepatic metabolism and biliary excretion**

- **FK-506 (Prograf)**
  - Binds **FK-binding protein**; actions similar to CSA but 10–100× more potent
  - Side effects: nephrotoxicity, mood changes; more GI and neurologic changes than CSA
  - Keeps trough 10–15

- **ATGAM**
  - Equine polyclonal antibodies directed against antigens on T cells (CD2, CD3, CD4, CD8, CD11/18)
  - Used for induction therapy
  - Complement dependent
  - Keeps peripheral T-cell count > 3

- **Thymoglobulin**
  - Rabbit polyclonal antibodies
  - Similar action as ATGAM

- **OKT3**
  - Monoclonal antibodies that block antigen recognition function of T cells by binding CD3, inhibiting T-cell receptor complex
  - Interferes with both class I and II MHC
  - Causes CD3 opsonization that is complement dependent
  - Used for severe rejection
  - Follows peripheral CD3 cells
  - Side effects: fever, chills, pulmonary edema, shock

- **Zenapax** – human monoclonal antibody against IL-2 receptors
  - Used with induction and to treat rejection

TYPES OF REJECTION
- **Hyperacute rejection (occurs within minutes to hours)**
  - Caused by preformed antibodies that should have been picked up by the crossmatch
  - Activates the complement cascade and thrombosis of vessels occurs
  - Tx: emergent retransplant

- **Accelerated rejection (occurs <1 week)**
  - Caused by sensitized T cells to donor antigens
  - Produces a secondary immune response
  - Tx: ↑ immunosuppression, pulse steroids, and possibly OKT3

- **Acute rejection (occurs 1 week to 1 month)**
  - Caused by T cells (cytotoxic and helper T cells)
  - Tx: ↑ immunosuppression, pulse steroids, and possibly OKT3

- **Chronic rejection (months to years)**
  - Partially a type IV hypersensitivity reaction (sensitized T cells)
  - Antibody formation also plays a role; leads to graft fibrosis and vascular damage
  - Monocytes and cytotoxic T cells have a role
  - Tx: ↑ immunosuppression or OKT3 – no really effective treatment

KIDNEY TRANSPLANTATION
- Can store kidney for 48 hours
- Need ABO type and crossmatch
- **UTI** – can still use kidney
- **Acute ↑ in creatinine (1.0–3.0)** – can still use kidney
- Mortality primarily from **stroke and MI**
- Attach to **iliac vessels**

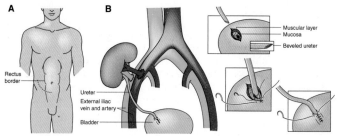

(A) Curvilinear iliac fossa incision used for the kidney transplant recipient procedure.
(B) Vascular anastomoses completed between the recipient external iliac artery and vein and donor renal artery and vein. Insets: Ureteral anastomosis performed using the external ureteroneocystostomy technique.

- **Complications**
  - **Urine leaks (#1)** – Tx: drainage and stenting usually first; may need reoperation
  - **Renal artery stenosis** – diagnose with ultrasound
    - Tx: PTA with stent
  - **Lymphocele** – most common cause of external compression
    - Tx: 1st **percutaneous drainage**; if that fails, then need **intraperitoneal marsupialization** (90% successful)
  - **Postop oliguria** – usually due to ATN (pathology shows hydrophobic changes)
  - **Postop diuresis** – usually due to urea and glucose
  - **New proteinuria** – suggestive of renal vein thrombosis
  - **Postop diabetes** – side effect of CSA, FK, steroids
  - **Viral infections** – CMV – Tx: ganciclovir; **HSV** – Tx: acyclovir

  - **Acute rejection** – usually occurs in 1st 6 months; pathology shows tubulitis or vasculitis with more severe form
  - **Kidney rejection workup** – usually for ↑ in Cr
    - Ultrasound with duplex (to rule out vascular problem and ureteral obstruction) and biopsy; empiric ↓ in CSA or FK (these can be nephrotoxic); pulse steroids
  - **Chronic rejection** – usually do not see until after 1 year; no good treatment
  - **5-year graft survival overall** – 70% (cadaveric 65%, living donors 75%)

- **Living kidney donors**
  - Most common complication – wound infection (1%)
  - Most common cause of death – fatal PE
  - The remaining kidney hypertrophies

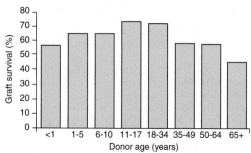

Kidneys transplanted from deceased pediatric donors aged 5 and below have lower graft survival rates than those from older pediatric and young adult donors. At the older extreme of age, graft survival rates are also lower.

LIVER TRANSPLANTATION
- Can store for 24 hours
- Contraindications to liver TXP – **current ETOH abuse, acute ulcerative colitis**
- **Chronic hepatitis** – most common reason for liver TXP in adults
- Criteria for emergent TXP – **stage III (stupor), stage IV (coma)**
- Patients with hepatitis B antigenemia can be treated with **HBIG (hepatitis B immunoglobulin) and lamivudine (protease inhibitor)** postoperatively
- **Hepatocellular CA** – if single tumor <5 cm or up to 3 tumors each <3 cm, can still consider TXP
- **Portal vein thrombosis** – not a contraindication to TXP
- **APACHE** score – best predictor of 1-year survival

- **Hepatitis C** – disease most likely to recur in the new liver allograft; reinfects essentially all grafts
- **Hepatitis B** – reinfection rate has been reduced to 20% with the use of HBIG

- **ETOH** – 20% will start drinking again (recidivism)
- **Macrosteatosis** – extracellular fat globules in the liver allograft
  - #1 predictor of primary nonfunction
  - If 50% of cross section is macrosteatatic in potential donor liver, there is a 50% chance of primary nonfunction

- Duct-to-duct anastomosis is performed
- Hepaticojejunostomy in kids
- Right subhepatic, right and left subdiaphragmatic drains
- Biliary system (ducts, etc.) depends on **hepatic artery** blood supply
- Most common arterial anomaly – **right hepatic coming off SMA**

- **Complications**
  - **Bile leak (#1)** – Tx: PTC tube and stent
  - **Primary nonfunction**
    - **1st 24 hours** – total bilirubin > 10, bile output < 20 cc/12 h, PT and PTT 1.5× normal
    - **After 96 hours** – hyperkalemia, mental status changes, ↑ LFTs, renal failure, respiratory failure
    - **Usually requires retransplantation**
  - **Hepatic artery thrombosis** – Tx: angio (potentially treated with angiography and balloon dilatation +/− stent), surgery, retransplantation
    - Hepatic vein thrombosis rare
  - **Abscesses** – most common from chronic hepatic artery thrombosis
  - **IVC stenosis** – edema, ascites, renal insufficiency
  - **Cholangitis** – get PMNs around portal triad, <u>not</u> mixed infiltrate

  - **Acute rejection** – T cell mediated against blood vessels
    - Clinical – fever, jaundice, ↓ bile output, change in bile consistency
    - Labs – leukocytosis, eosinophilia, ↑ LFTs, total bilirubin, and PT
    - Pathology – shows **portal lymphocytosis, endotheliitis (mixed infiltrate), and bile duct injury**
    - Usually occurs in 1st 2 months
  - **Chronic rejection** – disappearing bile ducts (antibody and cellular attack on bile ducts); gradually get bile duct obstruction with ↑ in alkaline phosphatase, portal fibrosis
    - Acute rejection most common predictor

- **Retransplantation rate** – 20%
- **5-year survival rate** – 70%

PANCREAS TRANSPLANTATION
- Need **donor celiac and SMA** for arterial supply
- Need **donor portal vein** for venous drainage
- Attach to iliac vessels
- Most use **enteric drainage** for pancreatic duct. Take second portion of duodenum from donor along with ampulla of Vater and pancreas, then perform anastomosis of donor duodenum to recipient bowel
- **Successful pancreas/kidney TXP** results in stabilization of retinopathy, ↓ neuropathy, ↑ nerve conduction velocity, ↓ autonomic dysfunction (gastroparesis), ↓ orthostatic hypotension
  - No reversal of vascular disease

- **Complications**
  - **Thrombosis (#1)** – hard to treat
  - **Rejection** – hard to diagnose if patient does not also have a kidney transplant
    - Can see ↑ glucose, amylase, or trypsinogen; fever, leukocytosis

HEART TRANSPLANTATION
- Can store for 6 hours
- Need ABO compatibility and crossmatch
- For patients with life expectancy <1 year
- Persistent pulmonary hypertension after heart transplantation
  - Tx: Flolan (PGI_2); inhaled nitric oxide, ECMO if severe
  - Associated with ↑ morbidity and mortality after heart TXP
- **Acute rejection** – shows <u>perivascular infiltrate</u> with ↑ grades of <u>myocyte inflammation and necrosis</u>
- **Chronic rejection** – progressive diffuse coronary **atherosclerosis**

LUNG TRANSPLANTATION
- Can store for 6 hours
- Need ABO compatibility and crossmatch
- For patients with life expectancy <1 year
- #1 cause of early mortality – **reperfusion injury**
- Indication for double-lung TXP – **cystic fibrosis**
- Exclusion criteria for using lungs – aspiration, moderate to large contusion, infiltrate, purulent sputum, PO_2 <350 on 100% FiO_2 and PEEP 5
- **Acute rejection** – perivascular lymphocytosis
- **Chronic rejection – bronchiolitis obliterans**

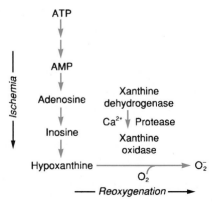

The classic pathway of superoxide anion generation by the metabolism of purines by xanthine oxidase. AMP, adenosine monophosphate; ATP, adenosine triphosphate.

OPPORTUNISTIC INFECTION

- **Viral** – CMV, HSV, VZV
- **Protozoan** – *Pneumocystis jiroveci* (*P. carinii*) pneumonia (reason for Bactrim prophylaxis)
- **Fungal** – *Aspergillus, Candida, Cryptococcus*

Hierarchy for Permission for Organ Donation from Next of Kin

1. Spouse
2. Adult son or daughter
3. Either parent
4. Adult brother or sister
5. Guardian
6. Any other person authorized to dispose of the body

INFLAMMATION PHASES

- **Injury** – leads to exposed <u>collagen</u>, <u>platelet-activating factor</u> release, <u>tissue factor</u> release from endothelium

- **Platelets bind** – release important growth factors (platelet-derived growth factor [<u>PDGF</u>]); leads to PMN, macrophage recruitment

- **Macrophages** – dominant role in wound healing, release important growth factors (PDGF) and cytokines (IL-1 and TNF-α)

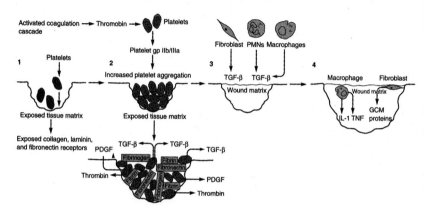

Establishment of a provisional wound matrix. (1) Platelets bind to the exposed wound matrix through interaction of beta-1 and beta-3 integrins and collagen, laminin, and fibrinonectin receptors. (2) After wounding, the coagulation cascade is activated, generating thrombin, which activates platelet glycoprotein (gp) IIb/IIIa and increases platelet aggregation. A provisional wound matrix is formed, made up of platelets, fibrin, fibrinogen, and fibronectin. The activated platelets in the wound generate transforming growth factor-beta (TGF-β), platelet-derived growth factor (PDGF), and thrombin. (3) TGF-β is strongly chemotactic for neutrophils, macrophages, and fibroblasts, recruiting these cells into the provisional wound matrix, where they are also subsequently activated by TGF-β. (4) Increasing concentrations of TGF-β result in macrophage activation, producing increased amounts of tumor necrosis factor-alpha (TGF-α) and interleukin-1 (IL-1). TGF-β also stimulates fibroblast production of extracellular matrix proteins. These reactions further enhance migration of macrophages and fibroblasts into the wound, facilitating repair.

GROWTH AND ACTIVATING FACTORS

- **PDGF** – similar effect as TGF-β
  - Chemotactic and activates inflammatory cells (PMNs and macrophages)
  - Chemotactic and activates fibroblasts → collagen and ECM proteins
  - Angiogenesis
  - Epithelialization
  - Chemotactic for smooth muscle cells
  - Has been shown to accelerate wound healing

- **EGF (epidermal growth factor)** – acts on similar receptors as TGF-β; less potent
  - Chemotactic and activates fibroblasts → collagen and ECM proteins
  - Angiogenesis – V-EGF stimulates angiogenesis and is involved in tumor metastasis
  - Epithelialization

- **FGF (fibroblastic growth factor)**
  - Chemotactic and activates fibroblasts → collagen and ECM proteins
  - Angiogenesis
  - Epithelialization

- **PAF (platelet-activating factor)** – not stored, generated by **phospholipase** in endothelium and other cells
  - Stimulates many types of inflammatory cells; chemotactic; ↑ adhesion molecules

- **Chemotactic factors**
  - For inflammatory cells – TGF-β, PDGF, IL-8, LTB-4, C5a and C3a, PAF
  - For fibroblasts – TGF-β, PDGF, EGF, FGF
- **Angiogenesis factors** – TGF-β, EGF, FGF, TGF-α, IL-8, hypoxia
- **Epithelialization factors** – TGF-β, PDGF, EGF, FGF, TGF-α

- **PMNs** – last 1–2 days in tissues (7 days in blood)
- **Platelets** – last 7–10 days
- **Lymphocytes** – involved in chronic inflammation (T cells) and antibody production (B cells)

- **TXA$_2$** and **PGI$_2$** – see Chap. 2

CELL TYPES IN TYPE I HYPERSENSITIVITY REACTIONS

- **Eosinophils**
  - Have IgE receptors that bind to allergen
  - Release major basic protein, which stimulates basophils and mast cells to release histamine
  - Eosinophils increased in parasitic infections
- **Basophils** – have IgE receptors
  - Main source of histamine in **blood;** not found in tissue
- **Mast cells** – primary cell in **type I hypersensitivity reactions**
  - Main source of histamine in **tissues** other than stomach

- **Histamine** – vasodilation, tissue edema, postcapillary leakage
  - Primary effectors in **type I hypersensitivity reactions** (allergic reactions)
- **Bradykinin** – vasodilation, increased permeability, pain, contraction of pulmonary arterioles
  - **Angiotensin-converting enzyme (ACE)** – inactivates bradykinin

NITRIC OXIDE

- Has arginine precursor
- Activates guanylate cyclase and increases cGMP, resulting in vascular smooth muscle dilation
- Is also called endothelium-derived relaxing factor (EDRF)
- **Endothelin** – vascular smooth muscle constriction

IMPORTANT CYTOKINES

- Main initial cytokine response to injury and infection is release of **TNF-α and IL-1**

- **Tumor necrosis factor-alpha (TNF-α)**
  - **Macrophages** – largest producers of TNF
  - Increases adhesion molecules
  - Overall, a procoagulant
  - Causes cachexia in patients with cancer
  - Activates neutrophils and macrophages → more cytokine production, cell recruitment
    - Can also cause myocardial depression

- Fever, hypothermia, tachycardia, ↑ cardiac output, ↓ SVRI → high concentrations can cause circulatory collapse and multisystem organ failure

IL-1
- Main source also macrophages; effects similar to TNF and synergizes TNF
- Responsible for **fever** (PGE_2 mediated in hypothalamus)
  - Raises thermal set point, causing fever
  - NSAIDs ↓ fever, reducing PGE_2 synthesis
- **Alveolar macrophages** – cause fever with atelectasis by **releasing IL-1**
- IL-1 also increases IL-6 production

IL-6
- ↑ **Hepatic acute phase proteins** (C-reactive protein, amyloid A)
- Lymphocyte activation

INTERFERONS
- Released by **lymphocytes** in response to <u>viral infection</u> or other stimulates
- Activate <u>macrophages, natural killer cells, and cytotoxic T cells</u>
- **Inhibit viral replication**

HEPATIC ACUTE PHASE RESPONSE PROTEINS
- IL-6 – most potent stimulus
- **Increased** – C-reactive protein (an opsonin, activates complement), amyloid A and P, fibrinogen, haptoglobin, ceruloplasmin, alpha-1 antitrypsin, alpha-1 antichymotrypsin and C3 (complement)
- **Decreased** – albumin and transferrin

CELL ADHESION MOLECULES
- **Selectins** – L-selectins, located on leukocytes, bind to <u>E- (endothelial) and P- (platelets) selectins</u>; rolling adhesion
- **Beta-2 integrins** (CD 11/18 molecules) – on leukocytes; bind ICAMs, etc., anchoring adhesion
- **ICAM, VCAM, PECAM, ELAM** – on endothelial cells, bind beta-2 integrin molecules located on leukocytes and platelets. These are also involved in transendothelial migration

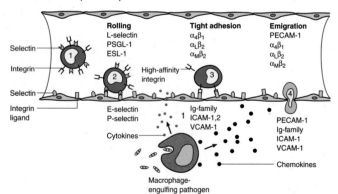

Leukocyte recruitment. (1) Circulating leukocytes express integrins in a low-affinity conformation. (2) Exposure to activated endothelium leads to rolling, which is mediated by L-selectin and P-selectin on the neutrophil and E-selectin on the endothelium. (3) Leukocyte exposure to cytokines released by macrophages phagocytosing pathogens induces a high-affinity integrin conformation. Tight leukocyte—endothelial adhesion involves integrin engagement with counterligand expressed on the endothelium. (4) Subsequent exposure to chemokines leads to diapedesis, which is further mediated by the family of β_1- and β_2-integrins.

COMPLEMENT

- **Classic pathway** (IgG or IgM) – antigen–antibody complex activates
  - **Factors C1, C2, and C4** – found only in the classic pathway
- **Alternative pathway** – endotoxin, bacteria, other stimuli activate
  - **Factors B, D, and P (properdin)** – found only in the alternate pathway
- **C3** – common to and is the convergence point for both pathways
- **Mg** – required for both pathways
- **Anaphylatoxins** – <u>C3a, C4a, C5a</u>; ↑ vascular permeability, smooth muscle contraction (bronchi); activate mast cells and basophils
- **Membrane attack complex** – C5b–9b
- **Opsonization** – C3b
- **Chemotaxis** – C3a and C5a

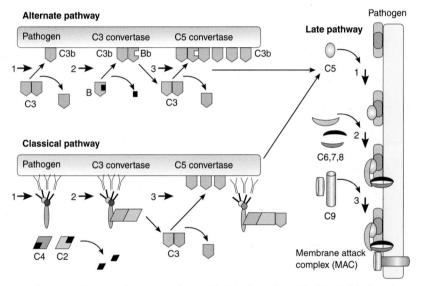

Complement pathways. Alternate pathway: (1) C3 is cleaved to C3b. (2) C3b binds and cleaves B to Bb to form C3 convertase (C3bBb). (3) Another C3b binds C3 convertase to form C5 convertase (C3bBbC3b). Classical pathway: (1) C1 binds immunoglobulin. (2) C1 binds and cleaves C4 and C2 to C4b and C2a to form C3 convertase (C4b2a). (3) C4b2a binds another C3b to generate C5 convertase (C4b2aC3b). Late pathway: (1) C5 convertase cleaves C5 to form C5b, which integrates into the plasmalemma. (2) C6–8 are recruited, forming the C5b–8 complex. (3) C5b–8 recruits numerous C9 subunits, which form a pore in the pathogen cell wall.

PROSTAGLANDINS

- **PGI$_2$ and PGE$_2$** – vasodilation, bronchodilation, ↑ permeability; inhibit platelets
- **PGD$_2$** – vasodilation, bronchoconstriction, ↑ permeability

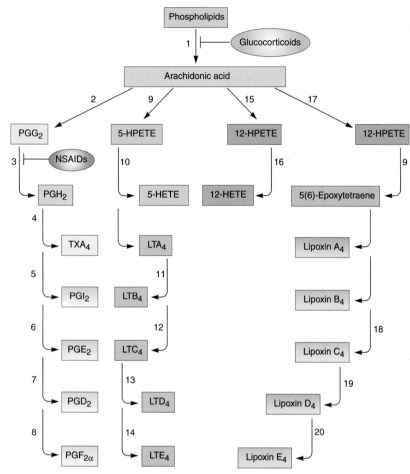

Eicosanoid production. (1) Phospholipases, (2) cyclooxygenase, (3) hydroperoxidase, (4) thromboxane synthetase, (5) prostacyclin synthetase, (6) E-isomerase, (7) D-isomerase, (8) F-reductase, (9) 5-lipoxygenase, (10) glutathione peroxidase, (11) hydrolase, (12) glutathione S-transferase, (13) γ-glutamyl transpeptidase, (14) cysteinyl glycanase, (15) 12-lipoxygenase, (16) peroxidase, (17) 15-lipoxygenase, (18) GSH-*cis*-11-*trans*-lipoxin A$_4$, (19) α-glutamyl transferase, and (20) dipeptidase.

- **NSAIDs** – inhibit cyclooxygenase (reversible)
- **Aspirin** – inhibits cyclooxygenase (irreversible), inhibits platelet adhesion by decreasing TXA$_2$
- **Steroids** – inhibit phospholipase, which converts phospholipids to arachidonic acid → inhibits inflammation

LEUKOTRIENES
- **LTC$_4$, LTD$_4$, LTE$_4$** – <u>slow-reacting substances of anaphylaxis</u>; bronchoconstriction, vasoconstriction followed by increased permeability (wheal and flare)
- **LTB$_4$** – chemotactic

CATECHOLAMINES
◼ Peak 24–48 hours after injury

◼ Norepinephrine released from sympathetic postganglionic neurons
◼ Epinephrine and norepinephrine released from adrenal medulla (neural response to injury)

Neuroendocrine response to injury – afferent nerves from site of injury stimulate CRF, ACTH, ADH, growth hormone, epinephrine, and norepinephrine release

Thyroid hormone – does *not* play a major note in injury

CXC chemokines – chemotaxis, angiogenesis, wound healing
   IL-8 and platelet factor 4 are CXC chemokines
   C = cysteine X $\rightarrow$ another amino acid

Oxidants Generated in Inflammation

$$O_2 + 1e^- \xrightarrow[\text{oxidase}]{\text{NADPH}} O_2^{\cdot-}$$ 　　　　　Superoxide anion

$$2H^+ + O_2^{\cdot-} + O_2^{\cdot-} \xrightarrow[\text{or superoxide dismutase}]{\text{spontaneous}} O_2 + H_2O_2$$ 　　　Hydrogen peroxide

$$H_2O_2 + + Fe^{2+} \rightarrow Fe^{3+} + OH^- + OH^{\cdot}$$ 　　　Hydroxyl radical

$$H_2O_2 + Cl^- + H^+ \xrightarrow{\text{myeloperoxidase}} H_2O + HOCl$$ 　　　Hypochlorous acid

$$R' RNH + HOCl \rightarrow H_2O + R'RNCl$$ 　　　Chloramines

Cellular Defenses Against Antioxidants

$$H_2O_2 + 2GSH \xrightarrow{\pm \text{ GSH peroxidase}} 2H_2O_2 + GSSG$$

$$ROOH + 2GSH \xrightarrow{\text{GSH peroxidase}} ROH + GSSG + H_2O$$

$$GSSG \xrightarrow[\text{GSH reductase}]{\text{NADPH}} 2GSH$$

$$O_2^{\cdot-} + O_2^{\cdot-} + 2H^+ \xrightarrow[\text{dismutase}]{\text{superoxide}} O_2 + H_2O_2$$

Catalase is also involved in reducing H_2O_2

Red blood cells – have some antioxidant properties (superoxide dismutase and catalase)
Reperfusion injury – **PMNs** are the primary mediator
Chronic granulomatous disease – NADPH-oxidase system enzyme defect in PMNs
   Results in ↓ superoxide radical (O_2^-) formation

CHAPTER 14. **WOUND HEALING**

WOUND HEALING PHASES
- **Inflammation** (days 1-10) – PMNs, macrophages; epithelialization 1-2 mm/day
- **Proliferation** (5 days-3 weeks) – fibroblasts, neovascularization, production of collagen, granulation tissue
- **Remodeling** (3 weeks-1 year) – type III collagen replaced with type I; decreased vascularity
  - Net amount of collagen does not change, although significant production and degradation occur
  - Collagen cross-linking occurs
- Peripheral nerves regenerate at **1 mm/day**

- **Order of cell arrival in wound**
  - **Platelets**
  - **PMNs**
  - **Macrophages**
  - **Fibroblasts**
  - **Lymphocytes**

- **Macrophages** are essential for wound healing (release of growth factors, cytokines, etc.)
- **Fibroblasts** – replace fibronectin-fibrin with **collagen**
- **Fibronectin** – chemotactic for macrophages; anchors fibroblasts
- **Thrombin and fibrin** – also act as growth factors for endothelial cells and fibroblasts
- **Predominant cell type by day**
  - **Days 0-2** – PMNs
  - **Days 3-4** – macrophages
  - **Days 5 and on** – fibroblasts
- **Platelet plug** – platelets and fibrin
- **Provisional matrix** – platelets, fibrin, and fibronectin
- **Accelerated wound healing** – reopening a wound results in quicker healing the 2nd time (as healing cells are already present there)

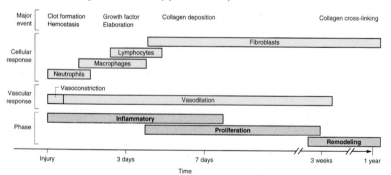

Time line of phases of wound healing with dominant cell types and major physiologic events.

PLATELET GRANULES
- **Alpha granules**
  - **Platelet factor 4** – aggregation
  - **Beta-thrombomodulin** – binds thrombin
  - **PDGF** – chemoattractant

- ■ **Dense granules** – adenosine, serotonin, and calcium
- ■ Platelet aggregation factors – **TXA$_2$, thrombin, platelet factor 4**
- ■ **Other factors released from platelets**
  - • **Platelet-activating factor**
  - • **Transforming growth factor-alpha**
  - • **Fibroblast growth factor**
  - • **Beta lysin** (antimicrobial)
  - • **PGE$_2$ and PGI$_2$** (vasodilators)
  - • **PGF$_2$** (vasoconstriction)

Epithelial integrity – most important factor in healing **open wounds (secondary intention)**
    <u>Migration</u> from wound edges, sweat glands, and hair follicles
    Dependent on granulation tissue
    Unepithelialized wounds leak serum and protein, promote bacteria

Tensile strength – most important factor in healing **closed incisions (primary intention)**
    Depends on collagen deposition and cross-linking of collagen
    Submucosa – strength layer of bowel
    Weakest time point for small bowel anastomosis – 3–5 days

Myofibroblasts (smooth muscle cell–fibroblast, communicate by gap junctions) –
    Involved in wound contraction and **healing by secondary intention**
Perineum has better wound contraction than leg

Collagen	
Type	**Description**
I	Most common type of collagen: skin, bone, and tendons <u>Primary collagen in a healed wound</u>
II	Cartilage
III	Increased in healing wound, also in blood vessels and skin
IV	Basement membranes
V	Widespread, particularly found in the cornea

- ■ **Alpha-ketoglutarate, vitamin C, oxygen, and iron** are required for <u>hydroxylation of proline</u> (prolyl hydroxylase) and subsequent <u>cross-linking of proline residues</u>
  - • Hydroxylysine also undergoes cross-linking
- ■ **Collagen** – has **proline every 3rd amino acid**; also has abundant **lysine**
- ■ **Scurvy** – vitamin C deficiency

- ■ **Tensile strength never equal to prewound (80%)**
  - • **Type III collagen** – predominant collagen type synthesized for days 1–2
  - • **Type I collagen** – predominant collagen type synthesized by days 3–4
  - • Type III replaced by type I collagen by 3 weeks
    - • **At 6 weeks,** wound is 80% of its final strength and 60% of its original strength
    - • **At 8 weeks,** wound reaches maximum tensile strength, which is 80% of its original strength
    - • Maximum collagen accumulation at 2–3 weeks after that → the amount of collagen stays the same but continued cross-linking improves strength
    - • **d-Penicillamine** – inhibits collagen cross-linking

- ▣ **Essentials for wound healing**
  - **Moist** environment (avoid desiccation)
  - **Oxygen delivery** – optimal fluids, no smoking, pain control, arterial reconstruction, supplemental oxygen
    - ◦ Want transcutaneous oxygen measurement (TCOM) > 25 mm Hg
  - **Avoid edema** – leg elevation, compression
  - **Remove necrotic tissue**

- ▣ **Impediments to wound healing**
  - **Bacteria > 10^5/cm^2** – ↓ oxygen content, collagen lysis, prolonged inflammation
  - **Devitalized tissue and foreign bodies** – retards granulation tissue formation and wound healing
  - **Cytotoxic drugs** – 5FU, methotrexate, cyclosporine, FK-506, etc., can impair wound healing
  - **Diabetes** – can contribute to poor wound healing by impeding the early-phase response
  - **Albumin < 3.0** – risk factor for poor wound healing
  - **Steroids** – prevent wound healing by inhibiting macrophages, PMNs, and collagen synthesis by fibroblasts; ↓ wound tensile strength as well
    - ◦ **Vitamin A** (25,000 IU qd) – counteracts effects of steroids on wound healing
  - **Wound ischemia**
    - ◦ Fibrosis
    - ◦ Pressure (sacral decubitus ulcers)
    - ◦ Poor arterial inflow
    - ◦ Poor venous outflow
    - ◦ Smoking
    - ◦ Radiation
    - ◦ Edema
    - ◦ Vasculitis

- ▣ **Diseases associated with abnormal wound healing**
  - **Osteogenesis imperfecta** – type I collagen defect
  - **Ehlers–Danlos syndrome** – 10 types identified, all collagen disorders
  - **Marfan's syndrome** – fibrillin (collagen) defect
  - **Epidermolysis bullosa** – excessive fibroblasts. Tx: phenytoin
  - **Scurvy**
  - **Pyoderma gangrenosum**

Diabetic foot ulcers – Charcot's joint (2nd MTP joint); secondary to neuropathy
  Pressure leads to ischemia
Leg ulcers – 90% of leg ulcers due to venous insufficiency. Tx: Unna boot, elastic wrap
Pressure sores – see Chap. 18
Scars – contain a lot of proteoglycans, hyaluronic acid, and water
  Scar revisions – wait for 1 year to allow maturation; may improve with age
  Infants heal with little or no scarring
Cartilage – contains no blood vessels
Denervation – has no effect on wound healing
Chemotherapy – has no effect on wound healing after 14 days
Keloids – autosomal dominant; dark skinned
  Collagen goes beyond original scar
  Tx: XRT, steroids, silicone, pressure garments
Hypertrophic scar tissue – dark skinned; flexor surfaces of upper torso
  Collagen stays within confines of scar
  Often occurs in burns or wounds that take a long time to heal
  Tx: steroids, silicone, pressure garments

1st peak for trauma deaths (0–30 minutes) – deaths due to lacerations of heart, aorta, brain, brainstem, spinal cord. Cannot really save these patients; death is too quick

2nd peak for trauma deaths (30 minutes–4 hours) – deaths due to head injury (#1) and hemorrhage (#2). These are the patients you can save with rapid assessment (golden hour)

3rd peak for trauma deaths (days to weeks) – deaths due to multisystem organ failure and sepsis

Blunt injury – 80% of all trauma; <u>liver</u> most commonly injured (some texts say spleen)

Kinetic energy = $\frac{1}{2} MV^2$, where M = mass, V = velocity

Falls – age and body orientation biggest predictors of survival. LD_{50} is 4 stories

Penetrating injury – <u>small bowel</u> most commonly injured (some texts say liver)

Hemorrhage – most common cause of death in 1st hour

    Blood pressure is usually OK until 30% of total blood volume is lost

Head injury – most common cause of death after reaching the ER alive

Infection – most common cause of death in the long term

Tongue – most common cause of upper airway obstruction → perform jaw thrust

Seat belts – small bowel perforations, lumbar spine fractures, sternal fractures

Saphenous vein at ankle – best site for cutdown for access

Diagnostic peritoneal lavage (DPL)

Used in hypotensive patients with blunt trauma

Positive if >10 cc blood, >100,000 RBCs/cc, food particles, bile, bacteria, >500 WBC/cc

Need laparotomy if DPL is positive

DPL needs to be supraumbilical if pelvic fracture present

DPL misses – retroperitoneal bleeds, contained hematomas

FAST scan (focused abdominal sonography for trauma)

Ultrasound scan used in lieu of DPL

Checks for blood in perihepatic fossa, perisplenic fossa, pelvis, and pericardium

Examiner dependent

Obesity can obstruct view

May not detect free fluid < 50–80 mL

Need laparotomy if FAST scan is positive

FAST scan misses – retroperitoneal bleeding, hollow viscous injury

Need a CT scan following blunt trauma in patients with <u>abdominal pain, need for general anesthesia, closed head injury, intoxicants on board, paraplegia, distracting injury, hematuria</u>

Patients requiring DPL that turned out negative will need an abdominal CT scan

CT scan misses – hollow viscous injury, diaphragm injury

Need laparotomy with peritonitis, evisceration, positive DPL, clinical deterioration, uncontrolled hemorrhage, free air, diaphragm injury, intraperitoneal bladder injury, positive contrast studies, specific renal, pancreas, and biliary tract injuries

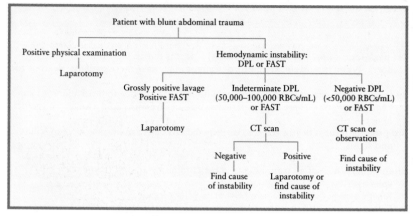

Diagnosis of blunt abdominal trauma.

Possible penetrating abdominal injuries (knife or low-velocity injuries) – local
exploration and observation if fascia not violated
Diagnostic laparoscopy to see if fascia was violated

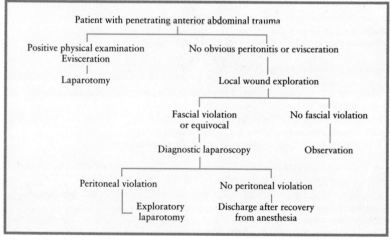

Diagnosis of low-velocity penetrating abdominal trauma.

Abdominal compartment syndrome
Occurs after massive fluid resuscitation, trauma, or abdominal surgery
Bladder pressure > 25–30
IVC compression is final common pathway for ↓ cardiac output
Gut malperfusion
Renal vein compression leading to ↓ urine output
Upward displacement of diaphragm affecting ventilation
Tx: decompressive laparotomy

Pneumatic antishock garment – controversial; use in patients with SBP < 50 and no
thoracic injury. Release compartments one at a time after reaching ER

ER thoracotomy

Blunt trauma – use only if pressure/pulse lost **in ER**

Penetrating trauma – use only if pressure/pulse lost **on way to ER or in ER**

Thoracotomy – open pericardium anterior to the phrenic nerve, cross-clamp the aorta, watch for the esophagus

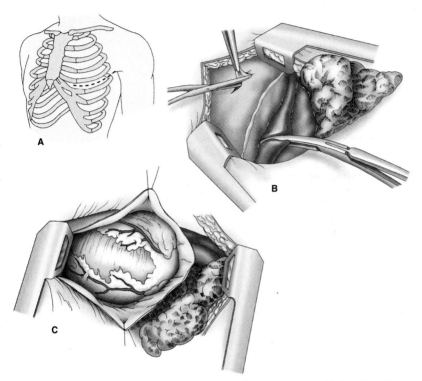

(A) Emergency department thoracotomies are performed through the fourth and fifth intercostal spaces using the anterolateral approach. *(B)* If the thoracotomy is performed for abdominal injury, the descending thoracic aorta is clamped. If blood pressure improved to >70 mm Hg, the patient is transported to the operating room for laparotomy. For patients in whom blood pressure does not reach 70 mm Hg, further treatment is futile. If the thoracotomy is performed for a cardiac injury, the pericardium is opened longitudinally and anterior to the phrenic nerve. *(C)* The heart can then be rotated out of the pericardium for repair. (From Johnson JL, Moore EE. Thoracic trauma. In: Fischer JE, Bland KI, et al., eds. *Mastery of Surgery*. 5th ed. Philadelphia: Lippincott Williams & Wilkins; 2007, with permission.)

Catecholamines – peak 24–48 hours after injury

ADH, ACTH, and glucagon – also ↑ after trauma (fight or flight response)

BLOOD TRANSFUSION

■ Type O blood (Universal donor) – contains no A or B antigens; males can receive Rh-positive blood; females who are prepubescent or of child-bearing age should receive Rh-negative blood

■ Type-specific blood (nonscreened, noncrossmatched) – can be administered relatively safely, but there may be effects from antibodies to minor antigens in the donated blood

Comparison of Blood Availability

Blood	Typing	Antibody Screen	Crossmatch	Time
Type O	No	No	No	Immediate
Type specific	Yes	No	No	<10 min
Type and screen	Yes	Yes	Yes	20–30 min
Type and crossmatch	Yes	Yes	Yes	45–60 min

HEAD INJURY (SEE ALSO CHAP. 41)
- **Glasgow Coma Scale (GCS)**
  - **Motor**
    - **6** – follows commands
    - **5** – localizes pain
    - **4** – withdraws from pain
    - **3** – flexion with pain (decorticate)
    - **2** – extension with pain (decerebrate)
    - **1** – no response
  - **Verbal**
    - **5** – oriented
    - **4** – confused
    - **3** – inappropriate words
    - **2** – incomprehensible sounds
    - **1** – no response
  - **Eye opening**
    - **4** – spontaneous opening
    - **3** – opens to command
    - **2** – opens to pain
    - **1** – no response
- **GCS score** – ≤ **14**: head CT; ≤ **10**: intubation; ≤ **8**: ICP monitor

Indications for Neurologic Imaging

Suspected skull penetration by a foreign body
- Discharge of cerebrospinal fluid (CSF), blood, or both from the nose
- Hemotympanum or discharge of blood or CSF from the ear
- Protracted unconsciousness
- Altered state of consciousness at the time of examination
- Focal neurologic signs or symptoms
- Any situation precluding proper surveillance
- Head injury plus additional trauma
- Possible head injury in the presence of additional pathologic findings, such as stroke
- Head injury with alcohol or drug intoxication

- **Epidural hematoma** – most commonly due to arterial bleeding from the **middle meningeal artery**
  - Head CT – shows lenticular (lens-shaped) deformity
  - Patients initially have loss of consciousness (LOC) → then lucid interval → then sudden deterioration (vomiting, restlessness, LOC)
  - Operate for significant neurologic degeneration or significant mass effect (shift > 5 mm)

- **Subdural hematoma** – most commonly from tearing of **venous plexus (bridging veins)** between dura and arachnoid
  - **Head CT** – shows crescent-shaped deformity
  - Operate for significant mass effect
  - **Chronic subdural hematomas** – usually in elderly after minor fall
    - Need drainage if >1 cm or causing significant symptoms

- **Intracerebral hematoma** – usually frontal or temporal
  - Can cause significant mass effect requiring operation
- **Cerebral contusions** – can be coup or contracoup
- **Traumatic intraventricular hemorrhage** – need ventriculostomy if causing hydrocephalus
- **Diffuse axonal injury** – shows up better on MRI than CT scan
  - Tx: supportive; may need craniectomy if ICP elevated
  - Very poor prognosis

- **Cerebral perfusion pressure (CPP)**
  - **CPP** = mean arterial pressure (MAP) *minus* intracranial pressure (ICP)
  - **Signs of elevated ICP** – ↓ ventricular size, loss of sulci, loss of cisterns
  - **ICP monitors** – indicated for GCS ≤ 8, suspected ↑ ICP, or patient with moderate to severe head injury and inability to follow clinical exam (e.g., is intubated)

  - **Supportive treatment for elevated ICP**
    - Normal ICP is 10; >20 needs treatment
    - Want CPP > 60
      - **Sedation and paralysis**
      - **Raise head of bed**
      - **Relative hyperventilation** for modest cerebral vasoconstriction (CO_2 30–35); do not want to overhyperventilate and cause cerebral ischemia from too much vasoconstriction
      - **Keep Na 140–150, serum Osm 295–310** – may need to use <u>hypertonic saline</u> at times (draws fluid out of brain)
      - **Mannitol** – load 1 g/kg, give 0.25 mg/kg q4h after that (draws fluid from brain)
      - **Barbiturate coma** – consider if above not working
      - **Ventriculostomy w/ CSF drainage (keep ICP < 20)**
      - **Craniotomy decompression** – if not able to get ICP down medically (can also perform Burr hole)
      - **Phenytoin** – given prophylactically to prevent seizures to most patients with traumatic brain injury
      - **Peak ICP** – occurs <u>48–72 hours after injury</u>
      - **Dilated pupil** – **temporal pressure** on the same side (CN III compression)

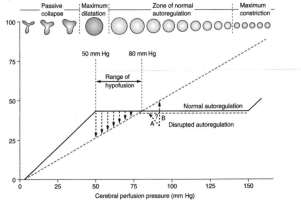

Cerebral pressure autoregulation. The normal relationship is indicated by the solid line with autoregulatory break points at 50 and 150 mm Hg. Two disrupted states are also diagrammed. Complete loss of autoregulation *(straight dashed line B)* results in a pressure-passive system wherein CBF (and CBV) increases linearly with CPP. The more common form of disruption is indicated by the sigmoid dashed line *(A)* where the major alteration is a right shift in the lower break point. The circles at the top of the figure represent the diameters of the resistance vessels in the normal situation. The area of the circles represents CBV. Shifting this relationship to the right by 30 mm Hg would represent the partially disrupted state. (© R.M. Chesnut.)

- **Basal skull fractures**
  - **Raccoon eyes** – anterior fossa fracture
  - **Battle's sign** – middle fossa fracture → can injure facial nerve
    - If acute, need exploration
    - If delayed, likely secondary to edema and exploration not needed
  - Can also have hemotympanum, CSF rhinorrhea/otorrhea, or injury to CN I, VII, and VIII
  - **Temporal skull fractures** – can injure CN VII and VIII
    - **Most common site of facial nerve injury** – geniculate ganglion
    - Temporal skull fractures most commonly associated with lateral skull or orbital blows
  - **Most skull fractures do <u>not</u>** require surgical treatment
    - Operate if significantly depressed (8–10 mm), contaminated, or persistent CSF leak not responding to conservative therapy
  - **CSF leaks** – treat expectantly

SPINE TRAUMA (SEE ALSO CHAP. 41)
- **Cervical spine**
  - C-1 burst (Jefferson fracture) – caused by axial loading
    - Tx: rigid collar
  - C-2 hangman's fracture – caused by distraction and extension
    - Tx: traction and halo
  - C-2 odontoid fracture
    - Type I – above base, stable
    - Type II – at base, unstable (will need fusion or halo)
    - Type III – extends into vertebral body (will need fusion or halo)
  - Facet fractures or dislocations – can cause cord injury; usually associated with hyperextension and rotation and with ligamentous disruption
- **Thoracolumbar spine**
  - 3 columns of the thoracolumbar spine
    - Anterior – anterior longitudinal ligament and anterior ½ of the vertebral body
    - Middle – posterior ½ of the vertebral body and posterior longitudinal ligament
    - Posterior – facet joints, lamina, spinous processes, interspinous ligament
  - If more than 1 column is disrupted, the spine is considered unstable
    - Compression (wedge) fractures usually involve the anterior column only and are considered stable
    - Burst fractures are considered unstable (>1 column) and require spinal fusion
  - **Upright fall** – at risk for calcaneus, lumbar, and wrist/forearm fractures
- MRI for neurologic deficits without bony injury to check for ligamentous injury
- **Indications for emergent surgical spine decompression**
  - Fracture or dislocation not reducible with distraction
  - Acute anterior spinal syndrome
  - Open fractures
  - Soft tissue or bony compression of the cord
  - Progressive neurologic dysfunction

MAXILLOFACIAL TRAUMA
- Facial nerve injuries need repair
- Fracture of temporal bone is most common cause of <u>facial nerve injury</u>
- Try to preserve skin and not trim edges with facial lacerations

Le Fort Classification of Facial Fractures

Type	Description	Treatment
I	Maxillary fracture straight across (−)	Reduction, stabilization, intramaxillary fixation (IMF) +/− circumzygomatic and orbital rim suspension wires
II	Lateral to nasal bone, underneath eyes, diagonal toward maxilla (/ \\)	Same as Le Fort I
III	Lateral orbital walls (- -)	Suspension wiring to stable frontal bone; may need external fixation

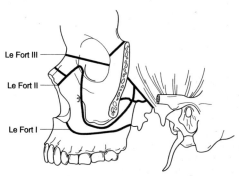

Le Fort classification system of maxillofacial fractures.

■ **Nasoethmoidal orbital fractures** – 70% have a CSF leak
  • Conservative therapy for 2 weeks
  • Can try epidural catheter to ↓ CSF pressure and help it close
  • May need surgical closure of dura to deal with leak
■ **Nosebleeds**
  • **Anterior** – packing
  • **Posterior** – can be hard to deal with; try balloon tamponade 1st
    • May need angioembolization of internal maxillary artery or ethmoidal artery
■ **Orbital blowout fractures** – patients with impaired upward gaze or diplopia with upward vision need repair, with restoration of orbital floor with bone fragments or bone graft
■ **Mandibular injury** – malocclusion #1 indicator of injury
  • Panorex film is often used to assess injury along with fine-cut facial CT scans with reconstruction
  • Most repaired with IMF (metal arch bars to upper and lower dental arches, 6–8 weeks) or open reduction and internal fixation (ORIF)
■ **Tripod fracture (zygomatic bone)** – ORIF for cosmesis

■ Patients w/ maxillofacial fractures are at high risk for cervical spine injuries

NECK TRAUMA
■ **Asymptomatic blunt** – neck CT scan
■ **Asymptomatic penetrating** – controversial; most common method below

Neck Zones	
Zone	**Method**
I	Clavicle to cricoid cartilage; need angiography, bronchoscopy, rigid esophagoscopy, barium swallow, pericardial window may be indicated. May need sternotomy to reach these lesions
II	Cricoid to angle of mandible. Exploration in OR
III	Angle of mandible to the base of skull. Need angio, laryngoscopy. May need jaw subluxation/digastric and sternocleidomastoid muscle release/mastoid sinus resection to reach vascular injuries in this location

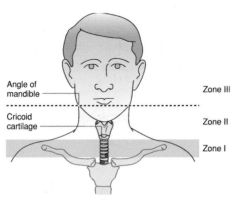

Zones of the neck. The junction of zones I and II is variously described as being at the cricoid cartilage or at the top of the clavicles. The important implication of a zone I injury is the greater potential for intrathoracic great vessel injury.

- **Symptomatic blunt or penetrating neck trauma** – shock, bleeding, expanding hematoma, losing or lost airway, subcutaneous air, stridor, dysphagia, hemoptysis, neurologic deficit
  - **Need neck exploration**

- **Esophageal injury**
  - Hardest neck injury to find
  - Rigid esophagoscopy and esophagogram – best combined modality (find essentially 95% of injuries when using both methods)
  - Contained injuries – can be observed
  - Noncontained injuries – if small injury, <24 hours, without significant contamination, and patient is stable → primary closure; otherwise make spit fistula and drain leak with chest tube
  - Always drain esophageal and hypopharyngeal repairs – 20% leak rate
  - Approach to esophageal injuries
    - Neck – **left side**
    - Upper ⅔ of thoracic esophagus – **right thoracotomy**
    - Lower ⅓ of thoracic esophagus – **left thoracotomy**

- **Laryngeal fracture and tracheal injuries**
  - **These are airway emergencies**
  - **Symptoms: crepitus, stridor, respiratory compromise**

- **Need to secure airway emergently in ER**
- Tx: primary repair, can use strap muscle for airway support; tracheostomy necessary for most to allow edema to subside and to check for stricture

- **Thyroid gland injuries** – control bleeding and drain
- **Recurrent laryngeal nerve injury** – can try to repair or can reimplant in cricoarytenoid muscle (hoarseness)
- **Shotgun injures to neck** – need angiogram and neck CT; esophagus/tracheal evaluation
- **Vertebral artery bleeds** – can ligate or embolize without sequela
- **Common carotid bleeds** – ligation will cause stroke in 20%

CHEST TRAUMA
- **Chest tube**
  - >1,500 cc after initial insertion, >250 cc/h for 3 hours, 2,500 cc/24 h, or bleeding with instability – all relative indications for thoracotomy in OR
  - Need to drain all of the blood (in <48 hours) to prevent fibrothorax, pulmonary entrapment, infected hemothorax
  - Unresolved hemothorax after 2 well-placed chest tubes → thoracoscopic or open drainage

- **Sucking chest wound**
  - Needs to be at least ⅔ the diameter of the trachea to be significant
  - Cover wound with dressing that has tape on three sides → prevents development of tension pneumothorax while allowing lung to expand with inspiration

- **Tracheobronchial injury**
  - Patient has worse oxygenation after chest tube placement
  - One of the very few indications in which clamping the chest tube may be indicated
  - Bronchial injuries are more common on **right**
  - May need to mainstem intubate patient on unaffected side
  - Dx: bronchoscopy
  - Tx: repair if large air leak and respiratory compromise or after 2 weeks of persistent air leak
  - **Right thoracotomy** for right mainstem, trachea, and proximal left mainstem injuries (avoids the aorta)
  - **Left thoracotomy** for distal left mainstem injuries

- **Esophageal injury** – see section "Neck Trauma"

- **Diaphragm**
  - Injuries are more likely to be found on **left** and to result from **blunt trauma**
  - CXR – see **air–fluid level** in chest from stomach herniation through hole (diagnosis can be made essentially with CXR)
  - Transabdominal approach if <1 week
  - Chest approach if >1 week
  - May need mesh

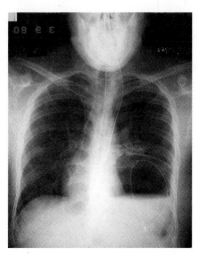

Chest roentgenogram demonstrating a nasogastric tube within the left chest (From Thal ER, Friese RS. Traumatic rupture of the diaphragm. In: Fischer JE, Bland KI, et al., eds. *Mastery of Surgery.* 5th ed. Philadelphia: Lippincott Williams & Wilkins; 2007, with permission.)

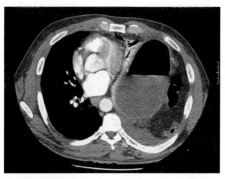

CT displaying intrathoracic herniation of abdominal contents. (From Thal ER, Friese RS. Traumatic rupture of the diaphragm. In: Fischer JE, Bland KI, et al., eds. *Mastery of Surgery.* 5th ed. Philadelphia: Lippincott Williams & Wilkins; 2007, with permission.)

■ **Aortic transection**
  • **Signs** – widened mediastinum, 1st rib fractures, apical capping, loss of aortopulmonary window, loss of aortic contour, left hemothorax, trachea deviation to right
  • Tear is usually at the **ligamentum arteriosum** (just distal to subclavian takeoff). Other areas include near the aortic valve and where the aorta traverses the diaphragm
  • CXR normal in 5% of patients with aortic tears – need aortic evaluation in patients with significant mechanism (head on car crash > 45 mph, fall >15 ft)
  • Dx: aortogram or CT angiogram of chest
  • Tx: need to **control blood pressure** with Nipride and esmolol
  • Operative approach – left thoracotomy with partial left heart bypass
  • Important to treat other life-threatening injuries 1st → patient with positive DPL or other life-threatening injury needs to have that addressed before the aortic transection
■ **Approach for specific injuries**
  • **Median sternotomy** – for injuries to ascending aorta, innominate artery, proximal right subclavian artery, innominate vein, proximal left common carotid

- **Left thoracotomy** – for injuries to left subclavian artery, descending aorta
- **Distal right subclavian artery** – midclavicular incision ½ resection of medial clavicle

- **Myocardial contusion** – V-tach and V-fib most common causes of death
  - Risk highest in 1st 24 hours
  - SVT – most common arrhythmia overall in these patients
  - Need monitoring

- **Flail chest** – ≥2 consecutive ribs broken at ≥2 sites → results in paradoxical motion
  - Underlying pulmonary contusion – biggest pulmonary impairment

- **Aspiration** – may not produce CXR findings immediately

- **Penetrating chest injury**
  - **Penetrating "box" injuries** – borders are clavicles, xiphoid process, nipples
    - **Need** pericardial window, bronchoscopy, esophagoscopy, barium swallow
  - **Penetrating chest wound outside "box"** without pneumothorax or hemothorax
    - Need chest tube if patient required intubation
    - Otherwise follow patient's CXRs
  - **Pericardial window** – if you find blood, need sternotomy to fix possible injury to heart; place pericardial drain
  - **Penetrating injuries anterior-medial to midaxillary line and below nipples**
    - Need laparotomy or laparoscopy
    - May also need evaluation for penetrating "box" injury depending on the exact location

- **Traumatic causes of cardiogenic shock** – cardiac tamponade (see Chap. 16), cardiac contusion, tension pneumothorax

- **Tension pneumothorax**
  - Hypotension, ↑ airway pressures, ↓ breath sounds, bulging neck veins, tracheal shift
  - Can see bulging diaphragm during laparotomy
  - Cardiac compromise secondary to ↓ venous return
  - Tx: chest tube

- **Sternal fractures** – these patients are at high risk for cardiac contusion

- **1st and 2nd rib fractures** – high risk for aortic transaction

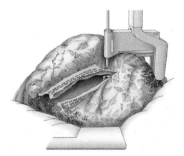

Pulmonary tractotomy. Dividing the pulmonary parenchyma between adjacent staple lines permits rapid direct access to injured vessels or bronchi along the tract of a penetrating injury. (From Johnson JL, Moore EE. Thoracic trauma. In: Fischer JE, Bland KI, et al. eds. *Mastery of Surgery.* 5th ed. Philadelphia: Lippincott Williams & Wilkins; 2007, with permission.)

PELVIC TRAUMA

- Pelvic fractures can be a major source of blood loss.
- If hemodynamically unstable with pelvic fracture and negative DPL, negative CXR, and no other signs of blood loss or reasons for shock → stabilize pelvis (C-clamp, external fixator, or sheet) and go to angio for embolization
- Patients at high risk for **GU and abdominal injuries**

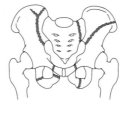

Type I: Unstable (crush)
Mortality: 20%–30%
Blood loss: >10 units
Complications: 60%–75%

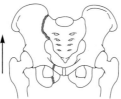

Type II: Unstable
Mortality: 8%–12%
Blood loss: 2–10 units
Complications: 30%–50%

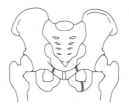

Type III: Stable.
Mortality: <5%
Blood loss: 1–4 units
Complications: 10%–20%

Classification of pelvic fractures with relative stability, mortality rates, and blood loss indicated.

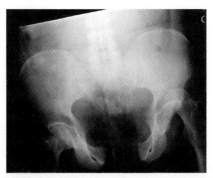

Wide pubic diastasis, characteristic of "open book" horizontally unstable pelvis (type B), with associated femoral head fracture and hip dislocation.

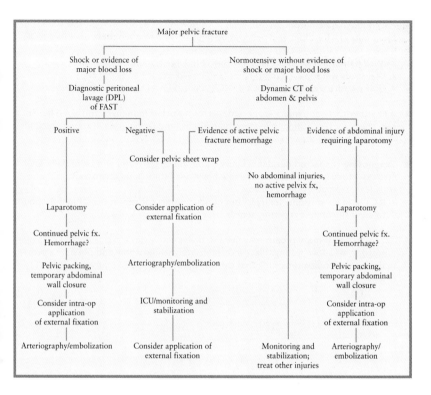

- **Anterior pelvic fractures** – more likely to have venous bleeding
- **Posterior pelvic fractures** – more likely to have arterial bleeding
- May need colostomy for open pelvic fractures with rectal tears and perineal lacerations
- Pelvic fracture repair itself may need to be delayed until other associated injuries are repaired
- **Penetrating injury pelvic hematomas** – open
- **Blunt injury pelvic hematomas** – leave unless expanding and patient unstable
  - If unstable, stabilize pelvic fracture, pack pelvis if in OR, and get patient to angiography embolization

DUODENAL TRAUMA
- Usually blunt from crush or deceleration injury
- **2nd portion of the duodenum** (descending portion, near ampulla of Vater) – most common area of injury
- Can also get tears near ligament of Treitz
- 70%–80% of injuries requiring surgery can be treated with **debridement and primary closure**
- Segmental resection with primary end-to-end closure possible with all **segments except second portion of the duodenum**
- 25% mortality in these patients because of associated **shock**
- **Fistulas** are the major source of morbidity

- **Paraduodenal hematomas** (usually in third portion of duodenum overlying spine in blunt injury) – for blunt and penetrating injuries need to open these up if in the OR

- **Missed hematomas** can present with high SBO 12–72 hours after injury
  - UGI study will show "stacked coins" or "coiled spring" appearance
  - Conservative treatment (TPN and NGT) cures 90% of these over 2–3 weeks

- If at laparotomy and injury suspected, perform **Kocher maneuver and open lesser sac**, check for <u>hematoma, bile, petechiae, sucus, and fat necrosis</u>. If found, need formal inspection of the entire duodenum

- **Diagnosing suspected duodenal injury** – abdominal CT with contrast initially. UGI contrast study best. CT scan may show bowel wall thickening, hematoma, air, contrast leak, retroperitoneal fluid/air
  - If CT scan is worrisome for injury but nondiagnostic, can repeat the CT in 8–12 hours to see if the finding is getting worse

- Tx: Try to get **primary repair**; may need to divert with <u>pyloric exclusion and gastrojejunostomy</u> to allow healing. Place a distal feeding jejunostomy and possibly a proximal draining jejunostomy tube that threads back to duodenal injury site. **Place drains**

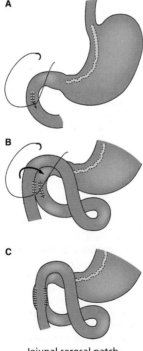

Jejunal serosal patch.

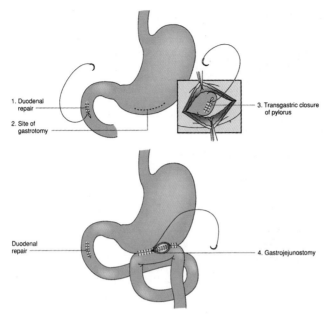

Pyloric exclusion for complex duodenal injury.

- If not enough duodenum is present for repair or is in 2nd portion of duodenum, need pyloric exclusion and gastrojejunostomy
  - Can then place jejunal patch over hole; may need Whipple procedure in future
  - Consider feeding and draining jejunostomies

- Trauma Whipple – rarely if ever indicated
- **Drains** – remove when patient tolerating diet without an increase in drainage
- **Fistulas** – often close with time
  - Tx: bowel rest, TPN, decompression, octreotide, fistulogram to rule out abscess, conservative management for 4-6 weeks. Consider distal obstruction

SMALL BOWEL TRAUMA
- Most common organ injured with penetrating injury
- These injuries can be hard to diagnose early if associated with blunt trauma
- **Occult small bowel injuries**
  - Abdominal CT scan showing **intra-abdominal fluid not associated with a solid organ injury, bowel wall thickening, or a mesenteric hematoma** is suggestive of injury
  - **Need close observation and possibly repeat abdominal CT** after 8–12 hours or so to make sure finding is not getting worse
  - Need to make sure patients with these nonconclusive findings can **tolerate a diet before discharge**
- Repair lacerations **transversely → avoids stricture**
- **Large lacerations** >50% of the circumference or results in lumen diameter, ⅓ normal – perform resection and reanastomosis
- **Multiple close lacerations** – just resect that segment
- **Mesenteric hematomas** – open if expanding or large (>2 cm)

COLON TRAUMA
- Most associated with penetrating injury
- Right and transverse colon – can perform primary reanastomosis
- Left colon – colostomy and Hartman's pouch or mucous fistula the safest procedure
- Paracolonic hematomas – both blunt and penetrating need to be opened
- 10% abscess rate after colon injury; 2% fistula rate, higher with primary repair

RECTAL TRAUMA
- Most associated with penetrating injury
- **High rectal**
  - **Extraperitoneal** – generally not repaired because of inaccessibility
    - Tx: presacral drainage and fecal diversion with colostomy; serial debridement
  - **Intraperitoneal** – Tx: repair defect, presacral drainage, fecal diversion with colostomy
- **Low rectal** (<5 cm) – can probably be repaired transanally

LIVER TRAUMA
- Lobectomy rarely necessary
- **Common hepatic artery** – can be ligated with collaterals through gastroduodenal artery
- **Hepatic lobar arteries** can be ligated without complication unless the patient is hypotensive, which could lead to liver ischemia
- **Pringle maneuver (clamping portal triad)** does not stop bleeding from **hepatic veins**

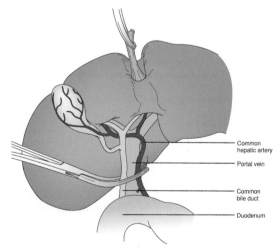

Pringle maneuver compression of the portal triad structures with a noncrushing vascular clamp for hepatic inflow control. If possible, clamp times should be limited to 15- to 20-minute intervals.

- **Atriocaval shunt** – for retrohepatic IVC injury, allows for control while performing repair

- **Perihepatic packing** – can pack severe penetrating liver injuries if patient becomes unstable in the OR. Go to the ICU and get the patient resuscitated and stabilized. Live to fight another day
- **Portal triad hematomas** – need to be explored

- **Common bile duct injury**
  - <50% of circumference – **repair over stent**
  - >50% or complex injury – **go with choledochojejunostomy**
  - May need intraoperative cholangiogram to define injury
  - 10% of duct anastomoses leak

- **Portal vein injury** – need to repair
  - May need to transect through the pancreas to get to the injury in the portal vein
  - Will need to perform distal pancreatectomy with that maneuver
  - Ligation of portal vein associated with 50% mortality

- **Omental graft** – can be placed in liver laceration to help with bleeding and prevent bile leaks
- **Leave drains with liver injuries**

- **Conservative management of blunt liver injuries**
  - **Has failed if** patient becomes unstable despite aggressive resuscitation, including 4 units of PRBCs (HR > 120 or SBP < 90) or requires >4 units of PRBCs to keep Hct > 25. **Go to OR**
  - **Active blush on abdominal CT or pseudoaneurysm** also indication for **OR**
    - If <u>posterior</u>, may be better off going to **angiogram** (when in doubt → OR)
    - If <u>anterior</u>, **go to OR**
  - **With conservative management, need bed rest for 5 days**

SPLEEN TRAUMA
- Fully healed after 6 weeks
- Postsplenectomy sepsis most common in 1st 5 years of life; greatest risk within 2 years of splenectomy
- Splenic salvage is associated with increased transfusions
- **Conservative management of blunt splenic injuries**
  - **Has failed if** patient becomes unstable despite aggressive resuscitation, including 2 units of PRBCs (HR > 120 or SBP ≤ 90) or requires >2 units of PRBCs to keep Hct > 25. **Go to OR**
  - **Active blush on abdominal CT or pseudoaneurysm** also indication for **OR**
  - **With conservative management, need bed rest for 5 days**
  - Threshold for splenectomy in **children** is much higher; hardly any children undergo splenectomy
  - Need immunizations after trauma splenectomy

PANCREATIC TRAUMA
- **Penetrating injury** – accounts for 80% of all pancreatic injuries
- **Blunt injury** – can result in pancreatic duct fractures, usually perpendicular to the duct

- Edema or necrosis of peripancreatic fat usually indicative of injury
- Pancreatic contusion – leave if stable, place drain

- **Distal pancreatic duct injury** – distal pancreatectomy, can take up to 80% of the gland

- **Pancreatic head injury that is not reparable** – place drains initially; delayed Whipple may be eventually necessary
- May be able to treat pancreatic duct injuries with ERCP and stent as opposed to resection

- Whipple vs. distal pancreatectomy based on duct injury in relation to the **SMA/SMV**
- Injuries to the right of the SMA/SMV treated with drains instead of Whipple initially

- Kocher maneuver helps evaluate the pancreas operatively
- **Leave drains with pancreatic injury**
- **Pancreatic hematoma** – both penetrating and blunt need to be opened

- Persistent or rising **amylase** may indicate missed pancreatic injury
- CT scans poor at diagnosing pancreatic injuries initially
  - Delayed signs – fluid, edema, necrosis
- Dx: ERCP good at picking up duct injuries and may be able to treat with stent

VASCULAR TRAUMA
- **Vascular repair performed before orthopaedic repair**
- **Major signs of vascular injury** – active hemorrhage, pulse deficit, expanding or pulsatile hematoma, distal ischemia, bruit, thrill → **go to OR for exploration** (some say angio 1st)
- **Moderate/soft signs of vascular injury** – history of hemorrhage, deficit of anatomically related nerve, large stable/nonpulsatile hematoma → **go to angio**
  - **ABI < 0.9** – go to angio
  - **Saphenous vein graft** – will be needed if segment > 2 cm missing
    - Use vein from the contralateral leg when fixing lower extremity arterial injuries (improves outflow)

  - Vein injuries that need repair – vena cava, femoral, popliteal, brachiocephalic, subclavian, and axillary
  - Transection of single artery in the calf in an otherwise healthy patient → ligate
  - Coverage of site of anastomoses with viable tissue and muscle important
  - Consider **fasciotomy** if ischemia > 4 hours – prevents compartment syndrome
  - **Compartment syndrome** – consider with pressures > 20 mm Hg or if clinical exam suggests elevated pressures
    - Pain → paresthesia → anesthesia → paralysis → poikilothermia → pulselessness (late finding)
    - Most commonly occurs after supracondylar humeral fractures, tibial fractures, crush injuries, or other injuries that result in a disruption and then restoration of blood flow

- **IVC** – primary repair if residual stenosis < 50% diameter of IVC; otherwise place saphenous vein or synthetic patch
  - Bleeding of IVC best controlled with proximal and distal pressure, <u>not</u> clamps → can tear it
  - Repair posterior wall injury through the anterior wall
  - May need to cut through the anterior IVC to get to posterior IVC injuries

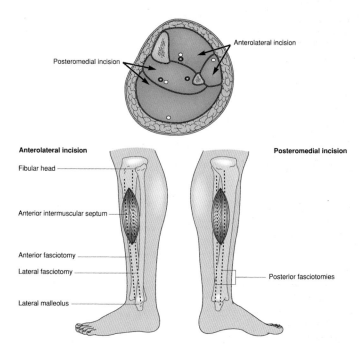

Surgical approach for four compartment fasciotomies through incisions on the medial and lateral aspects of the calf.

ORTHOPAEDIC TRAUMA (SEE ALSO CHAP. 42)
■ Can have >2 L blood loss from a femur fracture
■ Orthopaedic emergencies – pelvic fractures in unstable patients, spine injury with deficit, open fractures, dislocations or fractures with vascular compromise, compartment syndrome
■ Femoral neck fractures – high risk for avascular necrosis
■ Long bone fracture or dislocations with loss of pulse (or weak pulse) → immediate reduction of fracture or dislocation and reassessment of pulse:

Orthopaedic Trauma	Concomitant Nerve/Artery Injury
UPPER EXTREMITY	
Anterior shoulder dislocation	Axillary nerve
Posterior shoulder dislocation	Axillary artery
Proximal humerus	Axillary nerve
Midshaft humerus (or spiral humerus fracture)	Radial nerve
Distal (supracondylar) humerus	Brachial artery
Elbow dislocation	Brachial artery
Distal radius	Median nerve
LOWER EXTREMITY	
Anterior hip dislocation	Femoral artery
Posterior hip dislocation	Sciatic nerve
Distal (supracondylar) femur	Popliteal artery
Posterior knee dislocation	Popliteal artery
Fibula neck	Common peroneal nerve

Modified from Engelhardt SL, Winchell RJ. Definitive care phase: orthopedic and spinal injuries. In: Greenfield LJ, et al., eds. *Surgery: Scientific Principles and Practice.* 3rd ed. Philadelphia: Lippincott Williams & Wilkins; 2001:372.

- If pulse does not return → go to OR for vascular bypass or repair (some say proceed to angiography for diagnosis of location of injury and possible intervention)

- If pulse is weak → angiography

- All knee dislocations need to go to angiogram, unless pulse is absent, in which case some would just go to OR

RENAL TRAUMA
- Hematuria is best indicator of renal trauma
- All patients with hematuria need CT scan
- IVP can also be useful if going immediately to OR without abdominal CT scan → will identify presence of functional contralateral kidney, which could affect intraoperative decision making
- **Left renal vein** – can be ligated near IVC; has **adrenal and gonadal vein collaterals.** Right does <u>not</u>
- Anterior → posterior renal hilum structures – **vein, artery, pelvis**
- 95% of injuries are treated nonoperatively
- Not all urine extravasation injuries require operation
- **Indications for operation**
  - **Acutely** – ongoing hemorrhage with instability
  - **After acute phase** – major collecting system disruption, unresolving urine extravasation, severe hematuria
- With exploration, try to get control of the **vascular hilum 1st**
- Place **drains**, especially if collecting system is injured
- **Methylene blue dye** can be used at the end of the case to check for leak
- **When at exploration for another blunt injury or penetrating trauma**
  - **Blunt renal injury with hematoma** – leave unless preop CT/IVP shows no function or significant urine extravasation
  - **Penetrating renal injury with hematoma** – open unless preop CT/IVP shows good function without significant urine extravasation

- **Trauma to flank and IVP shows no uptake** – Tx: angiogram; can stent if flap present

BLADDER TRAUMA
- Hematuria best indicator of bladder trauma
- >95% associated with pelvic fractures
- Signs and symptoms – meatal blood, sacral or scrotal hematoma
- **Dx**: cystogram
- **Extraperitoneal bladder rupture** – cystogram shows starbursts
  - Tx: Foley 7–14 days
- **Intraperitoneal bladder rupture** – more likely in kids, cystogram shows leak
  - Tx: operation and repair of defect, followed by Foley drainage

URETERAL TRAUMA
- Hematuria unreliable → **IVP and retrograde urethrogram (RUG) best tests**

- **If large ureteral segment is missing** (>2 cm) and cannot perform reanastomosis:
  - **Upper ⅓ injuries and middle ⅓ injuries that won't reach bladder**
    - Temporize with **percutaneous nephrostomy** (tie off both ends of the ureter) if patient unstable. Can go with <u>ileal interposition or trans-ureteroureterostomy</u> later
    - If stable, most urologists would perform <u>trans-ureteroureterostomy</u>
  - **Lower ⅓ injuries** – reimplant in the bladder; may need bladder hitch procedure

- **If small ureteral segment is missing** (<2 cm), try to mobilize ends of ureter and perform **primary repair** over stent if in the upper or mid ureter or reimplant if in the lower ⅓ ureter
- One-shot IVP does not evaluate the ureters sufficiently
- IV indigo carmine or methylene blue can be used to check for leaks
- Blood supply is medial in the upper ⅔ of the ureter and lateral in the lower ⅓ of the ureter
- **Leave drains for all ureteral injuries**

URETHRAL TRAUMA
- **Hematuria or blood at meatus best sign**; free-floating prostate gland; usually associated with pelvic fractures
- No Foley if this injury is suspected
- **Urethrogram** best test
- Membranous portion at risk for transection
- **Significant tears** – Tx: suprapubic cystostomy and repair in 2–3 months (safest method)
  • High stricture and impotence rate if repaired early
- **Small, partial tears** – Tx: may get away with bridging urethral catheter across tear area and repair in 2–3 months
- **Genital trauma** – can get fracture in erectile bodies from vigorous sex
  • Need to repair the tunica and Buck's fascia
- **Testicular trauma** – get ultrasound to see if tunica albuginea is violated, then repair if necessary

PEDIATRIC TRAUMA
- Blood pressure is not a good indicator of blood loss in children – last thing to go
- Heart rate, respiratory rate, mental status, and clinical exam are best indicators of shock
- ↑ risk of **hypothermia** (↑ BSA compared with weight)
- ↑ risk of **head injury**

Normal Vital Signs by Age

Age Group	Pulse (beats/min)	SBP (mm Hg)	Respiratory Rate (breaths/min)
Infant (<1 yr)	160	80	40
Preschool (<5 yr)	140	90	30
Adolescent (>10 yr)	120	100	20

TRAUMA DURING PREGNANCY
- At all costs, **save the mother**
- Pregnant patients can have up to a ⅓ total blood volume loss without signs
- Estimate pregnancy based on **fundal height** (20 cm = 20 wk = umbilicus). Place fetal monitor
- Try to avoid CT scan with early pregnancy. If life-threatening and needed, get CT scan
- Ultrasound (FAST scan) may have a role in pregnant patients
- Check for vaginal discharge – blood, amnion. Check for effacement, dilation, fetal station
- **Maturity** – lecithin:sphingomyelin (LS) ratio >2:1; positive **phosphatidylcholine**
- **Placental abruption** > 50% results in almost 100% fetal death rate
  • >50% of all traumatic placental abruptions result in fetal demise
  • Signs of abruption – uterine tenderness, contractions, fetal HR < 120

- Can be caused by **shock (most common mechanism) or mechanical forces**
- **Kleihauer–Betke test** – test for fetal blood in the maternal circulation → sign of placental abruption

▪ **Uterine rupture** – more likely to occur in the <u>posterior fundus</u>
- If occurs after delivery of child, aggressive resuscitation even in the face of shock leads to the best outcome. The uterus will eventually clamp down after delivery; just have to aggressively resuscitate until then

▪ **Indications for C-section during exploratory laparotomy for trauma**
- Persistent maternal shock
- Pregnancy near term (>34 weeks) and mother with severe injuries
- Pregnancy a threat to the mother's life (hemorrhage, DIC)
- Mechanical limitation to life-threatening vessel injury
- Risk of fetal distress exceeds risk of immaturity
- Direct uterine trauma

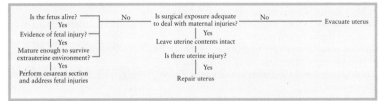

Assessment of the pregnant uterus during celiotomy.

Management of Hematomas

Hematoma	Penetrating Trauma	Blunt Trauma
Pelvic	Open	Leave
Paraduodenal	Open	Open
Portal triad	Open	Open
Retrohepatic	Leave if stable	Leave
Midline supramesocolic	Open	Open
Midline inframesocolic	Open	Open
Pericolonic	Open	Open
Perirenal	Open[a]	Leave[b]

[a]Unless preoperative CT scan or IVP shows no injury.
[b]Unless preoperative CT scan or IVP shows injury.

Zones of the Peritoneum

Zone	Location	Associated Injuries
1	Central retroperitoneum	Pancreaticoduodenal injuries or major abdominal vascular injury
2	Flank or perinephric area	Injuries to the genitourinary tract or to the colon (i.e., with penetrating trauma)
3	Pelvis	Pelvic fractures

Drains – leave drains with pancreatic, liver, biliary system, urinary, and duodenal injuries

Snakebites (symptoms depend on species) – shock, bradycardia, and arrhythmias can result
 Neuro symptoms leading to resp failure
 Tx; stabilize patient, anti-venin, tetanus shot

CHAPTER 16. CRITICAL CARE

CARDIOVASCULAR SYSTEM

Normal Values

Parameter	Value
Cardiac output (CO) (L/min)	4–8
Cardiac index (CI) (L/min)	2.5–4
Systemic vascular resistance (SVR)	800–1400
Systemic vascular resistance index (SVRI)	1500–2400
Pulmonary capillary wedge pressure (PCWP)	11 ± 4
Central venous pressure (CVP)	7 ± 2
Pulmonary artery (PA)	20–30/6–15
Mixed venous oxygen saturation (SvO2)	75 ± 5

- <u>MAP</u> = CO × SVR, <u>CI</u> = CO/BSA, <u>SVRI</u> = SVR × BSA

- <u>Kidney</u> gets 25% of CO, <u>brain</u> gets 15% of CO, heart gets 5%

- **Preload** – end-diastolic length, linearly related to end-diastolic volume (EDV) and filling pressure
- **Afterload** – resistance against the ventricle contracting (SVR)

- **Stroke volume** determined by <u>LVEDV, contractility, and afterload</u>
  - Stroke volume = LVEDV − LVESV
- **Ejection fraction** = stroke volume/EDV

- **EDV (end-diastolic volume)** – determined by preload and distensibility of the ventricle
- **ESV (end-systolic volume)** – determined by contractility and afterload

- Cardiac output increases with HR up to 120–150 beats/min, then starts to go down because of **decreased diastolic filling time**
- **Atrial kick** – accounts for 15%–30% of LVEDV

- **Anrep effect** – automatic increase in **contractility** secondary to ↑ **afterload**
- **Bowditch effect** – automatic increase in **contractility** secondary to ↑ HR

- Aortic mean and diastolic pressures are slightly greater than radial pressure
- Radial systolic pressures are slightly higher than mean aortic pressure

- **O_2 delivery** = CO × arterial O_2 content (CaO_2) = CO × (Hgb × 1.34 × O_2 saturation + 1 [P_{O_2} × 0.003])

- **O_2 consumption (VO_2)** = CO × (CaO_2 − CvO_2). CvO_2 = venous O_2 content
  - **Normal O_2 delivery-to-consumption ratio is 5:1.** CO increases to keep this ratio constant
  - O_2 consumption is usually <u>supply independent (consumption does not change until low levels of delivery are reached</u>

  - **Right shift on oxygen–Hgb dissociation curve (O_2 unloading)** – ↑ CO_2, ↑ temperature, ↑ ATP production, ↑ 2,3-DPG production, or ↓ pH
    - Normal p50 (O_2 at which 50% of O_2 receptors are saturated) = 27 mm Hg

- ↑ **SvO$_2$** (saturation of venous blood, normally 75% ± 5%) – occurs with ↑ shunting of blood or ↓ O$_2$ extraction (sepsis, cirrhosis, cyanide toxicity, hyperbaric O$_2$, hypothermia, paralysis, coma, sedation)
- ↓ **SvO$_2$** – occurs with ↑ O$_2$ extraction or ↓ O$_2$ delivery (↓ O$_2$ saturation, ↓ CO)

■ **Wedge** – may be thrown off by pulmonary hypertension, aortic regurgitation, mitral stenosis, mitral regurgitation, high PEEP, poor LV compliance

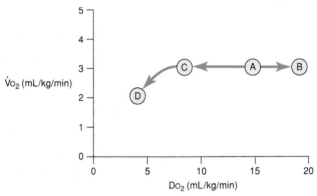

Normally *(A)*, systemic O$_2$ delivery is approximately 15 mL/kg/min and O$_2$ consumption is 3 mL/kg/min. Consumption becomes supply-dependent when delivery is very low *(C to D)*. Delivery increases in response to increased metabolism *(A to B)*. (From Bartlett RH, Anderson HL. Multiorgan failure. In: Zelenock GB, D'alecy LG, Fantone JC, et al., eds. *Clinical Ischemic Syndromes: Mechanisms and Consequences of Tissue Injury.* St. Louis, MO: Mosby; 1989:565, with permission.)

■ **Swan–Ganz catheter** – should be placed in **zone III** (lower lung)
  - **Hemoptysis after flushing Swan–Ganz catheter** – increase PEEP, which will tamponade the pulmonary artery bleed, mainstem intubate nonaffected side; can try to place Fogarty balloon down the affected side; may need thoracotomy and lobectomy
  - **Relative contraindications** – previous pneumonectomy, left bundle branch block
  - **Approximate Swan–Ganz catheter distances to wedge** – **R SCV** 45 cm, **R IJ** 50 cm, **L SCV** 55 cm, **L IJ** 60 cm
  - **Pulmonary vascular resistance** can be measured only by using a **Swan–Ganz catheter**

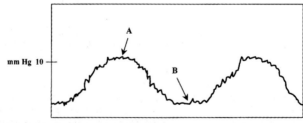

Pulmonary artery wedge tracing with the usual cyclical respiratory variations. Pulmonary artery wedge pressure should be measured at end-expiration. This corresponds to the peak of the wedge tracing for spontaneously breathing patients *(point A)* and the valley of the tracing for patients undergoing positive-pressure ventilation *(point B)*. (From Gangemi JJ, Cope JT, Peeler BB, Kron IL. Cardiovascular monitoring and support. In: Fischer JE, Bland KI, et al., eds. *Mastery of Surgery,* 5th ed. Philadelphia: Lippincott Williams & Wilkins; 2007, with permission).

- ↑ **ventricular wall tension and HR** are the primary determinants of <u>myocardial O_2</u> <u>consumption</u> → can lead to myocardial ischemia

- **Unsaturated bronchial blood** – empties into pulmonary veins; thus, LV blood is 5 mm Hg (Po_2) lower than pulmonary capillaries
- **Alveolar–arterial gradient** – 10–15 mm Hg normal in nonventilated patient
- Blood with the lowest venous saturation → coronary venous blood (30%)

SHOCK
- **Adrenal insufficiency**
  - **Acute** – cardiovascular collapse; characteristically **unresponsive to fluids and pressors**
  - **Chronic** – hyperpigmentation, weakness, weight loss, GI symptoms, ↑ K, ↓ Na, fever, hypotension
  - **Steroid potency**
    - 1× – cortisone, hydrocortisone
    - 5× – prednisone, prednisolone, methylprednisolone
    - 30× – dexamethasone

- **Neurogenic shock** – loss of sympathetic tone
  - <u>Usually have</u> ↓ HR, ↓ BP, warm skin
  - Tx: give volume 1st, then phenylephrine after resuscitation; give steroids for blunt spinal trauma with deficit

- **Hemorrhagic shock** – initial alteration is <u>↑ diastolic pressure</u>

- **Cardiac tamponade**
  - Causes decreased diastolic ventricular filling and hypotension
  - Beck's triad – hypotension, jugular venous distention, and muffled heart sounds
  - Echocardiogram shows **impaired diastolic filling of right atrium initially** (1st sign of cardiac tamponade)
  - Pericardiocentesis blood does not form clot
  - Tx: fluid resuscitation initially; need pericardial window or pericardiocentesis

Types of Shock

Shock	CVP and PCWP	CO	SVRI
Hemorrhagic	↓	↓	↑
Septic (hyperdynamic)[a]	↓, possibly ↑	↑	↓
Cardiogenic	↑	↓	↑
Neurogenic	↓	↓	↓
Hypoadrenal	↓, possibly ↑	↓	↓

[a]Severe septic shock that leads to cardiac dysfunction can cause a hypodynamic state, leading to ↓ CO and ↑ SVRI. (Modified from Maier RV. Shock. In: Greenfield LJ et al., eds. *Surgery: Scientific Principles and Practice.* 2nd ed. Philadelphia: Lippincott-Raven; 1997.)

- **Early sepsis triad** – hyperventilation, confusion, respiratory alkalosis
  - **Early gram-negative sepsis** – ↓ insulin, ↑ glucose (impaired utilization)
  - **Late gram-negative sepsis** – ↑ insulin, ↑ glucose (secondary to insulin resistance)
  - **Hyperglycemia** – often occurs just before patient becomes clinically septic
- **Activated protein C (Xigris)** – used for sepsis; mechanism is <u>fibrinolysis</u>

EMBOLI
- **Fat emboli**
  - Signs include petechia, hypoxia, and confusion (can also be similar to pulmonary embolism [PE])

- **Sudan red stain** may show fat in sputum and urine
- Most common with lower extremity (hip, femur) fractures/orthopaedic procedures
- **Pulmonary thromboemboli** – echo will show RV strain
  - Suspect PE with PA systolic pressures >40, ↓ Po_2 and Pco_2, respiratory alkalosis, chest pain, cough, dyspnea, ↑ HR
- **Air emboli** – place patient head down and roll to left (keeps air in RV and RA), then aspirate air out with central line or PA catheter to RA/RV

INTRA-AORTIC BALLOON PUMP (IABP)

- <u>Inflates</u> on **T wave (diastole)**; <u>deflates</u> on **P wave or start of Q wave (systole)**
- Aortic regurgitation contraindication
- Place tip of the catheter just distal to left subclavian (1–2 cm below the top of the arch)
- Used for cardiogenic shock (after CABG, MI) or in patients with refractory angina
- Decreases afterload (deflation during ventricular systole)
- Improves SBP (inflation during ventricular diastole), which **improves coronary perfusion**

RECEPTORS

- **Alpha-1** – vascular smooth muscle constriction; gluconeogenesis, glycogenolysis
- **Alpha-2** – venous smooth muscle constriction
- **Beta-1** – myocardial contraction and rate
- **Beta-2** – relaxes bronchial smooth muscle, relaxes vascular smooth muscle; increases insulin, glucagon, rennin
- **Dopamine receptors** – relax renal and splanchnic smooth muscle

CARDIOVASCULAR DRUGS

- **Dopamine (2–5 µg/kg/min initially, 20–50 mg/kg/min for high dose)**
  - 0–5 µg/kg/min – <u>dopamine receptors</u> (renal)
  - 6–10 µg/kg/min – <u>beta-adrenergic</u> (heart contractility)
  - >10 µg/kg/min – <u>alpha-adrenergic</u> (vasoconstriction and ↑ BP)

- **Dobutamine (3 µg/kg/min initially)**
  - 5–15 µg/kg/min – <u>beta-1</u> (↑ contractility mostly)
  - >15 µg/kg/min – <u>beta-2</u> (vasodilation, ↑ HR)

- **Milrinone**
  - Phosphodiesterase inhibitor (↑ cAMP)
  - Results in ↑ Ca flux and ↑ myocardial contractility
  - Also causes vascular smooth muscle relaxation and vasodilation
- **Phenylephrine**
  - Alpha-1, vasoconstriction

- **Norepinephrine (4 µg/min initially)**
  - <u>Low dose</u> – beta-1 (↑ contractility)
  - <u>High dose</u> – alpha-1 and alpha-2
  - Potent splanchnic vasoconstrictor

- **Epinephrine (2 µg/min initially)**
  - <u>Low dose</u> – beta-1 and beta-2 (↑ contractility and vasodilation)
    - Can ↓ BP at low doses
  - <u>High dose</u> – alpha-1 and alpha-2 (vasoconstriction)
    - ↑ cardiac ectopic pacer activity and myocardial O_2 demand

- **Isoproterenol (1–2 µg/min initially)**
  - Beta-1 and beta-2, ↑ HR and contractility, vasodilates
  - Side effects: extremely arrhythmogenic; ↑ heart metabolic demand (rarely used); may actually ↓ BP

■ **Vasopressin**
- V-1 receptors – vasoconstriction of vascular smooth muscle
- V-2 receptors (intrarenal) – water reabsorption at collecting ducts
- V-2 receptors (extrarenal) – mediate release of factor VIII and von Willebrand factor

■ **Nipride** – arterial and venous dilator
- **Cyanide toxicity** at doses >3 μg/kg/min for 72 hours; can check **thiocyanate levels** and signs of metabolic acidosis
- Tx: amyl nitrite, then sodium nitrite

■ **Nitroglycerin** – predominately venodilation, modest effect on coronaries; ↓ myocardial wall tension by ↓ preload

■ **Hydralazine** – α-blocker

PULMONARY SYSTEM
■ **Compliance** – (change in volume)/(change in pressure)
- <u>High compliance</u> means lungs easy to ventilate
- Pulmonary compliance ↓ in patients with ARDS, fibrotic lung diseases, reperfusion injury, pulmonary edema
■ **Aging** – ↓ FEV_1 and vital capacity, ↑ functional residual capacity (FRC)
■ **V/Q ratio** – highest in upper lobes, lowest in lower lobes

■ **Ventilator**
- <u>↑ PEEP</u> to improve oxygenation (alveoli recruitment) → **improves FRC**
- <u>↑ rate or volume</u> to ↓ CO_2
- **Normal weaning parameters** – negative inspiratory force (NIF) > 20, FiO_2 < 35%, PEEP 5 (physiologic), pressure support 5, RR < 24/min, HR < 120 beats/min, Po_2 > 60 mm Hg, Pco_2 < 50 mm Hg, pH 7.35–7.45, saturations > 93%, off pressors, follows commands, can protect airway

- **Pressure support** – ↓ the work of breathing (inspiratory pressure is held constant until minimum volume is achieved)
- **FiO_2 ≤ 60%** – prevents O_2 radical toxicity
- **Barotrauma** – high risk if plateaus >30 and peaks >50 → consider prophylactic chest tubes
- **PEEP** – improves FRC and compliance by keeping alveoli open → best way to improve oxygenation
- **Excessive PEEP complications** – ↓ RA filling, ↓ CO, ↓ renal blood flow, ↓ urine output, and ↑ pulmonary vascular resistance
- **High-frequency ventilation** – used a lot in kids; tracheoesophageal fistula, bronchopleural fistula
- **Inverse ratio ventilation** – helps reduce barotrauma (normal 1:2 I:E phase; go to 2:1)

■ **Pulmonary function measurements**
- **Total lung capacity (TLC)** – lung volume after maximal inspiration
  - TLC = FVC + RV
- **Forced vital capacity (FVC)** – maximal exhalation after maximal inhalation
- **Residual volume (RV)** – lung volume after maximal expiration (20% TLC)
- **Tidal volume (TV)** – volume of air with normal inspiration and expiration
- **Functional residual capacity (FRC)** – lung volume after normal exhalation
  - FRC = ERV + RV
  - Surgery (atelectasis), sepsis (ARDS), and trauma (contusion, atelectasis, ARDS) – all ↓ FRC

- **Expiratory reserve volume (ERV)** – volume of air that can be forcefully expired after normal expiration
- **Inspiratory capacity** – maximum air breathed in from FRC
- **FEV$_1$** – forced expiratory volume in 1 second (after maximal inhalation)
- **Minute ventilation** $= TV \times RR$
- **Restrictive lung disease** – $\downarrow$ TLC, $\downarrow$ RV, and $\downarrow$ FVC
  - FEV$_1$ can be normal or $\uparrow$
- **Obstructive lung disease** – $\uparrow$ TLC, $\uparrow$ RV, and $\downarrow$ FEV$_1$
  - FVC can be normal or $\downarrow$

- **Dead space** – normally to the level of the bronchiole (150 mL); $\uparrow$ with drop in cardiac output, PE, pulmonary HTN, ARDS, excessive PEEP; can lead to high **CO$_2$ buildup**
  - Area of lung that is ventilated but not perfused

- **COPD** – $\uparrow$ work of breathing due to prolonged expiratory phase
  - Work of breathing normally 2% of total body VO$_2$

- **ARDS** – mediated by cellular inflammatory processes, $\uparrow$ proteinaceous material, $\uparrow$ gradient, $\uparrow$ shunt
  - Most common cause is **sepsis**

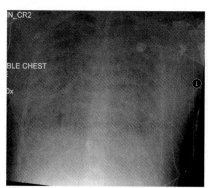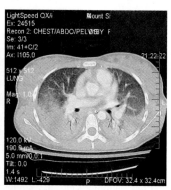

Characteristic chest radiograph *(A)* and CT scan *(B)* in a patient with severe ARDS following multiple trauma. (From Cheadle WG, Branson R, Franklin GA. Pulmonary risk and ventilatory support. In: Fischer JE, Bland KI, et al., eds. *Mastery of Surgery*, 5th ed. Philadelphia: Lippincott Williams & Wilkins; 2007, with permission.)

Diagnostic Criteria for Acute Lung Injury and Acute Respiratory Distress Syndrome[a]

Acute Lung Injury
Acute onset
Bilateral pulmonary infiltrates
Pao$_2$/Fio$_2$ $\leq$ 300
PAOP $<$ 18 mm Hg or no clinical evidence of LAH

Acute Respiratory Distress Syndrome
All the above criteria with Pao$_2$/Fio$_2$ $<$ 200

[a]Pao$_2$, arterial oxygen pressure; Fio$_2$, fractional inspired oxygen; PAOP, pulmonary artery occlusion pressure; LAH, left arterial hypertension. (Adapted from American-European Consensus Conference on ARDS, 1994)

- **SIRS** – mediated by TNF-α and IL-1; temperature >38°C or <36°C, RR >20/min, P_{CO_2} < 32 mm Hg, WBC > 12,000/µL or <4000/µL, HR >90 beats/min
- **Endotoxin (lipopolysaccharide – lipid A)** is the most potent stimulus for **SIRS.**

Definitions of Systemic Inflammatory Response Syndrome (SIRS), Sepsis, Sever Sepsis, Septic Shock, and Multisystem Organ Dysfunction (MOD)

SIRS   →   Sepsis   →   Severe Sepsis   →   Septic Shock   →   MOD

SIRS

- Temperature >38°C or <36°C
- Heart rate >90 beats/min
- White blood count >12,000/µL or <4,000/µL
- Respiratory rate >20/min or Pa_{CO_2} <32

Sepsis

- SIRS with clinical evidence of infection
- Sepsis with organ dysfunction

Septic shock

- Sepsis and arterial hypotension despite adequate volume resuscitation

MOD

- Progressive but reversible dysfunction of 2 or more organs arising from an acute disruption of normal homeostasis

From Awad SS, Gale SC. Multiple organ dysfunction syndrome: pathogenesis, management, and prevention. In: Fischer JE, Bland KI, et al., eds. *Mastery of Surgery*, 5th ed. Philadelphia: Lippincott Williams & Wilkins; 2007, with permission.

Diagnostic Criteria for Significant Organ Dysfunction[a]

Organ System	Criteria
Pulmonary	Need for mechanical ventilation; Pa_{O_2}:F_{IO_2} ratio <300 mm Hg for 24 hours
Cardiovascular	Need for inotropic drugs to maintain adequate tissue perfusion or CI <2.5 L/min/m^2
Kidney	Creatinine >2 times baseline on 2 consecutive days or need for renal replacement therapy
Liver	Bilirubin > 3 mg/dL on 2 consecutive days or PT > 1.5 control
Nutrition	10% reduction in lean body mass; albumin <2.0 g/dL or total lymphocyte count <1,000/µL
CNS	Glasgow Coma Scale score <10 without sedation
Coagulation	Platelet count <50,000/µL; fibrinogen <100 mg/dL or need for factor replacement
Host defenses	WBC <1,000/µL or invasive infection including bacteremia

[a]Pa_{O_2}, partial pressure of oxygen in arterial blood; F_{IO_2}, fraction of inspired oxygen; CI, cardiac index; PT, prothrombin time; WBC, white blood cell count. (From Awad SS, Gale SC. Multiple organ dysfunction syndrome: pathogenesis, management, and prevention. In: Fischer JE, Bland KI, et al., eds. *Mastery of Surgery*, 5th ed. Philadelphia: Lippincott Williams & Wilkins; 2007, with permission.)

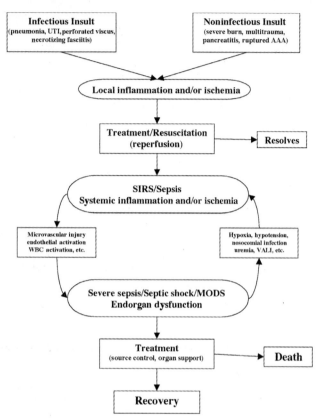

Pathophysiology of multisystem organ dysfunctions (MODS). UTI, urinary tract infection; AAA, abnormal aortic aneurysm; SIRS, systemic inflammatory response syndrome; WBC, white blood count; VALI, ventilator-associated lung injury. (From Cheadle WG, Branson R, Franklin GA. Pulmonary risk and ventilatory support. In: Fischer JE, Bland KI, et al., eds. *Mastery of Surgery*, 5th ed. Philadelphia: Lippincott Williams & Wilkins, 2007; with permission.)

■ **Aspiration** – pH <2.5 and volume >0.4 cc/kg associated with ↑ degree of damage
  • **Mendelson's syndrome – chemical pneumonitis from aspiration of gastric secretions**
  • **Most frequent site is the posterior portion of RUL and superior portion of RLL**

■ **Atelectasis** – bronchial obstruction and respiratory failure are the main causes
  • Most common cause of fever in first 48 hours after operation
  • Fever, tachycardia
  • Increased in patients with COPD, upper abdominal surgery, obesity
  • Tx: incentive spirometer

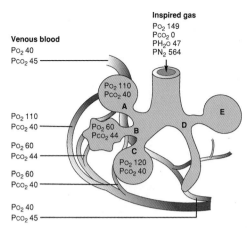

Inspired gas
Po$_2$ 149
Pco$_2$ 0
PH$_2$o 47
PN$_2$ 564

Venous blood
Po$_2$ 40
Pco$_2$ 45

Po$_2$ 110
Pco$_2$ 40
A

E

Po$_2$ 110
Pco$_2$ 40

Po$_2$ 60
Pco$_2$ 44
B

D

Po$_2$ 60
Pco$_2$ 44

C

Po$_2$ 60
Pco$_2$ 40

Po$_2$ 120
Pco$_2$ 40

Po$_2$ 40
Pco$_2$ 45

Variables affecting pulmonary gas exchange while air is breathed. In alveolus *A*, blood flow and ventilation are equal and normal. The values in the alveolus and the exiting blood represent the end of a normal resting exhalation. Alveolus *B* represents hypoventilation. Alveolus *C* represents diffusion block. Alveolus *D* represents collapse or transpulmonary shunt. Alveolus *E* is ventilated without blood flow.

▦ Lots of things can throw off a pulse oximeter → nail polish, dark skin, low-flow states, ambient light, anemia, vital dyes

▦ **Pulmonary vasodilation** – bradykinin, PGE$_1$, prostacyclin (PGI$_2$), nitric oxide
▦ **Pulmonary vasoconstriction** – histamine, serotonin, TXA$_2$, epinephrine, norepinephrine, **hypoxia**, acidosis
▦ **Alkalosis** – pulmonary vasodilator
▦ **Acidosis** – pulmonary vasoconstrictor
▦ **Pulmonary shunting** – occurs with nitroprusside (Nipride), nitroglycerin, and nifedipine

RENAL SYSTEM
▦ **Hypotension** – most common cause of postoperative renal failure
▦ 70% nephrons need to be damaged before renal dysfunction occurs
▦ **FeNa** = (urine Na/Cr)/(plasma Na/Cr) → best test for azotemia
▦ **Prerenal cause of acute renal failure** – FeNa <1%, urine Na <20, BUN/Cr ratio >20, urine osmolality >500 mOsm; otherwise consider renal cause of azotemia
▦ **Oliguria**
  • 1st – make sure patient is volume loaded (CVP 11–15 mm Hg)
  • 2nd – try diuretic trial → furosemide (Lasix)/butanamide
  • 3rd – dialysis if needed

▦ **Indications for dialysis** – fluid overload, ↑ K, metabolic acidosis, uremic encephalopathy, uremic coagulopathy, poisoning
▦ **Hemodialysis** – rapid, causes large volume shifts
▦ **CVVH** – slower, good for ill patients who cannot tolerate the volume shifts (septic shock, etc.)
  • Hct increases by 5–8 for each liter taken off

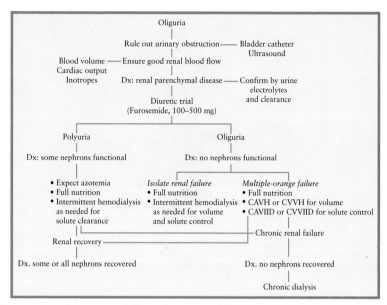

Management of acute renal failure. PD, peritoneal dialysis; CAVH, continuous arteriovenous hemofiltration; CAVHD, continuous arteriovenous hemodialysis.

Advantages of Intermittent Hemodialysis and Continuous Renal Replacement Therapy

Intermittent Hemodialysis	Continuous Renal Replacement Therapy
ADVANTAGES	
Lower risk of systemic bleeding	Better hemodynamic stability
Facilitates transport for other interventions	Fewer cardiac arrhythmias
More suitable for severe hyperkalemia	Improved nutritional support
Lower cost	Better pulmonary gas exchange
	Better fluid control
DISADVANTAGES	
Availability of dialysis staff	Greater vascular access problems
More difficult hemodynamic control	Higher risk of systemic bleeding
Inadequate dialysis dose (frequency)	Long-term immobilization of patient
Inadequate fluid control	More filter problems (rupture, clotting)
Inadequate nutritional support	Greater cost
Not suitable for patients with intracranial hypertension	
No removal of cytokines (theoretical)	
Potential complement activation by nonbiocompatible membranes	

Adapted from Lameire N, Van Biesen W, vanholder R. Acute renal failure. *Lancet* 2005;365:417–430.

■ **Renin**
- Released in response to ↓ pressure sensed by **juxtaglomerular apparatus** in kidney
- Also released in response to ↑ Na concentrations sensed by the **macula densa**
- Beta-adrenergic stimulation and hyperkalemia also cause release
- Converts angiotensinogen (synthesized in the liver) to angiotensin I
- **Angiotensin-converting enzyme (lung)** – converts angiotensin I to angiotensin II
- **Adrenal cortex** – releases aldosterone in response to angiotensin II
- **Distal convoluted tubule** – aldosterone acts here to reabsorb more water by ↑ Na/K
  - ATPase on membrane (potassium secreted)
- **Angiotensin II** – also vasoconstricts, increases HR, contractility, permeability, glycogenolysis, and gluconeogenesis; inhibits renin release

■ **Atrial natriuretic peptide (or factor)**
- Released from atrial wall with atrial distention
- Inhibits Na and water resorption in the collecting ducts
- Also a **vasodilator**

■ **Antidiuretic hormone (ADH; vasopressin)**
- Released by posterior pituitary gland when osmolality is high
- Acts on collecting ducts for water resorption
- Also a **vasoconstrictor**

■ Efferent limb of kidney controls GFR
■ **Renal toxic drugs**
- **NSAIDs** – cause renal damage by **inhibiting prostaglandin synthesis,** resulting in renal arteriole vasoconstriction
- **Aminoglycosides** – direct tubular injury and later renal vasoconstriction
- **Myoglobin** – direct tubular injury
  - Tx: alkalinize urine
- **Contrast dyes** – direct tubular injury
  - Tx: premedicate with *N*-acetylcysteine and volume

BRAIN DEATH
■ **Precludes diagnosis** – uremia, temperature <30°C, BP <70/40 mm Hg, desaturation with apnea test, drugs (phenobarbital, pentobarbital), metabolic derangements
■ Must exist for 6–12 hours → unresponsive to pain, absent caloric oculovestibular reflexes, absent oculocephalic reflex, positive apnea test, no corneal reflex, no gag reflex, fixed and dilated pupils
■ **EEG** – electrical silence; **MRA**—can be used → will show no blood flow to brain
■ **Apnea test** – disconnected from ventilation; CO_2 >60 mm Hg or increase in CO_2 by 20 is a positive test for apnea. If arterial pressure drops to <60 or patient desaturates, the test is terminated
■ **Can still have deep tendon reflexes with brain death**

OTHER CONDITIONS
■ **Carbon monoxide**
- Can falsely ↑ oxygen saturation reading on pulse oximeter
- Binds hemoglobin directly (creates carboxyhemoglobin)
- Can usually correct with 100% oxygen on ventilator (displaces carbon monoxide); may need hyperbaric O_2 if really high
- Abnormal carboxyhemoglobin >10%; in smokers >20%
■ **Methemoglobinemia** (from nitrites such as Hurricaine spray; nitrites bind Hgb) – **O_2 saturation reads 85%**
- Tx: methylene blue

- **Critical illness polyneuropathy** – motor $>$ sensory neuropathy; occurs with sepsis; can lead to failure to wean from ventilation
- **Xanthine oxidase** – in endothelial cells, forms toxic oxygen radicals with reperfusion, involved in reperfusion injury
  - Also involved in the metabolism of purines and breakdown to uric acid
- **DKA** – nausea and vomiting, thirst, polyuria, abdominal pain, $\uparrow$ glucose, $\uparrow$ ketones, $\downarrow$ Na, $\uparrow$ K
  - Tx: insulin and eventually glucose, so patient does not bottom out, isotonic solutions, K^+ (although initial K will be high, it will be driven back into cells by insulin), HCO_3^- for pH $<$ 7.25
- **ETOH withdrawal** – HTN, tachycardia, delirium, seizures after 48 hours
  - Tx: thiamine, folate, Mg, K, B_{12}, PRN lorazepam (Ativan)
- **ICU (or hospital) psychosis** – generally occurs after third postoperative day and is frequently preceded by lucid interval
  - Need to rule out metabolic (hypoglycemia, DKA, hypoxia, hypercarbia, electrolyte imbalances) and organic (MI, CVA) causes

CHAPTER 17. BURNS

Burn Classification

Degree	Description
1st	Sunburn (epidermis)
2nd	
Superficial dermis (papillary)	Painful to touch; blebs and blisters; hair follicles intact; blanches
Deep dermis (reticular)	Decreased sensation; loss of hair follicles (need skin grafts)
3rd	Leathery feeling (charred parchment); down to subcutaneous fat
4th	Down to bone, into adjacent adipose or muscle tissue

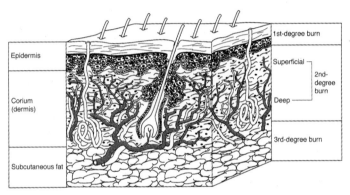

Schematic depiction of the skin.

ADMISSION CRITERIA[1]

- 2nd- and 3rd-degree burns >10% BSA in patients aged <10 or >50 years
- 2nd- and 3rd-degree burns >20% BSA in all other patients
- 2nd- and 3rd-degree burns to significant portions of hands, face, feet, genitalia, perineum, or skin overlying major joints
- 3rd-degree burns >5% in any age group
- Electrical and chemical burns
- Concomitant inhalational injury, mechanical traumas, preexisting medical conditions
- Injuries in patients with special social, emotional, or long-term rehabilitation needs
- Suspected child abuse or neglect

- Deaths highest in children and elderly (trouble getting away)
- Scald burns – most common
- Flame burns – more likely to come to hospital and be admitted
- **Assessing percentage of body surface burned (rule of 9s)**
  - Head = 9, arms = 18, chest = 18, back = 18, legs = 36, perineum = 1
  - Can also use patient's palm to estimate injury (palm = 1%)

[1]Modified from Feliciano DV, et al. *Trauma*. 3rd ed. Stamford, CT: Appleton & Lange; 1996:937.

- **Parkland formula**
  - For burns ≥ 20% – give 4 cc/kg × % burn in first 24 hours; give ½ in first 8 hours
  - Use lactated Ringer's solution (LR) in first 24 hours
    - Urine output best measure of resuscitation (0.5–1.0 cc/kg/h in adults, 2–4 cc/kg/h in children < 6 months)
  - Parkland formula can grossly underestimate volume requirements with inhalational injury, ETOH, electrical injury, postescharotomy
  - **Important to use LR in first 24 hours**
    - Colloid (albumin) in 1st 24 hours shown to ↑ pulmonary/respiratory complications → can use colloid after 24 hours

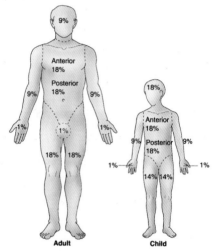

Estimating burn size accurately is essential for care of the burn patient. The rule of nines provides a simple algorithm for calculating the burned surface area.

- **Escharotomy indications (perform within 4–6 hours)**
  - Circumferential burns
  - Low temperature; weak pulse; ↓ capillary refill, ↓ pain sensation, and ↓ neurologic function in extremity → may need fasciotomy if compartment syndrome suspected
  - Problems ventilating patient with significant chest torso burns

Risk Factors for Burn Injuries
Alcohol or drug use
Age (very young/very old)
Smoking
Low socioeconomic status
Occupation
Violence
Epilepsy

CHILD ABUSE
- Accounts for 15% of burn injuries in children

Important Points of History and Exam that Suggest Abuse or Neglect

HISTORY
Delayed presentation for medical care
Conflicting histories
Previous injuries

SUSPICIOUS BURN PATTERNS
Sharply demarcated margins
Uniform depth
Absence of splash marks
Stocking or glove patterns
Flexor sparing
Dorsal location of contact injury of the hands
Very deep localized contact injury

LUNG INJURY
- Caused by carbonaceous materials and smoke, <u>not</u> heat
- **Risk factors for airway injury** – ETOH, trauma, closed space, rapid combustion, extremes of age, delayed extrication
- **Signs and symptoms of possible airway injury** – facial burns, wheezing, carbonaceous sputum
- **Indications for intubation** – upper airway stridor or obstruction, worsening hypoxemia, can occur with massive volume resuscitation
- **Pneumonia** – most common infection in burn wound patients
  - Also most common cause of **death** after inhalation injury

UNUSUAL BURNS
- **Acid and alkali burns** – copious water irrigation
  - Alkalis produce deeper burns than acid due to <u>liquefaction necrosis</u>
  - Acid burns produce <u>coagulation necrosis</u>
- **Hydrofluoric acid burns** – spread calcium on wound
- **Powder burns** – wipe away before irrigation
- **Tar burns** – cool, then wipe away with a lipophilic solvent
- **Electrical burns** – cardiac monitoring
  - Can cause rhabdomyolysis and compartment syndrome
  - Other complications – polyneuritis, quadriplegia, transverse myelitis, cataracts, liver necrosis, intestinal perforation, gallbladder perforation, pancreatic necrosis
- **Lightning** – cardiopulmonary arrest secondary to electrical paralysis of brainstem

1ST WEEK – EARLY EXCISION OF BURNED AREAS
- **Cardiac output in severely burned patients** – first have ↓ CO for 24–48 hours, then have ↑ CO (ebb and flow phases following burn)
- **Caloric need: 25 kcal/kg/day + (30 kcal × % burn)**
- **Protein need: 1 g/kg/day + (3 g × % burn)**
- **Glucose** – best source of nonprotein calories in patients with burns
  - Burn wounds use glucose in an obligatory fashion
- **Try to excise burn wounds in** <72 hours
  - Used for deep 2nd- and 3rd-degree burns
  - Viability is based on color, texture, punctate bleeding after removal

- **Skin grafts contraindicated** if culture is positive for **beta-hemolytic strep or bacteria >10^5**

- **Autografts (split-thickness [STSG] or full-thickness [FTSG])** – <u>best</u>
  - ↓ infection, desiccation, protein loss, pain, water loss, heat loss, and RBC loss
  - ↑ granulation tissue and improve survival
- **Split-thickness grafts** should be 12–15 mm (include epidermis and part of the dermis)

- **Homografts** (allografts; cadaveric skin) – not as good as autografts
  - Can be a good temporizing material; last 2–4 weeks
  - Allografts vascularize and are eventually rejected at which time they must be replaced
- **Xenografts** (porcine) – not as good as homografts; last 2 weeks; these do not vascularize
- **Dermal substitutes** – not as good as homografts or xenografts
- **Wounds to face, palms, soles, and genitals should be deferred for the 1st week**

- **For each burn wound incision** – <1 L blood loss, <20% of skin excised, <2 hours in OR
  - Patients can get extremely sick if too much time is spent in OR

- **Meshed grafts** – back, flank, trunk, arms, and legs
  - **Reasons to delay autografting** – infection, not enough skin, patient septic or unstable, do not want to create any more donor sites with concomitant blood loss
  - **Most common reason for skin graft loss** – seroma or hematoma formation under graft
    - Need to apply pressure dressing (cotton balls) to the skin graft to prevent seroma and hematoma buildup underneath the graft
  - **STSGs** are more likely to survive – graft not as thick so easier for imbibition and subsequent revascularization to occur
  - **FTSGs** have less wound contraction – good for areas such as the palms and back of hands
- **Burn scar hypopigmentation and irregularities** can be improved with dermal abrasion thin split-thickness grafts

2ND TO 5TH WEEKS – SPECIALIZED AREAS ADDRESSED, ALLOGRAFT REPLACED WITH AUTOGRAFT
- **Face** – topical antibiotics for 2 weeks, full-thickness grafts for unhealed areas (nonmeshed)
- **Hands**
  - **Superficial** – ROM exercises, splint in functional position if too much edema
  - **Deep** – immobilize for 7 days after operation, then physical therapy. May need wire fixation of joints if unstable or open. Treat with full-thickness grafts
- **Palms** – try to preserve specialized palmar attachments. Splint hand in extension for 1 week. Graft in week 2 with full-thickness nonmeshed autograft graft
- **Genitals** – antibiotics for 2 weeks. Graft unhealed areas (can use meshed)

BURN WOUND INFECTIONS
- Usually apply **bacitracin or Neosporin** immediately after burns
- <u>No</u> role for prophylactic IV antibiotics
- **Pseudomonas** is most common organism in burn wound infection, followed by
  - *Staphylococcus*, *E. coli*, and *Enterobacter*
- More common in burns > **30% BSA**
- Topical agents have decreased incidence of burn wound bacterial infections
- *Candida* infections have increased incidence secondary to topical antimicrobials
- Granulocyte chemotaxis and cell-mediated immunity are impaired in burn patients

- **Silvadene (silver sulfadiazine)** – <u>can cause neutropenia and thrombocytopenia</u>
  - Do not use in patients w/ sulfa allergy
  - Limited eschar penetration
  - Ineffective against some *Pseudomonas* species and other GNRs; effective for *Candida*
  - Methemoglobinemia – contraindicated in patients with G6PD deficiency

- **Silver nitrate** – <u>can cause electrolyte imbalances</u> → hyponatremia and hypochloremia, hypocalcemia and hypokalemia
  - Discoloration
  - Limited eschar penetration
  - Ineffective against some *Pseudomonas* species and GPCs

- **Sulfamylon (mafenide sodium)** – <u>painful</u> application
  - <u>Metabolic acidosis</u> due to carbonic anhydrase inhibition (↓ renal conversion of $H_2CO_3 \rightarrow H_2O + CO_2$) – can cause hypersensitivity reactions
  - **Good eschar penetration**; good for burns overlying **cartilage**
  - Broadest spectrum against *Pseudomonas* and GNRs

- **Signs of burn wound infection** – peripheral edema, 2nd- to 3rd-degree burn conversion, hemorrhage into scar, erythema gangrenosum, green fat, black skin around wound, rapid eschar separation, focal discoloration
- **Burn wound sepsis** – usually due to *Pseudomonas*
- **HSV** – most common viral infection in burn wounds
- $<10^5$ **organisms** – <u>not</u> a burn wound infection
- Best way to detect burn wound infection (and differentiate from colonization) – **biopsy of wound**

COMPLICATIONS AFTER BURNS

- **Seizures** – usually iatrogenic and related to Na concentration; can also be benzodiazepine withdrawal
- **Peripheral neuropathy** – secondary to small vessel injury and demyelination
- **Ectopia** – from contraction of burned adnexa. Tx: eyelid release
- **Eyes** – fluorescein staining to find injury. Tx: topical fluoroquinolone or gentamycin
- **Corneal abrasion** – Tx: topical antibiotics
- **Symblepharon** – eyelid stuck to conjunctiva. Tx: release with glass rod
- **Heterotopic ossification of tendons** – Tx: physical therapy; may need surgery
- **Fractures** – Tx: often get external fixation to allow for treatment of burns
- **Curling's ulcer** – gastric ulcer that occurs with burns
- **Marjolin's ulcer** – highly malignant squamous cell CA that arises in chronic nonhealing burn wounds or unstable scars
- **Hypertrophic scar**
  - Usually occurs 3–4 months after injury secondary to ↑ neovascularity
  - More likely to be deep thermal injuries that take >3 weeks to heal, heal by contraction and epithelial spread, or heal across flexor surfaces
  - Wait 1–2 years before scar modification
  - Tx: grafting, steroids, silicone, compression

OTHER SERIOUS SKIN INJURIES

- **Toxic epidermal necrolysis (TEN; variant of erythema multiforme major) and staphylococcal scalded skin syndrome**
  - <u>Epidermal–dermal separation</u> seen
  - Caused by a variety of drugs (Dilantin, Bactrim, penicillin) and viruses
  - Tx: supportive; need to prevent wound desiccation with topical antimicrobials and xenografts

- Antibiotics if due to *Staphylococcus aureus*
- **No** steaids

■ **Stevens–Johnson syndrome (erythema multiforme)** – less severe form of TEN
  - Hypersensitivity reaction – <u>subepidermal bullae, epidermal cell necrosis, dermal edema</u>
  - Caused by a variety of drugs (Dilantin, Bactrim, penicillin) and viruses
  - Tx: supportive; need to prevent wound desiccation with topical antimicrobials and xenografts
  - **No** steaids

CHAPTER 18. PLASTICS, SKIN, AND SOFT TISSUES

SKIN
- **Epidermis** – primarily cellular
  - **Keratinocytes** – main cell type in epidermis; originate from basal layer; provide mechanical barrier
  - **Melanocytes** – neuroectodermal origin (neural crest cells); in basal layer of epidermis
    - Have dendritic processes that transfer melanin to neighboring keratinocytes via melanosomes
    - Density of melanocytes is the same among races; difference is in production
- **Dermis** – primarily structural proteins for the epidermis
- **Langerhans cells**
  - Act as antigen-presenting cells (MHC class II)
  - Originate from bone marrow
  - Have a role in contact hypersensitivity reactions (type IV)
- **Sensory nerves**
  - **Pacinian corpuscles** – pressure
  - **Ruffini's endings** – warmth
  - **Krause's end-bulbs** – cold
  - **Meissner's corpuscles** – tactile sense
- **Eccrine sweat glands** – aqueous sweat (thermal regulation, usually hypotonic)
- **Apocrine sweat glands** – milky sweat
  - Highest concentration of glands in palms and soles; most sweat is the result of sympathetic nervous system via acetylcholine

- **Lipid-soluble drugs** – ↑ skin absorption
- **Type I collagen** – predominant type; 70% weight of dermis; gives tensile strength
- **Tension** – resistance to stretching (collagen)
- **Elasticity** – ability to regain shape (branching proteins that can stretch to 2× normal length)
- **Cushing's striae** – caused by loss of tensile strength and elasticity

GRAFTS
- **Split-thickness skin grafts (STSGs)**
  - Include all of the epidermis and part of the dermis
  - Donor site skin regenerated from hair follicles and skin edges on split-thickness grafts
- **STSGs** are more likely to survive → graft not as thick so easier for imbibition and subsequent revascularization to occur
- Full-thickness skin grafts – have less wound contraction → good for areas such as the palms and back of hands
- **Imbibition (osmotic)** – blood supply to skin graft for days 0–3
- **Neovascularization** – starts around day 3
  - Poorly vascularized beds are unlikely to support skin grafting → tendon, bone without periosteum, XRT areas
- **Pedicled or anastomosed free flap necrosis – venous thrombosis** most common cause
- **Tissue expansion** occurs by local recruitment, thinning of the dermis and epidermis, mitosis
- **TRAM flaps**
  - Complications – flap necrosis, ventral hernia, bleeding, infection, abdominal wall weakness

- Rely on superior epigastric vessels
- **Periumbilical perforators most important determinant of TRAM flap viability**

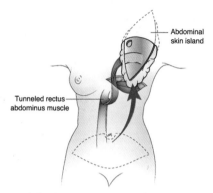

Transverse rectus abdominus myocutaneous (TRAM) flap reconstruction.

Stage	Description	Treatment
Pressure Sores		
I	Erythema and pain, no skin loss	
II	Partial skin loss with yellow debris	Local treatment, keep pressure off
III	Full-thickness skin loss, subcutaneous tissue exposure	Sharp debridement; will likely need myocutaneous flap
IV	Usually involves bony cortex	Myocutaneous flaps

After Deziel DJ, et al. *Rush University Review of Surgery.* 3rd ed. Philadelphia, PA: WB Saunders; 2000:598.

UV RADIATION
- Damages DNA and repair mechanisms
- Both a promoter and initiator
- Melanin single best factor for protecting skin from UV radiation
- **UV-B** – responsible for chronic sun damage

MELANOMA
- Represents only 3%–5% of skin CA but accounts for 65% of the deaths
- **Risk factors for melanoma**
  - **Dysplastic, atypical, or large congenital nevi** – 10% lifetime risk for melanoma
  - **Familial BK mole syndrome** – almost 100% risk of melanoma
  - **Xeroderma pigmentosum**
  - Fair complexion, easy sunburn, intermittent sunburns, previous skin CA, previous XRT
- 10% of melanomas familial
- **Most common melanoma site on skin** – back in men, legs in women
- **Prognosis worse** for men, ulcerated lesions, ocular and mucosal lesions
- **Signs of transformation** – color change, angulations, indentation/notching, enlargement, darkening, bleeding, ulceration
- Originates from **neural crest cells** (melanocytes) in basal layer epidermis
- Blue color → most ominous
- **Lung** – most common location for distant melanoma metastases
- Most common metastasis to <u>small bowel</u> – **melanoma**

▓ **Dx:**
- **<2 cm lesion** – excisional biopsy (tru-cut core needle biopsy) unless cosmetically sensitive area – need resection **w/** margins if pathology comes back as melanoma
- **>2 cm lesions or cosmetically sensitive area** – incisional biopsy (or punch biopsy), will need to resect w/ margins if pathology shows melanoma

▓ **Types**
- **Lentigo maligna** – least aggressive, minimal invasion, radial growth 1st usual; elevated nodules
- **Superficial spreading melanoma** – most common, intermediate malignancy; originates from nevus/sun-exposed areas
- **Nodular** – most aggressive; most likely to have metastasized at time of diagnosis; deepest growth at time of diagnosis; vertical growth 1st; bluish black with smooth borders; occurs anywhere on the body
- **Acral lentiginous** – very aggressive; palms/soles of African Americans
- **Melanoma in situ or thin lentigo maligna** – 0.5-cm margins OK
- Staging – need CXR and LFTs; examine all possible draining lymph nodes
- Tx: for all stages, resection of primary tumor with appropriate margins
- Alpha-interferon, IL-2, and tumor vaccines can be used for systemic disease

▓ **Nodes**
- Always need to resect clinically positive nodes with melanoma
- Perform sentinel lymph node biopsy if nodes clinically negative and tumor ≥ 1 mm deep
- **Involved nodes** usually nontender, round, hard, 1–2 cm
- All stage III tumors need full lymph node dissection
- Need to include superficial parotidectomy for anterior head and neck melanomas

▓ **Axillary node melanoma with no other primary** – Tx: complete axillary node dissection

▓ **Resection of metastases** has provided some patients with long disease-free interval and is the best chance for cure

▓ **Isolated metastases** (i.e., lung or liver) that can be resected with a low-risk procedure should probably undergo resection

American Joint Commission on Cancer Melanoma Staging System, TNM Definitions

PRIMARY TUMOR
TX: Cannot be assessed (shave biopsy, regressed lesion)
T0: Unknown primary
Tis: In situ melanoma
T1: †1.0 mm Breslow thickness
    a. Without education
    b. With ulceration or Clark level IV or V
T2: 1.01–2.0 mm
    a. Without ulceration
    b. With ulceration
T3: 2.01–4.0 mm
    a. Without ulceration
    b. With ulceration
T4: >4.0 mm
    a. Without ulceration
    b. With ulceration

(continued)

American Joint Commission on Cancer Melanoma Staging System, TNM Definitions (*continued*)

REGIONAL LYMPH NODE INVOLVEMENT

Nx: Cannot be assessed (previously removed)
N0: No regional node metastasis
N1: Metastasis in one regional node
    a. Micrometastasis (diagnosed by SLNB or elective lymph node dissection)
    b. Macrometastasis (clinically palpable or found on imaging studies, confirmed
       histologically, or gross extracapsular extension)
N2: Metastasis in two or three regional nodes
    a. Micrometastasis
    b. Macrometastasis
    c. In-transit or satellite metastasis without nodal metastasis
N3: Metastasis ‡4 regional nodes, matted nodes, or in-transit or satellite metastasis with
positive metastatic nodes

DISTANT METASTASIS

MX: Cannot be assessed
M0: No distant metastasis
M1a: Distant skin, subcutaneous, or lymph node metastasis with normal LDH
M1b: Lung metastasis with normal LDH
M1c: All other distant metastasis or any distant site with elevated LDH

SLNB, sentinel lymph node biopsy; LDH, lactate dehydrogenase.

Clark's Levels for Melanoma

Level	Description
I	Epidermis basement membrane intact
II	Papillary dermis through basement membrane
III	Junctional dermis between papillary and reticular dermis
IV	Reticular dermis
V	Fat

Melanoma Margins

Depth	Margin Needed
<1 mm	1 cm
1–4 mm	2 cm
>4 mm	2–3 cm

Survival of AJC Clinical Stage I and II Melanoma Patients Relative to Tumor Location

Thickness (mm)	7.5-Yr Survival Rate (%)				
	Extremities	Hands or Feet	Head and Neck	Trunk	BANS
<0.85	100	100	100	100	98
0.85–1.69	100	100	100	97	78
1.7–3.64	86	60	64	77	58
≥3.65	83	0	65	12	33

BANS, upper back, posterolateral arm, posterior and lateral neck, and posterior scalp.
Modified from Chang AE, et al. Cutaneous neoplasms. In: Greenfield LJ, et al., eds. *Surgery: Scientific Principles and Practice.*
3rd ed. Philadelphia: Lippincott Williams & Wilkins; 2001.

BASAL CELL CARCINOMA
- **Most common malignancy in United States**; 4× more common than squamous cell skin CA
- 80% on head and neck
- Originates from epidermis – basal epithelial cells and hair follicles
- **Pearly appearance, rolled borders**
- **Pathology – peripheral palisading of nuclei and stromal retraction**
- Slow, indolent growth
- Ulcerative, rare metastases, deep invasion, occasionally dark
- Regional adenectomy for clinically positive nodes
- **Morpheaform type** – most aggressive; has **collagenase** production
- Tx: 0.3–0.5-cm margins
  - XRT and chemotherapy – may be of limited benefit for inoperable disease or metastases; neuro, lymphatic, or vessels invasion

SQUAMOUS CELL CARCINOMA
- Overlying erythema, papulonodular with crust and ulceration
- May have surrounding induration and satellite nodules
- Usually red-brown; can have a pearly appearance
- Metastasizes more frequently than basal cell CA but less common than melanoma
- Can develop in postradiation areas or in old burn scars
- **Risk factors** – actinic keratoses, xeroderma pigmentosum, Bowen's disease, atrophic epidermis, arsenics, hydrocarbons (coal tar), chlorophenols, nitrates, HPV, immunosuppression, sun exposure, fair skin, XRT exposure, previous skin CA

- Risk factors for metastasis – poorly differentiated, greater depth, recurrent lesions, immunosuppression
- Tx: 0.5–1.0-cm margins for low risk
  - Can treat high risk with Mohs surgery (margin mapping using conservative slices; <u>not</u> used for melanoma) when trying to minimize area of resection (i.e., lesions on face)
  - **Regional adenectomy for clinically positive nodes**
  - XRT and chemotherapy – may be of limited benefit for inoperable disease or metastases; neuro, lymphatic, or vessels invasion

SOFT TISSUE SARCOMA
- **Most common soft tissue sarcomas – #1 malignant fibrous histiosarcoma**, #2 liposarcoma
- 50% arise from extremities; 50% in children (arise from embryonic mesoderm)
- Most sarcomas are large, grow rapidly, and are painless

- Symptoms: asymptomatic mass (most common presentation), GI bleeding, bowel obstruction, neurologic deficit
- CXR – to r/o lung mets
- MRI before biopsy to r/o vascular, neuro, or bone invasion

- **Biopsy**
  - **Excisional biopsy** if mass < 4 cm
  - **Longitudinal incisional biopsy** for masses > 4 cm (may need to eventually resect biopsy skin site if biopsy shows sarcoma)
- **Hematogenous spread**, not to lymphatics → <u>metastasis to nodes is rare</u>
  - **Lung** – most common site for metastasis

- **Staging based on grade**, not size or nodes
- **Tx**: Want at least **3-cm margins and at least 1 uninvolved fascial plane** → try to perform limb-sparing operation
  - **Place clips** to mark site of likely recurrence → will XRT these later
  - **Postop XRT** – for high-grade tumors, close margins, or tumors > 5 cm
  - **Chemotherapy is doxorubicin based**
  - Tumors > 10 cm may benefit from preop XRT and chemotherapy → may allow limb-sparing resection
  - **Isolated sarcoma metastases** without other evidence of systemic disease (i.e., lung or liver) can be resected and are the best chance for survival; otherwise can palliate with XRT
  - Midline incision favored for pelvic and retroperitoneal sarcomas
  - With resection, try to preserve motor nerves and retain or reconstruct vessels

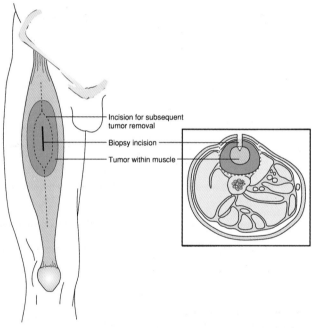

Incision for subsequent tumor removal

Biopsy incision

Tumor within muscle

Technique for biopsy of an extremity soft-tissue mass suspected of being a sarcoma. The incision should be oriented along the long axis of the extremity, at the point where the lesion is closest to the surface, and situated so that it can be readily excised along with the tumor if a diagnosis of sarcoma is made. There should be no raising of flaps or disturbance of tissue planes superficial to the tumor. The mass should not be enucleated within the pseudocapsule; rather, incisional biopsy leaving the bulk of the lesion undisturbed should be carried out. Before wound closure, hemostasis should be achieved to avoid a hematoma, which could disseminate tumor cells through normal tissue planes. Drains are not used routinely.

Relative Frequency of Histologic Types of Soft Tissue Sarcomas in Adults (All Sites)	
Histologic Type	Percentage
Malignant fibrous histiocytoma	25.9
Liposarcoma	17.7
Leiomyosarcoma	14.8
Fibrosarcoma	6.6
Neurofibrosarcoma	4.0
Synovial sarcoma	3.6
Rhabdomyosarcoma	3.6
Angiosarcoma	2.9
Extraskeletal chondrosarcoma	1.2
Malignant mesenchymoma	1.0
Extraskeletal osteosarcoma	0.6
Unclassified	5.4
Other	12.7

Modified from Lawrence W Jr, Donegan WI, Natarajan A, et al. Adult soft tissue sarcomas: a pattern of care survey of the American College of Surgeons. *Ann Surg.* 1987;205:349.

- **Poor prognosis overall**
  - Delay in diagnosis
  - Difficulty with total resection
  - Difficulty getting XRT to pelvic tumors
  - 40% 5-year survival rate with complete resection

- **Head and neck sarcomas** – can occur in the pediatric population (usually rhabdomyosarcoma)
  - Hard to get margin because of proximity to vital structures
  - Postop XRT for positive or close margins as negative margins may be impossible to obtain

- **Visceral and retroperitoneal sarcomas** – most commonly are leiomyosarcomas and liposarcomas
  - Ability to completely remove the tumor the most important prognostic factor in visceral and retroperitoneal sarcomas

- **Risk factors**
  - **Asbestos** – mesothelioma
  - **PVC and arsenic – angiosarcoma**
  - **Other risk factors – XRT, chlorophenols, pesticides**
  - **Chronic lymphedema** – associated with lymphangiosarcoma

- **Kaposi's sarcoma** – vascular sarcoma
  - Can involve skin, mucous membranes, or GI tract
  - Associated with immunocompromised state
  - Rarely a cause of death in AIDS; 15–20-year survival; slow growing
  - Tx: XRT or intralesional vinblastine for local disease; systemic chemotherapy for disseminated disease
  - Surgery for intestinal hemorrhage

- **Childhood rhabdomyosarcoma**
  - #1 soft tissue sarcoma in kids
  - Head/neck, genitourinary, extremities and trunk (poorest prognosis)

- **Embryonal** subtype – most common
- **Alveolar** subtype – worst prognosis
- Tx: surgery; doxorubicin-based chemotherapy

■ **Bone sarcomas**
  - Most are metastatic at the time of diagnosis
  - **Osteosarcoma**
    - Increased incidence around the knee
    - Originates from **metaphyseal cells**
    - Usually in children
  - Usually need to take the joint, followed by reconstruction; may require amputation

■ **Genetic syndromes for soft tissue tumors**
  - Neurofibromatosis – CNS tumors, peripheral sheath tumors, pheochromocytoma
  - Li–Fraumeni syndrome – childhood rhabdomyosarcoma, many others
  - Hereditary retinoblastoma – also includes other sarcoma
  - Tuberous sclerosis – angiomyolipoma
  - Gardner's syndrome – familial adenomatous polyposis and intra-abdominal desmoids

OTHER CONDITIONS
■ **Xanthoma** – yellow, contains histiocytes. Tx: excision
■ **Warts (verruca vulgaris)** – viral origin, contagious, autoinoculable, can be painful
  - Tx: liquid nitrogen initially
■ **Lipomas** – common but rarely malignant; back, neck, between shoulders
■ **Neuromas** – can be associated with neurofibromatosis and von Recklinghausen's disease
  - Café-au-lait spots, axillary freckling, optic nerve gliomas, CNS tumors
■ **Keratoses**
  - **Actinic keratosis** – premalignant, in sun-damaged areas; need excisional biopsy if suspicious
  - **Seborrheic keratosis** – <u>not</u> premalignant; trunk on elderly; can be dark
  - **Arsenical keratosis** – associated with squamous cell carcinoma
■ **Merkel cell carcinoma** – are **neuroendocrine**
  - Aggressive regional and systemic spread; patients have red to purple papulonodule/indurated plaque
  - Have **neuron-specific enolase (NSE), cytokeratin, and neurofilament protein**
■ **Glomus cell tumor**
  - Painful tumor composed of blood vessels and nerves
  - **Benign**; most common in the terminal aspect of the digit
  - Tx: tumor excision
■ **Hutchinson's freckle** – in elderly, often on face; premalignant, not aggressive
■ **Lip lacerations** – important to line up vermillion border
■ **Desmoid tumors** – usually benign; occur in fascial planes
  - **Anterior abdominal wall (most common location)** desmoids can occur during or following pregnancy; can also occur after trauma or surgery
  - **Intra-abdominal desmoids** associated with Gardner's syndrome and retroperitoneal fibrosis
  - High risk of local recurrences; no distant spread
  - Tx: surgery or chemotherapy/XRT if vital structure involved
■ **Bowen's disease** – SCCA in situ; 10% turn into invasive SCCA
  - Tx: excision with negative margins usual (exception includes peri-anal region)

- **Keratoacanthoma**
  - Rapid growth, rolled edges, crater filled with keratin
  - Is not malignant but can be confused with SCCA
  - Involutes spontaneously over months
  - Always biopsy these to be sure
  - If small, excise; if large, biopsy and observe
- **Hyperhydrosis** – ↑ sweating, especially noticeable in the palms. Tx: sympathectomy if refractory
- **Hidradenitis** – infection of the apocrine sweat glands, usually in axilla and groin regions
  - Staph/strep most common organisms
  - Tx: antibiotics, improved hygiene 1st; may need surgery
- **Benign cysts**
  - **Epidermal inclusion cyst** – most common; have completely mature epidermis with creamy keratin material
  - **Trichilemmal cyst** – in scalp, no epidermis
  - **Ganglion cyst** – over tendons, usually over wrist; filled with collagenous material
  - **Dermoid cyst** – midline abdominal and sacral lesions, occiput and nose; found along body fusion planes
  - **Pilonidal cyst** – congenital coccygeal sinus with ingrown hair; gets infected and need to be excised
- **Keloids** – autosomal dominant; dark skin
  - Collagen goes beyond original scar
  - Tx: XRT, steroids, silicone, pressure garments
- **Hypertrophic scar tissue** – dark skin; flexor surfaces of upper torso
  - Collagen stays within confines of scar
  - Often occurs in burns or wounds that take a long time to heal
  - Tx: steroids, silicone, pressure garments

ANATOMY AND PHYSIOLOGY

▓ **Anterior neck triangle** – sternocleidomastoid muscle, sternal notch, inferior border of the digastric muscle; contains the **carotid sheath**

▓ **Posterior neck triangle** – posterior border of the sternocleidomastoid muscle, trapezius muscle, and the clavicle; contains the **spinal accessory nerve and the brachial plexus**

▓ **Phrenic nerve** – on anterior scalene muscle

▓ **Parotid glands** – secrete mostly serous fluid

▓ **Sublingual glands** – secrete mostly mucin

▓ **Submandibular glands** – 50/50

▓ In larynx, the false vocal cords are superior to the true vocal cords

▓ Trachea has U-shaped cartilage and a posterior portion that is membranous

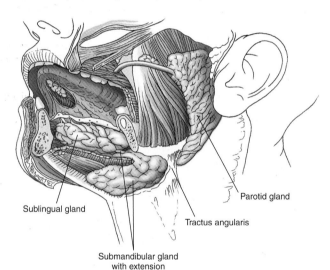

Sublingual gland

Parotid gland

Tractus angularis

Submandibular gland
with extension

Major salivary glands. The lateral view, illustrating the tractus angularis and submandibular gland with extension under the mylohyoid muscle and the sublingual gland. (From Byers RM. Operations involving the submandibular and sublingual salivary glands. In: Fischer JE, Bland KI, et al., eds. *Mastery of Surgery.* 5th ed. Philadelphia: Lippincott Williams & Wilkins; 2007, with permission.)

▓ **Vagus nerve** – runs between IJ and carotid arteries

▓ **Phrenic nerve** – runs on top of the anterior scalene muscle

▓ **Trigeminal nerve** – ophthalmic, maxillary, mandibular branches
  • Gives sensation to most of face
  • Mandibular branch – taste to anterior ⅔ of tongue, floor of mouth, and gingiva

▓ **Facial nerve** – temporal, zygomatic, buccal, marginal mandibular, and cervical branches
  • Motor function to face

▓ **Glossopharyngeal nerve** – sensory to posterior tongue
  • Motor to stylopharyngeus
  • Injury affects swallowing

- **Hypoglossal nerve** – motor to all of tongue except palatoglossus
- Tongue deviates to side of injury
- **Recurrent laryngeal nerve** – innervates all of larynx except cricothyroid muscle
- **Superior laryngeal nerve** – innervates the cricothyroid muscle
- **Frey's syndrome** – occurs after parotidectomy; injury of **auriculotemporal nerve** that then cross-innervates with sympathetic fibers to sweat glands of skin
  - Symptom: gustatory sweating

- **Thyrocervical trunk** – "**STAT**": **s**uprascapular artery, **t**ransverse cervical artery, **a**scending cervical artery, inferior **t**hyroid artery
- **External carotid artery** – 1st branch is superior thyroid artery
- **Trapezius flap** (spinal accessory nerve, shoulder shrug) – based on transverse cervical artery
- **Pectoralis major** – based on thoracoacromial artery

- **Torus palatini** – congenital bony mass on upper palate of mouth. Tx: nothing
- **Torus mandibular** – similar to above but on the anterior lingual surface of the mandible

- **Radical neck dissection** (RND) – takes accessory nerve (CN XII), sternocleidomastoid, internal jugular, omohyoid, submandibular gland, sensory nerves C2–C5, cervical branch of facial nerve, and ipsilateral thyroid
  - Most morbidity occurs from accessory nerve resection
- **Modified radical neck dissection** (MRND) – takes omohyoid, submandibular gland, sensory nerves C2–C5, cervical branch of facial nerve, ipsilateral thyroid
  - No mortality difference compared with RND

Progressive Signs and Symptoms Indicating Head and Neck Cancer	
Odynophagia	Nasal obstruction
Dysphagia	Epistaxis
Weight loss	Facial pain
Loose dentition	Cranial neuropathies
Oral fetor	Secondary infections
Trismus	Aspiration
Otalgia	Fistulization
Neck mass	Hemorrhage
Serous otitis media	Airway obstruction

ORAL CAVITY CANCER

- **Most common cancer of the oral cavity, pharynx, and larynx** – squamous cell CA
  - **Biggest risk factors** – tobacco and ETOH
  - **Erythroplakia** – considered more premalignant than leukoplakia

- **Oral cavity includes** mouth floor, anterior ⅓ of tongue, gingiva, hard palate, anterior tonsillar pillars, and lips
- **SCCA** – most common cancer of oral cavity
- Lower lip – most common site for oral cavity CA
- **Survival rate lowest for hard palate tumors – hard to resect**

- **Oral cavity CA increased in patients with Plummer–Vinson syndrome** (glossitis, cervical dysphagia from esophageal web, spoon fingers, iron-deficiency anemia)

- ■ **Treatment**
  - **Wide resection of tumor if ≤2 cm (T1)**, need 1–2 cm margins
  - **MRND** for tumors > 2 cm or if clinically positive nodes
  - **Postop XRT** for advanced lesions (>2 cm, positive margins, nerve/vascular/ lymphatic invasion)

- ■ **Lip CA** – lower lip CA more common than upper due to sun exposure
  - May need **flaps** if more than ½ of the lip is removed
  - Lesions along the **commissure are most aggressive**

- ■ **Tongue CA** – can still operate with jaw invasion

- ■ **Verrucous ulcer** – well-differentiated tumor of the cheek
  - Not aggressive
  - Tx: full cheek resection +/− flap; no MRND

- ■ **Cancer of maxillary sinus** – Tx: maxillectomy

PHARYNGEAL CANCER
- ■ **Nasopharyngeal SCCA** – EBV; Chinese; presents with nose bleeding or obstruction
  - Goes to **posterior (deep) cervical neck nodes**
  - Tx: **XRT primary; MRND** for tumors > 2 cm or clinically positive nodes; postop chemo for advanced stage
  - **Children** – lymphoma #1 tumor of nasopharynx. Tx: chemotherapy
  - **Papilloma** – most common benign neoplasm of nose/paranasal sinuses

- ■ **Oropharyngeal SCCA** – neck mass, sore throat
  - Goes to **posterior (deep) cervical neck nodes**
  - Tx: **XRT or surgery; MRND** for tumors > 2 cm or if clinically positive nodes

- ■ **Tonsillar CA** – ETOH, tobacco, males; SCCA most common; asymptomatic until large; 80% have lymph node metastases at time of diagnosis
  - Tx: tonsillectomy best way to biopsy; XRT mainstay

- ■ **Hypopharyngeal SCCA** – hoarseness; early metastases
  - Goes to **anterior cervical nodes**
  - Tx: **usually surgery** (laryngectomy), **MRND, postop XRT**

- ■ **Nasopharyngeal angiofibroma** – benign tumor
  - Presents in males < 20 years (obstruction or epistaxis)
  - Extremely vascular
  - Tx: angiography and embolization (usually internal maxillary artery), followed by resection

LARYNGEAL CANCER
- ■ Hoarseness, aspiration, dyspnea, dysphagia
- ■ Can preserve larynx in some cases of cancer (glottis free of tumor and mobile)
- ■ Take **ipsilateral thyroid lobe** with MRND
- ■ Papilloma – most common benign lesion of larynx

- ■ **Supraglottic SCCA** – early nodal spread to submental/submandibular areas
  - Small – Tx: **XRT or conservative surgery**
  - Large – Tx: **laryngectomy, MRND, postop XRT**

■ **Glottic SCCA** – nodal spread to anterior cervical chain
  • Small – Tx: **XRT or laser**, chordectomy with recurrence
  • Large – Tx: **laryngectomy, MRND, postop XRT**
  • **Fixed cords require laryngectomy**
■ **Subglottic SCCA** – early nodal to anterior cervical chain and metastatic spread
  • Small – Tx: **XRT or conservative surgery**
  • Large – Tx: **laryngectomy, MRND, postop XRT**

SALIVARY GLAND CANCERS
■ Parotid, submandibular, sublingual, and minor salivary glands

■ Submandibular or sublingual tumors – can present as a neck mass or swelling in the floor of the mouth

■ **Mass in large salivary gland** → more likely mass is <u>benign</u>
■ **Mass in small salivary gland** → more likely mass is <u>malignant</u>, although the parotid gland is the most frequent site for malignant tumor

■ **Malignant tumors**
  • **Mucoepidermoid CA** – #1 malignant tumor of the salivary glands
    • Wide range of aggressiveness
  • **Adenoid cystic CA** – #2 malignant tumor of the salivary glands; #1 malignant salivary tumor of the minor salivary glands
    • Long, indolent course; propensity to invade nerve roots

  • Often present as a painful mass but can also present with facial nerve paralysis or lymphadenopathy
  • Lymphatic drainage to the intraparotid nodes and the anterior cervical chain nodes

  • Tx for both: **resection of salivary gland (parotidectomy); prophylactic MRND and postop XRT if high grade or SCCA**
    • If in parotid, need to take whole lobe; try to preserve facial nerve
    • Other tumors – adenocarcinoma, SCCA, lymphoma

> **General Principles for Surgical Treatment of Salivary Gland Malignancies**
>
> Malignant tumors of the parotid gland warrant total parotidectomy.
> The facial nerve should be sacrificed only for direct tumor invasion or for preexisting facial paralyses.
> Patients with high-grade tumors should undergo elective neck dissection if there is no clinical neck disease or a modified neck dissection for palpable adenopathy.
> Postoperative radiotherapy is indicated for all high-grade tumors; close margins; recurrent disease; skin, bone, nerve, or extraparotid involvement; positive nodes; or unresectable disease.

■ **Benign tumors**
  • **Pleomorphic adenoma** (mixed tumor) – #1 benign tumor of the salivary glands
  • **Malignant degeneration in 5%**
    • Tx: superficial parotidectomy

- If malignant degeneration, need total parotidectomy; if high grade also need MRND
- **Warthin's tumor** – #2 benign tumor of the salivary glands
  - Males, bilateral in 10%
  - Tx: superficial parotidectomy
- Often present as a painless mass

- Most common injured nerve with parotid surgery – **greater auricular nerve** (numbness over lower portion of auricle)
- For submandibular gland resection – need to find <u>mandibular branch of facial nerve, lingual nerve, hypoglossal nerve</u>
- Most common salivary gland tumor in children – **hemangiomas**

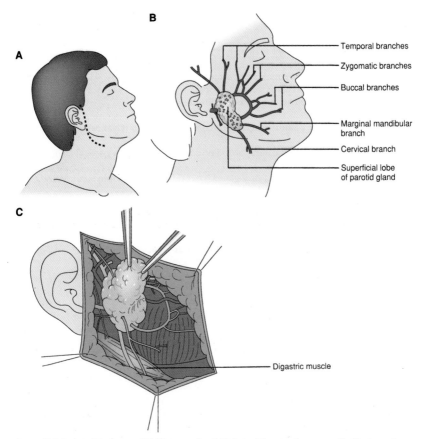

Superficial parotidectomy. *(A)* The standard Blair incision or the cosmetically superior face-lift incision can be used. *(B)* Branches of the facial nerve course between the superficial and deep lobes of the parotid *(C)*. The main trunk of the facial nerve is identified 8 mm deep to the tympanomastoid suture line and at the same level as the digastric muscle.

EAR

- **Cauliflower ear** – undrained hematomas that organize and calcify; need to be drained to avoid this
- **Chemodectomas** – vascular tumor of middle ear (paraganglionoma). Tx: surgery +/− XRT
- **Acoustic neuroma** – CN VIII, tinnitus, hearing loss, unsteadiness; can grow into cerebellar/pontine angle. Tx: craniotomy and resection; XRT is alternative to surgery
- **Cholesteatoma** – epidermal inclusion cyst of ear; slow growing but erode as they grow; present with conductive hearing loss and clear drainage from ear. Tx: surgical excision
- **Pinna lacerations** – need suture through involved cartilage
- **Ear SCCA** – 20% metastasize to parotid gland. Tx: parotidectomy, MRND for positive nodes or large tumors, XRT
- **Rhabdomyosarcoma** – most common childhood aural malignancy (although rare) of the middle or external ear

NOSE

- **Nasal fractures** – set after swelling decreases
- **Septal hematoma** – need to drain to avoid infection and necrosis of septum
- **CSF rhinorrhea** – usually a cribriform plate fracture (CSF has **tau protein**)
  - Repair of facial fractures may help leak; may need contrast study to help find leak
  - Tx: conservative 2–3 weeks; try epidural catheter, may need transethmoid repair
- **Epistaxis**
  - 90% anterior and can be controlled with packing
  - Consider internal maxillary artery or ethmoid artery ligation (direct or angiographically) for persistent posterior bleeding despite packing/balloon

NECK AND JAW

- **Radicular cyst** – local excision or curettage; lucent on x-ray
- **Ameloblastoma** – slow-growing malignancy; soap bubble appearance on x-ray; can have metastases. Tx: wide local excision
- **Osteogenic sarcoma** – poor prognosis. Tx: multimodality approach that includes surgery
- **Maxillary jaw fractures** – most treated with wire fixation
- **TMJ dislocations** – treated with closed reduction
- **Lip numbness** – inferior alveolar nerve damage

- **Stensen's duct laceration** – repair over catheter stent
  - Ligation can cause painful parotid atrophy and facial asymmetry
- **Suppurative parotitis** – usually in elderly patients; occurs with dehydration; staph most common organism
  - Tx fluids, salivation, antibiotics; drainage if abscess develops or patient not improving
  - Can be life-threatening
- **Sialoadenitis** – acute inflammation of the salivary gland related to a stone in the duct; most calculi near orifice
  - Recurrent sialoadenitis is thought to be due to ascending infection from the oral cavity
  - Gland excision may eventually be necessary for recurrent disease
  - 80% of the time affects the submandibular or sublingual glands
  - Tx: incise duct and remove stone

ABSCESSES
- **Peritonsillar abscess** – older kids (>10 years)
  - Symptoms: trismus, odynophagia; usually does <u>not</u> obstruct airway
  - <u>Tx</u>: needle aspiration 1st, then drainage through tonsillar bed if no relief in 24 hours
    - May need to intubate to drain; will self-drain with swallowing once opened

- **Retropharyngeal abscess** – younger kids (<10 years)
  - Symptoms: fever, odynophagia, drool; is an **airway emergency**
  - Can occur in elderly with Pott's disease
  - <u>Tx</u>: intubate the patient in a calm setting; drainage through posterior pharyngeal wall; will self-drain with swallowing once opened

- **Parapharyngeal abscess** – all age groups; occurs with dental infections, tonsillitis, pharyngitis
  - Morbidity comes from vascular invasion and mediastinal spread via prevertebral and retropharyngeal spaces
  - <u>Tx</u>: drain through lateral neck to avoid damaging internal carotid and internal jugular veins; need to leave drain in

- **Ludwig's angina** – acute infection of the floor of the mouth, involves **mylohyoid muscle**
  - Most common cause is dental infection of the mandibular teeth
  - May rapidly spread to deeper structures and cause airway obstruction
  - Tx: airway control, surgical drainage, antibiotics

ASYMPTOMATIC HEAD AND NECK MASSES
- **Preauricular tumors**
  - All lumps near ear are parotid tumors until proved otherwise
  - Diagnosis is usually made after superficial lobectomy
  - 80% of all salivary tumors are in parotid
  - 80% of parotid tumors are benign
  - 80% of benign parotid tumors are pleomorphic adenomas – 5% malignant degeneration
  - **Most common distant metastases for head and neck tumors → lung**
    - Tx: **chemotherapy**
- **Posterior neck masses** – if no obvious malignant epithelial tumor, considered to have Hodgkin's lymphoma until proved otherwise. Need FNA or open biopsy

- **Neck mass workup**
  - 1st – history and exam, laryngoscopy, antibiotics if thought to be inflammatory, FNA if hard
  - 2nd – panendoscopy with multiple random biopsies, neck and chest CT
  - 3rd – still cannot figure it out → perform excisional biopsy; need to be prepared for MRND
  - Adenocarcinoma suggests breast, GI, or lung primary
- **Epidermoid CA found in cervical node without known primary**
  - 1st – panendoscopy with random biopsies
  - 2nd – CT scan
  - 3rd – still cannot find primary → ipsilateral MRND, ipsilateral tonsillectomy, bilateral XRT

OTHER CONDITIONS
- **Esophageal foreign body** – dysphagia; most just below the cricopharyngeus (95%)
  - Dx: **rigid EGD** under anesthesia
  - Perforation risk increases with <u>length of time in the esophagus</u>

- **Fever and pain** after EGD for foreign body → CXR and Gastrografin followed by barium swallow to rule out perforation
- **Laryngeal foreign body** – coughing; emergent cricothyroidotomy as a last resort may be needed to secure airway
- **Lip lacerations** – apposition of the vermillion border is key. Layered closure is preferred
- **Sleep apnea** – associated with MIs, arrhythmias, and death
  - More common in obese and those with micrognathia/retrognathia → have snoring and excessive daytime somnolence
  - Tx: CPAP, uvulopalatopharyngoplasty, hyoid suspension, or permanent trach
- **Prolonged intubation** – can lead to subglottic stenosis, which is treated with laser, dilatation, possible excision
- **Tracheostomy** – consider in patients who will require intubation for >7–14 days
  - Decreases secretions, provides easier ventilation, decreases pneumonia risk
- **Tracheo-innominate fistula** – occurs after tracheostomy, can have rapid exsanguination
  - **Tx**: place finger in trach hole and hold pressure → median sternotomy
  - This complication is avoided by keeping tracheostomy above the 3rd tracheal ring
- **Median rhomboid glossitis** – failure of tongue fusion. Tx: none necessary
- **Cleft lip** (primary palate) – involves lip, alveolus, or both
  - Repair at 10 weeks, 10 lb, Hgb 10. Repair nasal deformities at same time
  - May be associated with poor feeding
- **Cleft palate** (secondary palate) – involves hard and soft palates; may affect speech and swallowing if not closed soon enough; may affect maxillofacial growth if closed too early → repair at 12 months
- **Hemangioma** – most common benign head and neck tumor in adults
- **Mastoiditis** – infection of the mastoid cells; can destroy bone
  - Rare; results as a complication of untreated acute supportive otitis media
  - Ear pushed forward
  - Tx: antibiotics, may need emergency mastoidectomy
- **Epiglottitis**
  - Rare since immunization against *H. influenzae* type B
  - Mainly in children aged 3–5
  - Symptoms: stridor, drooling, leaning forward position, high fever, throat pain, thumbprint sign on lateral neck film
  - Can cause airway obstruction
  - Tx: early control of the airway; antibiotics
- **Kaposi's sarcoma** – oral and pharyngeal mucosa are the most common sites
  - Can get odynophagia and dysphagia; bleeding
  - Primary goal usually is palliation
  - **Most common neoplasm in patients with AIDS**
  - Tx: XRT, intratumor vinblastine

ANATOMY AND PHYSIOLOGY

■ **Hypothalamus** – releases TRH, CRH, GnRH, GHRH, and dopamine into median eminence; passes through neurohypophysis on way to adenohypophysis
■ **Dopamine** – inhibits prolactin secretion
■ **Posterior pituitary (neurohypophysis)**
  • **ADH** – supraoptic nuclei, regulated by osmolar receptors in hypothalamus
  • **Oxytocin** – paraventricular nuclei in hypothalamus
■ Neurohypophysis does not contain cell bodies
■ **Anterior pituitary (80% of gland, adenohypophysis)**
  • ACTH, TSH, GH, LH, FSH, and prolactin
  • Does not have its own direct blood supply; passes through neurohypophysis 1st

■ **Bitemporal hemianopia** – pituitary mass compressing optic nerve (CN II) at chiasm
■ **Nonfunctional tumors** – almost always macroadenomas; present with mass effect and decreased ACTH, TSH, GH, LH, FSH. Tx: transsphenoid resection
■ **Contraindications to transsphenoid approaches** – suprasellar extension, massive lateral extension, dumbbell-shaped tumor
■ TSH- and FSH-/LH-secreting tumors may respond to **bromocriptine**

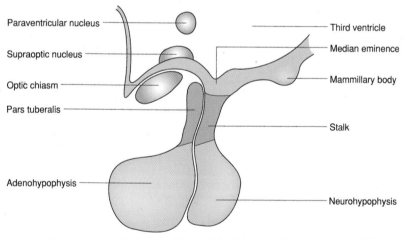

Paraventricular nucleus
Supraoptic nucleus
Optic chiasm
Pars tuberalis
Adenohypophysis

Third ventricle
Median eminence
Mammillary body
Stalk
Neurohypophysis

Schematic diagram of the pituitary and floor of the third ventricle as seen in a midline sagittal view. Anterior is to the left.

PROLACTINOMA

■ **Most common pituitary adenoma**
■ Mostly microadenomas
■ Most patients do not need surgery. Prolactin is usually >150 in these patients
■ Symptoms: galactorrhea, irregular menses, ↓ libido, infertility, ↓ vision
■ Tx: bromocriptine for most, or transsphenoidal resection for failure of medical management
  • Macroadenomas – resection with hemorrhage, visual loss, wants pregnancy, CSF leak
  • Microadenomas – resection if bromocriptine unsafe or ineffective (is OK in pregnancy)

ACROMEGALY (GROWTH HORMONE)

- Symptoms: HTN, DM, gigantism
- GH > 10 in 90%, usually macroadenomas
- Preoperative octreotide may be helpful (inhibits release of GH)
- Can be life-threatening secondary to cardiac symptoms (valve dysfunction, cardiomyopathy)
- Higher remission rate for microadenomas
- Symptoms: hypertension, diabetes mellitus, gigantism
- Dx: elevated IGF-1, growth hormone > 5—10
- Tx: transsphenoidal resection; XRT and bromocriptine can be used for primary or secondary therapy

OTHER CONDITIONS

- **Sheehan's syndrome**
  - Postpartum **trouble lactating – usually 1st sign**
  - Can also have amenorrhea, adrenal insufficiency, and hypothyroidism
  - Due to **pituitary ischemia** following hemorrhage and hypotensive episode
- **Craniopharyngioma** – calcified cyst, remnants of Rathke's pouch
  - Symptoms: most frequently presents with endocrine abnormalities, visual disturbances, headache, hydrocephalus
  - Tx: surgery, XRT
  - Diabetes insipidus – frequent complication postoperatively
- **Bilateral pituitary masses** – check axis; if OK, probably metastases
- **Nelson's syndrome**
  - Occurs after bilateral adrenalectomy; ↑ CRH causes pituitary enlargement, resulting in amenorrhea, visual problems (bitemporal hemianopia)
  - Also get hyperpigmentation from **beta-MSH** (melanocyte-stimulating hormone), a peptide byproduct of ACTH
  - Tx: steroids
- **Waterhouse—Friderichsen syndrome** – adrenal gland hemorrhage that occurs after meningococcal sepsis infection; can lead to adrenal insufficiency

Superior adrenal – inferior phrenic artery
Middle adrenal – aorta
Inferior adrenal – renal artery
Left adrenal vein goes to left renal vein
Right adrenal vein goes to inferior vena cava

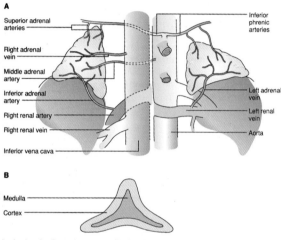

(A) Arterial (dark shaded) and venous (light shaded) anatomy of the adrenal glands.
(B) Schematic showing outer adrenal cortex (light shaded) and inner adrenal medulla
(dark shaded).

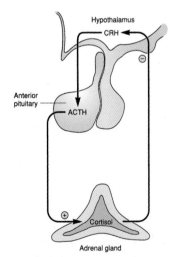

Schematic of hypothalamic–pituitary–adrenal axis for cortisol. Regulatory feedback
relationships are designated with arrows.

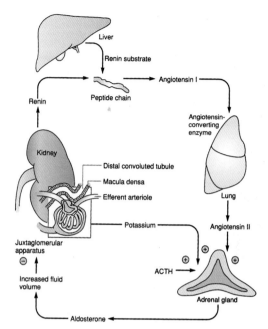

Regulatory relationships of renin, the angiotensins, and their sites of production and enzymatic conversion.

ASYMPTOMATIC ADRENAL MASS

- 1%–2% of abdominal CT scans show incidentaloma (5% are metastases or primary adrenal tumors)
- Benign adenomas are common
- Adrenals are also common sites for metastases
- Surgery is indicated if mass **has ominous characteristics (nonhomogenous)** or is **>4–6 cm, functioning, or enlarging**
- Need to follow up very 3 months for 1 year, then yearly
- Dx: serum K, urine metanephrines/VMA/catecholamines, urinary hydroxycorticos-teroids, plasma renin and aldosterone levels if HTN or ↓ K; CXR, stool guaiac and colonoscopy, mammogram
  - Anterior approach for adrenal CA resection

Common metastases to adrenal – lung CA (#1), breast CA, melanoma, renal CA
Cancer history with asymptomatic adrenal mass – need biopsy

ADRENAL CORTEX

- From mesoderm – remember GFR = salt, sugar, sex steroids
- **Glomerulosa** – aldosterone; **fasciculata** – glucocorticoids; **reticularis** – androgens/estrogens
- Cholesterol → progesterone → androgens/cortisol/aldosterone
- All zones have **21- and 11-beta hydroxylase**
- No innervation to the cortex
- Medulla receives innervation from the splanchnic nerves
- Lymphatics drain to subdiaphragmatic and renal lymph nodes
- Corticotropin-releasing hormone (CRH) is released from the hypothalamus and goes to anterior pituitary gland
- ACTH is released from the anterior pituitary gland and causes the release of cortisol

- Cortisol has a diurnal peak at 4–6 a.m.
- Aldosterone stimulates renal sodium resorption and secretion of potassium, hydrogen ion, and ammonia
- Aldosterone secretion is stimulated by **angiotensin II and hyperkalemia, and to some extent ACTH**
- **Excess estrogens and androgens** by adrenals – almost always cancer
- **Congenital adrenal hyperplasia (enzyme defect in cortisol synthesis)**
  - **21-Hydroxylase deficiency** (90%) – most common; precocious puberty in males, virilization in females
    - ↑ 17-OH progesterone leads to ↑ production of testosterone
    - **Is salt wasting (↓ sodium and ↑ potassium) and causes hypotension**
    - Tx: cortisol, genitoplasty
  - **11-Hydroxylase deficiency** – precocious puberty in males, virilization in females
    - ↑ 11-Deoxycortisone
    - **Is salt saving** (deoxycortisone acts as a mineralocorticoid) and causes **hypertension**
    - Tx: cortisol, genitoplasty
  - **17-Hydroxylase deficiency** – ambiguous genitalia in males at birth; salt saving

- **Hyperaldosteronism (Conn's syndrome)**
  - **Symptoms**: HTN secondary to sodium retention without edema; hypokalemia; also have weakness, polydipsia, and polyuria
  - **Primary disease (low renin)** – adenoma (80%–90%)→ #1 cause of primary hyperaldosteronism, hyperplasia (10%–20%), ovarian tumors (rare), cancer (rare)
  - **Secondary disease (high renin)** – more common than primary disease; CHF, renal artery stenosis, liver failure, pregnancy, diuretics, Bartter's syndrome (renin-secreting tumor)
  - **Dx for primary hyperaldosteronism**
    - Urine aldosterone after salt load best (will stay high)
    - ↓ serum K, ↑ urine K, ↑ serum Na, metabolic alkalosis
    - Plasma renin activity will be low
    - Aldosterone:renin ratio > 20
  - **Localizing studies** – MRI, NP-59 scintigraphy (shows hyperfunctioning adrenal tissue; differentiates adenoma from hyperplasia; 90% accurate); adrenal venous sampling if others nondiagnostic
    - **Tx: adenoma** resection has good results with adrenalectomy
      - **Hyperplasia** – seldom cured (↑ morbidity with bilateral resection)
        - Try medical **therapy** first with hyperplasia using spironolactone, calcium channel blockers, and potassium
        - If bilateral **resection** is performed (usually done for refractory hypokalemia), patient will need fludrocortisone postoperatively

- **Hypocortisolism (adrenal insufficiency, Addison's disease)**
  - #1 cause – **withdrawal of exogenous steroids**
  - #1 primary disease – **autoimmune disease**
  - Also caused by pituitary disease, infection, adrenal hemorrhage, adrenal metastasis, surgical resection or injury
  - Get ↓ cortisol and aldosterone
  - **Dx**: ↓ serum Na, ↑ serum K, ACTH stimulation test
  - **Acute adrenal insufficiency** – hypotension, fever, lethargy, abdominal pain, ↓ glucose, ↓ mental status, nausea and vomiting, ↑ K
  - Tx: dexamethasone, fluids, and ACTH stimulation test (measure cortisol level after test)

- **Hypercortisolism (Cushing's syndrome)**
  - Most commonly **iatrogenic**

- Dx:
  - 1st – 24-hour urine cortisol (most sensitive test)
  - 2nd – low-dose overnight dexamethasone suppression test; look to see whether it suppresses cortisol production (measure in urine). If cortisol is low, the diagnosis is Cushing's disease (the pituitary adenoma was suppressed). If cortisol remains high, go to 3rd
  - 3rd – measure serum ACTH. If high, have either ectopic ACTH or pituitary tumor that was not suppressed with low-dose overnight dexamethasone suppression test, go to 4th. If low ACTH, patient has cortisol-secreting tumor (i.e., adrenal tumor or adrenal hyperplasia)
  - 4th – if serum ACTH high → high-dose overnight dexamethasone suppression test (positive = pituitary origin, negative = ectopic origin of ACTH). In 20% you still cannot tell; go to 5th
  - 5th – CRH test → pituitary adenomas will increase ACTH; ectopic producers will have no change in ACTH
  - MRI useful. NP-59 scintography localizes adrenal tumors and can help differentiate them from hyperplasia
- **Pituitary adenoma (Cushing's disease)**
  - **#1 noniatrogenic cause of Cushing's syndrome** → 70%–80% of cases
  - Cortisol should be suppressed with either low- or high-dose dexamethasone suppression test
  - Mostly **microadenomas**
  - Need petrosal sampling to figure out which side; MRI can also help
  - Vertical incisions to find adenoma
  - Tx: most tumors removed with transsphenoidal approach; unresectable or residual tumors treated with XRT
- **Ectopic ACTH**
  - **#2 noniatrogenic** cause of Cushing's syndrome
  - Most commonly from small cell lung CA
  - Cortisol is <u>not</u> suppressed with either low- or high-dose dexamethasone suppression test
  - Chest and abdominal CT can help localize
  - Tx: resection of primary if possible; medical suppression or bilateral adrenalectomy for inoperable lesions
- **Adrenal adenoma**
  - **#3 noniatrogenic** cause of Cushing's syndrome
  - ↓ ACTH, unregulated steroid production; does not suppress
  - Tx: adrenalectomy
- **Adrenocortical carcinoma** – rare cause of Cushing's syndrome
  - Tx: radical adrenalectomy; debulking can help patients and prolong survival
- **Adrenal hyperplasia** (macro or micro)
  - Tx: bilateral adrenalectomy

- **Medical therapy** for ectopic ACTH production or adrenocortical cancer with residual or metastatic disease after resection
  - **Ketoconazole and metyrapone** – inhibit steroid formation
  - **Aminoglutethimide** – inhibits cholesterol conversion
  - **Op-DDD (mitotane)** – adrenal-lytic, used for metastatic disease

- **Bilateral adrenalectomy** – may be needed in patients with ectopic ACTH from tumor that is unresectable or from pituitary adenoma that cannot be found
- Need to remember to <u>give steroids postoperatively</u>

■ **Adrenocortical carcinoma**
- Bimodal distribution (before age 5 and in the 5th decade); more common in females
- **50% are functioning tumors** – cortisol, aldosterone, sex steroids

- Children display virilization 90% of the time (precocious puberty in boys, virilization in females)
- Feminization in men; masculinization in women can occur
- Symptoms: abdominal pain, weight loss, weakness
- 80% have advanced disease at the time of diagnosis
- Tx: radical adrenalectomy; mitotane for residual or recurrent disease
- 20% 5-year survival rate

ADRENAL MEDULLA

- **From ectoderm neural crest cells**
- Catecholamine production – **tyrosine → dopa → dopamine → norepinephrine → epinephrine**

- **Tyrosine hydroxylase** – rate-limiting step (tyrosine to dopa)
- **PNMT** – enzyme that converts norepinephrine → epinephrine (requires methylation)
  - **Enzyme is found only in adrenal medulla** (exclusive producers of epinephrine)
- **Only adrenal pheochromocytomas will produce epinephrine**
- **MAO** (monoamine oxidase) – converts norepinephrine to normetanephrine, epinephrine to metanephrine; VMA produced from these
- **Extra-adrenal rest of neural crest tissue can exist**, usually in the retroperitoneum, most notably in the organ of Zuckerkandl

- **Pheochromocytoma** (chromaffin cells)
  - Rare; usually slow growing; arise from sympathetic ganglia or ectopic neural crest cells
  - **10% rule** – malignant, bilateral, in children, familial, extra-adrenal
  - Can be associated with MEN IIa, MEN IIb, von Recklinghausen's disease, tuberous sclerosis, Sturge–Weber disease
  - **Right-sided** predominance
  - **Extra-adrenal tumors more likely malignant**
  - Symptoms: HTN (frequently **episodic**), headache, diaphoresis, palpitations
  - **Dx: urine metanephrines and VMA** – breakdown products of epi and norepinephrine
    - **VMA most sensitive**
    - **MIBG** scan (norepinephrine analogue) – can help identify location if having trouble finding tumor
    - **Clonidine suppression test** – tumor does not respond, keeps catecholamines ↑
    - **No venography** → can cause hypertensive crisis
    - CT/MRI can help localize tumors
    - Not able to localize → still proceed with laparotomy

  - **Preoperatively: volume replacement, α-blocker first** (phenoxybenzamine → avoids hypertensive crisis); then β-blocker if patient has tachycardia or arrhythmias
    - Need to be careful with β-blocker and give after α-blocker → can precipitate **hypertensive crisis** (unopposed alpha stimulation) and **heart failure** in patients with cardiomyopathy

  - **Tx**: check for other tumors at resection; ligate adrenal veins first to avoid spilling catecholamines during tumor manipulation
    - Debulking helps symptoms in patients with unresectable disease
    - **Metyrosine** – inhibits tyrosine hydroxylase causing ↓ synthesis of catecholamines
    - Should have Nipride, Neo-Synephrine, and anti-arrhythmic agents (e.g., amiodarone) ready during the time of surgery

  - **Postop conditions** – persistent hypertension, hypotension, hypoglycemia, bronchospasm, arrhythmias, intracerebral hemorrhage, CHF, MI
  - **Other sites of pheochromocytomas** – vertebral bodies, opposite adrenal gland, bladder, aortic bifurcation

- Most common site of extramedullary tissue – **organ of Zuckerkandl (inferior aorta near bifurcation)**
- **Falsely elevated VMA** – coffee, tea, fruits, vanilla, iodine contrast, labetalol, α- and β-blockers
- **Extramedullary tissue** – responsible for **medullary CA of thyroid and extra-adrenal pheochromocytoma**

■ **Ganglioneuroma** – rare, benign, asymptomatic tumor of neural crest origin in the adrenal medulla or sympathetic chain

Indications for Adrenalectomy

Unilateral adrenalectomy
Aldosteronoma
Cortisol-secreting adenoma (Cushing's syndrome or subclinical Cushing)
Unilateral pheochromocytoma (sporadic or familial)
Virilizing or feminizing tumors
Nonfunctioning unilateral tumor
    Size > 4–5 cm
    Imaging features atypical for adenoma, myelolipoma, or cyst
    Adrenocortical carcinomas
    Solitary unilateral adrenal metastasis
Bilateral adrenalectomy
Bilateral pheochromocytomas
Cushing's syndrome from:
    Bilateral nodular adrenal hyperplasia
    Ectopic ACTH-producing tumor unresponsive to primary therapy
Cushing's disease (pituitary tumor) unsuccessfully treated by surgery or radiation

ACTH, adrenocorticotropic hormone.
From Brunt LM, Cohen MS. Adrenalectomy – open and minimally invasive. In: Fischer JE, Bland KI, et al., eds. *Mastery of Surgery.* 5th ed. Philadelphia: Lippincott Williams & Wilkins; 2007, with permission.

Diagnosis and Preoperative Preparation of Common Adrenal Tumors

Tumor Type	Biochemical Diagnosis	Preoperative Preparation
Pheochromocytoma	Plasma fractionated metanephrines and/or 24-h urinary catecholamines and metanephrines	α-Receptor blockade; β-blockade only if persistent tachycardia or epinephrine-secreting tumor
Aldosteronoma	Plasma aldosterone concentration (PAC) and plasma renin activity (PRA); urinary aldosterone and potassium (on high-salt diet)	Replete hypokalemia, control hypertension
Cushing's syndrome from cortical adenoma	24-h urine-free cortisol; overnight low-dose DMST; plasma ACTH	Perioperative stress steroids
Adrenal cortical carcinoma	24-h urine cortisol, plasma DHEA level	None unless tumor is cortisol secreting
Incidentaloma	Low-dose DMST, plasma fractionated metanephrines or urine catecholamines and metanephrines; PAC and PRA if hypertensive or hypokalemic	None unless biochemical screen positive

ACTH, adrenocorticotropic hormone; DHEA, dehydroepiandrosterone; DMST, dexamethasone suppression set.
From Brunt LM, Cohen MS. Adrenalectomy – open and minimally invasive. In: Fischer JE, Bland KI, et al., eds. *Mastery of Surgery.* 2nd ed. Philadelphia: Lippincott Williams & Wilkins; 2007, with permission.

CHAPTER 22. **THYROID**

ANANTOMY AND PHYSIOLOGY

- From the 1st and 2nd pharyngeal pouches
- **Thyrotropin-releasing factor (TRF)** – released from the hypothalamus; acts on the anterior pituitary gland and causes release of TSH
- **Thyroid-stimulating hormone (TSH)** – released from the anterior pituitary gland; acts on the thyroid gland to release T3 and T4 (through a mechanism that involves ↑ cAMP)
- TRF and TSH release are controlled by T3 and T4 through a negative feedback loop

- **Superior thyroid artery** – 1st branch off external carotid artery
- **Inferior thyroid artery** – off thyrocervical trunk; supplies inferior and superior parathyroids
  - Ligate close to thyroid to avoid injury to parathyroid glands with thyroidectomy
- **Ima artery** – occurs in 1%, arises from the innominate or aorta and goes to the isthmus

- **Superior and middle thyroid veins** – drain into internal jugular vein
- **Inferior thyroid vein** – drains into innominate vein

- **Nonrecurrent laryngeal nerve** – in 2%–3%; more common on the right
- **Superior laryngeal nerve**
  - Motor to cricothyroid muscle
  - Runs lateral to thyroid lobes
  - Tracks close to superior thyroid artery but is variable
  - Injury results in **loss of projection and easy voice fatigability** (opera singers)
- **Recurrent laryngeal nerves** (RLNs)
  - Motor to all of larynx except cricothyroid muscle
  - Run posterior to thyroid lobes in the tracheoesophageal groove
  - Can track with inferior thyroid artery but are variable
  - Left RLN loops around aorta; right RLN loops around right subclavian (or innominate) artery
  - Injury results in **hoarseness**; bilateral injury can **obstruct airway** → needs emergency tracheostomy
  - **The right nerve** is more likely <u>not</u> to be recurrent compared with the left
  - Risk of injury for nonrecurrent laryngeal nerve injury during thyroid surgery

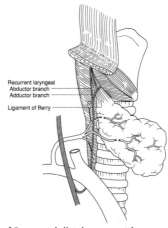

The ligament of Berry and distal recurrent laryngeal nerves.

- **Ligament of Berry** – posterior medial suspensory ligament close to RLNs; careful dissection
- **Thyroglobulin** – stores T3 and T4 in colloid
  - Plasma T4:T3 ratio is 15:1; T3 more active form (is tyrosine + iodine)
  - Most T3 produced in periphery by T4 to T3 conversion by peroxidases
- **Peroxidases** link (or separate) tyrosine and iodine
- **Thyroid-binding globulin** – thyroid hormone transport; T3 and T4 also bind albumin
- **TSH** – most sensitive indicator of gland function
- **Tubercles of Zuckerkandl** – most lateral, posterior extension of thyroid tissue
  - Rotate medially to find RLNs
  - This portion is left behind with subtotal thyroidectomy because of proximity to RLNs
- **Parafollicular C cells** – produce **calcitonin**
- **Resin T3 uptake** – measures free T3 by having it bind resin
  - ↑ resin uptake → hyperthyroidism or ↓ TBG
  - ↓ uptake → hypothyroidism or ↑ TBG
- **Thyroxine treatment** – TSH levels should fall to 50%; osteoporosis long-term side effect
- **Postthyroidectomy stridor** – open neck and remove hematoma emergently → can result in airway compromise

THYROID STORM

- Symptoms: ↑ HR, fever, numbness, irritability, vomiting, diarrhea, high-output cardiac failure (most common cause of death)
- Most common after surgery in patient with undiagnosed **Graves' disease**
- Can also be precipitated by anxiety, excessive palpation of the gland, adrenergic stimulants
- Tx: β-blockers, PTU, Lugol's solution (KI), cooling blankets, oxygen, glucose, fluid
  - Emergent thyroidectomy rarely indicated
- **Wolff–Chaikoff effect** – very effective for patients in thyroid storm
  - Patient given high doses of iodine (Lugol's solution, potassium iodide), which inhibits TSH action on thyroid and inhibits organic coupling of iodide, resulting in less T3 and T4 release

ASYMPTOMATIC THYROID NODULE

- **1st Thyroid function tests**
  - If elevated, give thyroxine; nodule should regress within 6 months
  - If not elevated, proceed with fine-needle aspiration (FNA)
- **2nd FNA**
  - **Determinant in 75%–90%** → follow appropriate treatment
    - Shows follicular cells → thyroidectomy or lobectomy (5%–10% malignancy risk)
    - Shows thyroid CA → thyroidectomy or lobectomy and appropriate treatment (see the following text)
    - Shows cyst fluid → drain fluid
      - If it recurs → thyroidectomy or lobectomy
    - Shows colloid tissue → most likely colloid goiter; low chance of malignancy (<1%)
      - Tx: thyroxine; thyroidectomy or lobectomy if it enlarges
  - **Indeterminant in 10%–25%** → get radionuclide study
    - **Hot nodule** → thyroxine for 6 months; if size does not ↓, perform **lobectomy**
- **Cold nodule** → thyroidectomy or lobectomy (more likely malignant than hot nodule)
  - 85% of thyroid nodules are benign
  - Thyroid nodules have a female predominance
- **Goiter**
  - Any abnormal enlargement
  - Most identifiable cause is iodine deficiency
    - Tx: iodine replacement

- Diffuse enlargement without evidence of functional abnormality = nontoxic colloid goiter
  - Tx: try to suppress with thyroxine; ^{131}I (may be ineffective), thioamides, subtotal thyroidectomy or lobectomy on side of goiter if medical treatment ineffective
- **Substernal goiter**
  - Usually secondary (vessels originate from superior and inferior thyroid arteries)
  - Primary substernal goiter – rare (vessels originate from innominate artery)
    - Tx: try to suppress with thyroxine
    - ^{131}I (may be ineffective), thioamides, subtotal thyroidectomy or lobectomy on side of goiter if medical treatment ineffective
- **Mediastinal thyroid tissue** – most likely from acquired disease with inferior extensions of a normally placed gland

ABNORMALITIES OF THYROID DESCENT
- **Pyramidal lobe** – occurs in 10%, extends from the isthmus toward the thymus
- **Lingual thyroid**
  - Thyroid tissue that persists in the area of the foramen cecum at the base of the tongue
  - Symptoms: dysphagia, dyspnea, dysphonia
  - 2% malignancy risk
  - Tx: thyroxine suppression; abolish with ^{131}I or resection if it is enlarged or suggestive of cancer, or if it does not shrink after medical therapy
  - Is the only thyroid tissue in 70% of patients who have it
- **Thyroglossal duct cyst**
  - Classically moves upward with swallowing
  - Susceptible to infection and may be premalignant
  - Tx: resection → need to take midportion or all of hyoid bone along with the thyroglossal duct cyst

HYPERTHYROIDISM TREATMENT
- **Propylthiouracil (PTU) and methimazole** – good for young patients, small goiters, mild T3 and T4 elevation
- **PTU (thioamides)**
  - Inhibits peroxidases and prevents DIT and MIT coupling
  - Side effects: **aplastic anemia or agranulocytosis** (rare)
- **Methimazole**
  - Inhibits peroxidases and prevents DIT and MIT coupling
  - Side effects: **cretinism** in newborns (crosses placenta) and **aplastic anemia or agranulocytosis** (rare)
- **Radioactive iodine (^{131}I)**
  - Good for patients who are poor surgical risks or unresponsive to PTU
  - ^{131}I should not be used in children or during pregnancy → can traverse placenta
- **Thyroidectomy**
  - Good for large glands, cold nodules in toxic glands, toxic multinodular goiters not responsive to medical therapy, toxic adenomas not responsive to medical therapy, pregnant patients not controlled with medical therapy
  - Best time to operate is 2nd trimester (↓ risk of teratogenic events and premature labor)
  - Subtotal thyroidectomy can leave patient euthyroid

CAUSES OF HYPERTHYROIDISM
- **Graves' disease** (toxic diffuse goiter)
  - Women; exophthalmos, pretibial edema, atrial fibrillation, heart dysfunction, heat intolerance, thirst, ↑ appetite, weight loss, sweating, palpitations
  - Most common cause of hyperthyroidism (80%)

- Caused by **IgG antibodies to TSH receptor** (long-acting thyroid stimulator, thyroid-stimulating immunoglobulin)
- If large, can get cervical compression syndromes
- Dx: ↑ ^{123}I uptake (thyroid scan) diffusely in thyrotoxic patient with goiter; LATS level, decreased TSH, increased T3 and T4
- Tx: **thioamides** (70% recurrence), ^{131}I (10% recurrence), **subtotal thyroidectomy** (10% recurrence), or **total thyroidectomy** with thyroxine replacement if medical therapy fails
- Medical therapy usually manages hyperthyroidism
- **Unusual to have to operate** on these patients unless in setting of suspicious nodule
  - **Preop preparation**: PTU or methimazole until euthyroid, β-blocker, 1 week before surgery, Lugol's solution for 10–15 days to decrease friability and vascularity (start only after euthyroid)
  - **Operation**: bilateral subtotal or total thyroidectomy
  - Indications for surgery: noncompliant patient, recurrence after medical therapy, children, pregnant women not controlled with medical therapy, or concomitant suspicious thyroid nodule

■ **Toxic multinodular goiter**
- Most common cause of thyroid enlargement
- Women; age > 50 years, normal thyroid function tests
- Symptoms: cardiac symptoms, weight loss, insomnia, airway compromise; symptoms can be precipitated by contrast dyes

- Usually nontoxic 1st
- Caused by hyperplasia secondary to chronic low-grade TSH stimulation
- Tx: ^{131}I and thioamides; ^{131}I can be less effective in some (inhomogeneous uptake by gland); subtotal thyroidectomy if medical treatment ineffective
- **Unusual to have to operate** on these patients unless in setting of suspicious nodule

■ **Single toxic nodule**
- Women; younger; can cause cervical compression
- >3 cm usually symptomatic
- Dx: thyroid scan
- 20% of hot nodules eventually cause symptoms
- Thought to function autonomously
- Tx: ^{131}I and thioamides; lobectomy if medical treatment ineffective

■ **Rare causes of hyperthyroidism** – trophoblastic tumors, TSH-secreting pituitary tumors

CAUSES OF THYROIDITIS
■ **Hashimoto's disease**
- **Most common cause of hypothyroidism in adults**
- Enlarged gland, painless, chronic thyroiditis
- Women; history of childhood XRT
- Can cause thyrotoxicosis in the acute early stage
- Caused by both **humeral and cell-mediated autoimmune disease** (microsomal and thyroglobulin antibodies)
- Goiter secondary to **lack of organification of trapped iodide inside gland**
- Pathology shows a **lymphocytic infiltrate**
- Tx: **thyroxine** 1st line; **partial thyroidectomy** if continues to grow despite thyroxine, if nodules appear, or compression symptoms occur
- Frequently no surgery is necessary for Hashimoto's disease

■ **Bacterial thyroiditis (rare)**
- Usually secondary to **contiguous spread**
- Normal thyroid function tests, fever, dysphagia, tenderness
- Upper respiratory tract infection (URI) symptoms most common precursor (staph/strep)
- Tx: **antibiotics**
  - May need **lobectomy** to rule out cancer in patients with unilateral swelling and tenderness
  - May need total thyroidectomy for persistent inflammation

■ **De Quervain's thyroiditis**
- Can be associated with hyperthyroidism initially
- **Viral URI**, tender thyroid, sore throat, mass, weakness, fatigue
- More common in women
- Elevated ESR
- Tx: **steroids and ASA**
  - May need **lobectomy** to rule out cancer in patients with unilateral swelling and tenderness
  - May need total thyroidectomy for persistent inflammation

■ **Riedel's fibrous struma** (rare)
- Woody, fibrous component that can involve adjacent strap muscles and carotid sheath
- Can resemble thyroid CA or lymphoma (need biopsy)
- Disease frequently results in hypothyroidism and compression symptoms
- Associated with sclerosing cholangitis, fibrotic diseases, methysergide treatment, and retroperitoneal fibrosis
- Tx: **steroids and thyroxine**
  - May need isthmectomy or tracheostomy
  - If resection needed, watch for RLNs

THYROID CANCER
■ Most common endocrine malignancy in the United States
■ **Follicular cells on FNA** – 5%–10% chance of malignancy (unable to differentiate between follicular cell adenoma, follicular cell hyperplasia, normal thyroid tissue, and follicular cell CA on FNA)
■ **Worrisome for malignancy** – solid, solitary, cold, slow growing, hard; male, age > 50, previous neck XRT, MEN IIa or IIb
■ **Sudden growth** – could be hemorrhage into previously undetected nodule or malignancy
■ Patients can also present with voice **changes and dysphagia**
■ **Thyroid adenomas** – need to be differentiated from carcinomas → require lobectomy
■ **Follicular adenomas** – colloid, embryonal, fetal → no increase in cancer risk
- Still need lobectomy to prove it is adenoma

■ **Papillary thyroid carcinoma**
- Most common (80%–90%) thyroid CA
- Least aggressive, slow growing, has the best prognosis
- Young adults, women, children
- Risk factors: childhood XRT (very ↑ risk) → most common tumor following neck XRT
- Older age (>40–50 years) predicts a worse prognosis

- **Lymphatic spread 1st** but is not prognostic
- **Prognosis based on local invasion**
- Rare metastases – **lung most common**

- **Children are more likely to be node positive** (70%–80%) than are adults (10%–20%)
- Large, firm nodules in children are worrisome
- Many are **multicentric**
- Pathology - **psammoma bodies** (calcium) **and Orphan Annie nuclei**

- Tx: minimal/incidental (<1 cm) → **lobectomy**
  - **Total thyroidectomy** for bilateral lesions, multicentricity, history of XRT, positive margins, tumors > 1 cm
  - **Clinically positive cervical nodes** – need ipsilateral MRND
  - **Extrathyroidal tissue involvement** – need ipsilateral MRND
  - **Metastatic disease, residual local disease, positive lymph nodes, or capsular invasion** → ^{131}I 6 weeks after surgery
  - **XRT** only for unresectable disease not responsive to ^{131}I
- Do not give thyroid replacement until <u>after</u> treatment with ^{131}I → will suppress uptake
- 95% 5-year survival rate; death secondary to local disease

- **Enlarged lateral neck lymph node** that shows normal-appearing thyroid tissue is **papillary thyroid CA with lymphatic spread**
  - Tx: total thyroidectomy and MRND

■ **Follicular thyroid carcinoma**
- **Hematogenous spread** (**bone** most common) → 50% have metastatic disease at the time of presentation
- More aggressive than thyroid papillary cell CA
- Older adults (50–60s), women
- FNA shows just **follicular cells** – 10% chance of malignancy; need thyroidectomy

- Tx: **lobectomy** → if pathology shows **adenoma or follicular cell hyperplasia**, nothing else needed
  - **If follicular CA** → total thyroidectomy for lesions > 1 cm or extrathyroidal disease
  - **Clinically positive cervical nodes** – need ipsilateral MRND
  - **Extrathyroidal tissue involvement** – need ipsilateral MRND
  - **Patients with lesions > 1 cm or extrathyroidal disease (or capsular invasion)** – ^{131}I 6 weeks after surgery
  - **If microinvasive** (<1 cm), has rare nodal spread (<10%), and is usually incidental finding on pathology → as long as margins are negative, lobectomy is probably all that is needed
  - 70% 5-year survival rate; prognosis based on stage

■ **Medullary thyroid carcinoma**
- Can be associated with MEN IIa or IIb
- **Usually the 1st manifestation of MEN IIa and IIb**
- Tumor arises from **parafollicular C cells (which secrete calcitonin)**
- **C-cell hyperplasia** considered premalignant
- **Pathology** – shows **amyloid** deposition
- **Gastrin** can be used to test for medullary thyroid CA → causes an ↑ in calcitonin
- ≠ **calcitonin** – can cause <u>flushing and diarrhea</u>
- Need to screen for <u>hyperparathyroidism and pheochromocytoma</u>

- ≠ **lymphatic spread** – most have involved nodes at time of diagnosis
- **Early metastases to lung, liver, and bone**

- Tx: **total thyroidectomy with central neck node dissection**
  - **MRND** if patient has clinically positive nodes (bilateral MRND if both lobes have tumor) or if extrathyroidal disease present
  - Prophylactic thyroidectomy and central node dissection in MEN IIa or IIb patients at age 2
  - Liver and bone metastases prevent attempt at cure
  - XRT may be useful for unresectable local and distant metastatic disease
- May be useful to **monitor calcitonin levels for disease recurrence**
- More aggressive than follicular and papillary CA
- 50% 5-year survival rate; prognosis based on presence of regional and distant metastases

■ **Hürthle cell carcinoma**
- Most are benign (Hürthle cell adenoma); presents in older patients
- Early nodal spread if malignant
- Metastases go to bone and lung
- Tx: total thyroidectomy; MRND for clinically positive nodes

■ **Anaplastic thyroid cancer**
- Elderly patients with long-standing goiters
- Most aggressive thyroid CA
- Rapidly lethal (0% 5-year survival rate); usually beyond surgical management by diagnosis
- Tx: total thyroidectomy for the rare lesion that can be resected
- Can perform palliative thyroidectomy for compressive symptoms or give palliative chemotherapy or XRT

XRT effective for papillary, follicular, medullary, and Hürthle cell thyroid CA
^{131}**I effective** for papillary and follicular thyroid CA only
  Can cure bone and lung metastases
  Done 6 weeks after surgery
  Indications
      Recurrent thyroid papillary or follicular CA
      Primary inoperable tumors due to local invasion
      Papillary thyroid CA with extrathyroidal disease
      Follicular thyroid CA > 1 cm or with extrathyroidal disease
        Patients with papillary or follicular cell CA with metastases → need to perform total thyroidectomy to facilitate uptake of ^{131}I to the metastatic lesions
  Side effects: sialoadenitis, GI symptoms, infertility, bone marrow suppression, parathyroid dysfunction, leukemia
TSH levels highest 4–6 weeks after thyroidectomy – best time for ^{131}I scan for metastatic disease
Thyroxine – can help suppress TSH and slow metastatic disease
  Administered only after ^{131}I therapy has finished
      Lymphoma and squamous cell CA – very rare causes of thyroid CA

CHAPTER 23. PARATHYROID

ANATOMY AND PHYSIOLOGY

- **Superior parathyroids – 4th pouch**; associated with thyroid complex
  - Lateral to recurrent laryngeal nerves (RLNs), posterior surface of superior portion of gland, above inferior thyroid artery
- **Inferior parathyroids – 3rd pouch**; associated with thymus
  - Medial to RLNs, more anterior, below inferior thyroid artery
  - Inferior parathyroids have more variable location and are more likely to be ectopic
  - Occasionally are found in the **tail of the thymus** (most common ectopic site) and can migrate to the anterior mediastinum
  - Other ectopic sites – intrathyroid, mediastinal, near tracheoesophageal groove
- 90% have all 4 glands
- **Inferior thyroid artery** – blood supply to **both superior and inferior parathyroid glands**

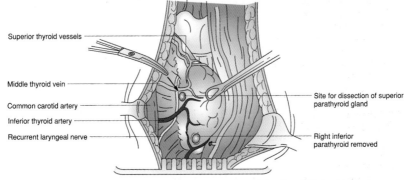

Lateral view of the right side of the neck after rotation of the thyroid lobe. The important anatomic landmarks are emphasized.

- **PTH** – ↑ serum Ca
  - ↑ kidney Ca reabsorption in the distal convoluted tubule, ↓ kidney PO_4 absorption
  - ↑ osteoclasts in bone to release Ca (and PO_4^-)
  - ↑ vitamin D production in kidney (↑ 1-OH hydroxylation) → ↑ Ca-binding protein in intestine → ↑ intestinal Ca reabsorption

- **Vitamin D** – ↑ intestinal Ca and PO_4 absorption by increasing **calcium-binding protein**

- **Calcitonin** – ↓ serum Ca
  - ↓ bone Ca resorption (osteoclast inhibition)
  - ↑ urinary Ca and PO_4 excretion

- **Normal Ca level**: 8.5–10.5 (ionized 4.4–5.5)
- **Normal PTH level**: 5–40 pg/mL
- **Normal PO_4 level**: 2.5–5.0
- **Normal Cl^- level**: 98–107

- Most common cause of hypoparathyroidism is **previous thyroid surgery**

PRIMARY HYPERPARATHYROIDISM

- PRAD-1 oncogene increases the risk for adenomas
- Women, older age
- Due to autonomously high PTH
- Dx: ↑ Ca, ↓ phosphorus; Cl^- to phosphorus ratio > 33, ↑ renal cAMP, HCO_3^- secreted in urine
- Can get **hyperchloremic metabolic acidosis**
- **Osteitis fibrosa cystica (brown tumors)** – bone lesions from Ca resorption; characteristic of hyperparathyroidism
- Most patients **have no symptoms** – ↑ Ca found on routine lab work for some other problem or on checkup
- Symptoms: muscle weakness, myalgia, nephrolithiasis, pancreatitis, PUD, depression, bone pain, pathologic fractures, mental status changes, constipation, nausea and vomiting, anorexia
- Hypertension can result from renal impairment

Diagnostic Workup for Primary Hyperparathyroidism

Take careful history, including records or medications, symptoms, prior head and neck radiotherapy, and other endocrinopathies in the patient and the patient's family.
Establish elevated calcium through 2 or 3 determinations.
Order a chest radiograph and search for bony metastases, sarcoidosis, and pulmonary tumors.
Order an excretory urogram and search for nephrolithiasis and, rarely, renal tumors.
Order a serum protein electrophoresis to rule out multiple myeloma.
Order a 24-hour urinary calcium determination (i.e., benign familial hypocalciuric hypercalcemia).
Rule out multiple endocrine neoplasia (usually multiple endocrine neoplasia type I).
Check the absolute or relative elevation of the parathyroid hormone level.

From Smith SL, Van Heerden JA. Conventional parathyroidectomy for primary hyperparathyroidism. In: Fischer JE, Bland KI, et al., eds. *Mastery of Surgery*. 5th ed. Philadelphia: Lippincott Williams & Wilkins, 2007, with permission.

- **Indications for surgery** – symptomatic disease or asymptomatic disease with Ca > 13, ↓ Cr clearance, kidney stones, substantially ↓ bone mass

- **Single adenoma** – occurs in 80% of patients
- **Multiple adenomas** – occur in 4% of patients
- **Diffuse hyperplasia** – occurs in 15%; patients with MEN I or IIa have 4-gland hyperplasia
- **Parathyroid adenocarcinoma** – very rare; can get very high Ca levels

- **Treatment**
  - **Adenoma** – resection; inspect other glands to rule out hyperplasia or multiple adenomas
  - **Parathyroid hyperplasia**
    - Do not biopsy all glands → risks hemorrhage and hypoparathyroidism
    - Resect 3½ glands or total parathyroidectomy and autoimplantation
  - **Parathyroid CA** → need radical parathyroidectomy (need to take ipsilateral thyroid)
  - **Pregnancy** – surgery in 2nd trimester; ↑ risk of stillbirth if not resected

- **Intraop frozen section** → can confirm that the tissue taken was indeed parathyroid
- **Intraop PTH levels** → can help determine if the causative gland is removed (PTH should go to <½ of the preop value); PTH half-life is 10 minutes

- **Missing gland** – check inferiorly in thymus tissue (most common ectopic location), near carotids, vertebral body, superior to pharynx, thyroid
- **Still cannot find gland** – close and follow PTH; if PTH still ↑, get parathyroid scan to localize
  - Some say perform thyroidectomy on the side in which only one gland was found
- **At reoperation for missing gland,** most common location for the gland is normal anatomic position

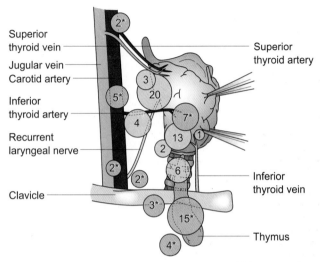

Location of parathyroid tumors missed on initial exploration but identified on subsequent operation.

- **Postop hypocalcemia** – caused by bone hunger, hypomagnesemia, failure of parathyroid remnant or graft
- **Persistent hyperparathyroidism (1%)** – most commonly due to missed adenoma remaining in the neck
- **Recurrent hyperparathyroidism** – occurs after a period of hypocalcemia or normo-calcemia
  - Can be due to new adenoma formation
  - Can be due to tumor implants at the original operation that have now grown
  - Need to consider recurrent parathyroid CA
- **Reoperation** associated with ↑ risk of RLN injury, permanent hypoparathyroidism

- Hypocalcemia postop
  - Bone hunger – normal PTH, decreased HCO_3^-
  - Aparathyroidism – decreased PTH, normal HCO_3^-

- **Sestamibi-technetium-99**
  - Will have preferential uptake by the overactive parathyroid gland
  - Good for picking up adenomas but not 4-gland hyperplasia
  - Best for trying to pick up ectopic glands

SECONDARY HYPERPARATHYROIDISM
- Seen in patients with renal failure
- ↑ PTH in response to low Ca

- Most do <u>not</u> need surgery (90%)
- Ectopic calcification and osteoporosis can occur
- Tx: control diet PO_4, PO_4-binding gel, ↓ aluminum, Ca supplement, vitamin D, Ca in dialysate
  - Surgery for bone pain (most common indication; 80%–90% get relief), fractures, or pruritus (80%–90% get relief)
  - Surgery involves total parathyroidectomy with autotransplantation or subtotal parathyroidectomy

TERTIARY HYPERPARATHYROIDISM
- Renal disease now corrected with transplant but still overproduces PTH
- Has similar lab values as primary hyperparathyroidism (hyperplasia)
- Tx: subtotal (3½ glands) or total parathyroidectomy with autoimplantation

FAMILIAL HYPERCALCEMIC HYPOCALCIURIA
- Patients have ↑ serum Ca and ↓ urine CA (should be ↑ if hyperparathyroidism)
- Caused by defect in PTH receptor in distal convoluted tubule of the kidney that causes ↑ resorption of Ca
- Dx: Ca 9–11, normal PTH (30–60), ↓ urine Ca
- Tx: nothing (Ca generally not that high in these patients); **no parathyroidectomy**

PSEUDOHYPOPARATHYROIDISM
- Because of defect in PTH receptor in the kidney, does not respond to PTH

PARATHYROID CANCER
- Rare cause of hypercalcemia
- 50% 5-year survival rate
- Mortality is due to hypercalcemia
- ↑ Ca, PTH, and alkaline phosphatase (can have extremely high Ca levels)
- **Lung** most common location for metastases
- Tx: wide en bloc excision (parathyroidectomy and ipsilateral thyroidectomy)
- Recurrence in 50%

MULTIPLE ENDOCRINE NEOPLASIA SYNDROMES
- Derived from APUD cells
- Neoplasms can develop synchronously or metachronously
- Autosomal dominant, 100% penetrance, variable expressivity

- **MEN I**
  - **Parathyroid hyperplasia**
    - Usually the first part to become symptomatic; urinary symptoms
    - Tx: 4-gland resection with autotransplantation
  - **Pancreatic islet cell tumors**
    - Gastrinoma #1
    - 50% multiple, 50% malignant – major morbidity of syndrome
  - **Pituitary adenoma**
    - Prolactinoma #1
  - Need to correct hyperparathyroidism 1st

- **MEN IIa**
  - **Parathyroid hyperplasia**
  - **Pheochromocytoma**
    - Very often bilateral, nearly always benign

- **Medullary CA of thyroid**
  - Nearly all patients; diarrhea most common symptom; often bilateral
  - #1 cause of death in these patients
  - Usually 1st part to be symptomatic
- Need to correct pheochromocytoma 1st

- **MEN IIb**
  - **Pheochromocytoma**
    - Very often bilateral, nearly always benign
  - **Medullary CA of thyroid**
    - Nearly all patients; diarrhea most common symptoms; often bilateral
    - #1 cause of death in these patients
    - Usually 1st part to be symptomatic
  - **Mucosal neuromas**
  - **Marfan's habitus, musculoskeletal abnormalities**
  - Need to correct pheochromocytoma 1st

- **MEN I** – MENIN gene
- **MEN II** – RET proto-oncogene

Disease Phenotypes Related to Mutation of the RET Proto-Oncogene

Phenotype	Clinical Features	Prevalence (%)
MEN 2A (60%)	Medullary thyroid carcinoma	100
	Pheochromocytoma	10–60
	Hyperparathyroidism	5–20
MEN 2B (5%)	Medullary thyroid carcinoma	100
	Pheochromocytoma	50
	Marfanoid habitus	100
	Mucosal neuromas (gut) and ganglioneuromatosis	100
FMTC (35%)	Medullary thyroid carcinoma	100

MEN 2A, multiple endocrine neoplasia type 2A; MEN 2B, multiple endocrine neoplasia type 2B; FMTC, familial medullary thyroid carcinoma.

CAUSES OF HYPERCALCEMIA
- Malignancy
  - Hematologic (25%) – lytic bone lesions
  - Nonhematologic (75%) – cancers that release PTHrp (small cell lung CA, breast CA)
- Hyperparathyroidism
- Hyperthyroidism
- Familial hypercalcemic hypocalciuria
- Immobilization
- Granulomatous disease (sarcoidosis or tuberculosis)
- Excess vitamin D
- Milk–alkali syndrome (excessive intake of milk and calcium supplements)
- Thiazide diuretics

Mithramycin – inhibits osteoclasts (used with malignancies or failure of conventional treatment); has hematologic, liver, and renal side effects

Hypercalcemic crisis – usually secondary to another surgery
Tx: fluids, furosemide, dialysis

Breast CA metastases to bone – release **PTHrp; can cause hypercalcemia**
Small cell lung CA and other nonhematologic cancers can do this as well → this is not due to bone destruction
Associated with ↑ urinary cAMP (from action of PTHrp on kidney)

Hematologic malignancies – these can cause bone destruction; can also ↑ Ca and urinary cAMP will be low

ANATOMY AND PHYSIOLOGY
■ **Breast development**
   • Breast formed from ectoderm milk streak
   • **Estrogen** – duct development (double layer of columnar cells)
   • **Progesterone** – lobular development
   • **Prolactin** – synergizes estrogen and progesterone
■ **Cyclic changes**
   • **Estrogen** – ↑ breast swelling, growth of glandular tissue
   • **Progesterone** – ↑ maturation of glandular tissue; withdrawal causes menses
   • **FSH, LH surge** – cause ovum release
   • After menopause, lack of estrogen and progesterone results in atrophy of breast tissue
■ **Nerves**
   • **Long thoracic nerve** – innervates **serratus anterior;** injury results in winged scapula
      • **Lateral thoracic artery** to serratus anterior
   • **Thoracodorsal nerve** – innervates **latissimus dorsi;** injury results in weak arm pull-ups and adduction
   • **Thoracodorsal artery** to latissimus dorsi
   • **Medial pectoral nerve** – innervates pectoralis major and pectoralis minor
   • **Lateral pectoral nerve** – pectoralis major only
   • **Intercostobrachial nerve** – lateral cutaneous branch of the 2nd intercostal nerve; provides sensation to medial arm and axilla; encountered just below axillary vein when performing axillary dissection
      • Can transect without serious consequences
■ Branches **of internal thoracic artery, intercostal arteries, thoracoacromial artery, and lateral thoracic artery** supply breast

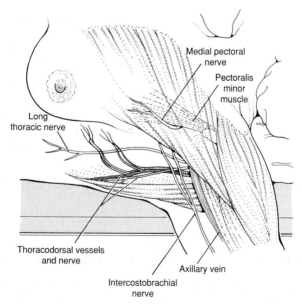

Major neurovascular structures to be preserved in an axillary dissection.

- **Batson's plexus** – valveless vein plexus that allows direct hematogenous metastasis of breast CA to spine
- **Lymphatic drainage**
  - 97% is to the axillary nodes
  - 1%–2% is to the internal mammary nodes
  - Any quadrant can drain to the internal mammary nodes
  - Supraclavicular nodes – considered M1 disease
  - Primary axillary adenopathy – **#1 lymphoma**
- **Cooper's ligaments** – suspensory ligaments; divide breast into segments
  - Breast CA involving these strands can dimple the skin

BENIGN BREAST DISEASE

- **Abscesses** – usually associated with breast-feeding. *S. aureus* most common, strep
  - Tx: incision and drainage; discontinue breast-feeding; ice, heat, breast pump, antibiotics
- **Infectious mastitis** – most commonly associated with breast-feeding
  - ***S. aureus* most common**; in nonlactating women can be due to chronic inflammatory diseases (actinomyces, tuberculosis, syphilis) or autoimmune disease (SLE)
  - May need to rule out necrotic cancer – need incisional biopsy including the skin
- **Periductal mastitis (mammary duct ectasia or plasma cells mastitis)**
  - Dilated mammary ducts, inspissated secretions, marked periductal inflammation
  - Symptoms: noncyclical mastodynia, nipple retraction, creamy discharge from nipple; can have sterile subareolar abscess
  - Patients have a history of difficulty with breast-feeding
  - Tx: if typical creamy discharge is present that is not bloody and not associated with nipple retraction, may be able to reassure; otherwise need to rule out malignancy
- **Galactocele** – breast cysts filled with milk; occurs with breast-feeding
  - Tx: ranges from aspiration to incision and drainage
- **Galactorrhea** – can be caused by ↑ prolactin (pituitary prolactinoma), OCPs, TCAs, phenothiazines, metoclopramide, alpha-methyl dopa, reserpine
  - Is often associated with amenorrhea
- **Gynecomastia** – 2-cm pinch; can be associated with cimetidine, spironolactone, marijuana; idiopathic in most
  - Tx: will likely regress; may need to resect if cosmetically deforming or causing social problems

- **Neonatal breast enlargement** – due to circulating maternal estrogens; will regress
- **Accessory breast tissue (polythelia)** – can present in axilla (most common location)
- **Accessory nipples** – can be found from axilla to groin (most common breast anomaly)
- **Breast asymmetry** – common
- **Breast reduction** – ability to lactate frequently compromised
- **Poland's syndrome** – hypoplasia of chest wall, amastia, hypoplastic shoulder, no pectoralis muscle
- **Mastodynia** – pain in breast; rarely represents breast CA; H and P and get bilateral mammogram
  - Tx: danazol, OCPs, NSAIDs, evening primrose oil, bromocriptine
  - Discontinue caffeine, nicotine, methylxanthines
  - **Cyclic mastodynia** – pain before menstrual period; most commonly from fibrocystic disease
  - **Continuous mastodynia** – continuous pain, most commonly represents acute or subacute infection
    - Continuous mastodynia more refractory to treatment than cyclic mastodynia

- **Mondor's disease** – superficial vein thrombophlebitis of breast; feels cordlike, can be painful
  - Associated with trauma and strenuous exercise
  - Usually occurs in lower outer quadrant
  - Tx: NSAIDs
- **Fibrocystic disease**
  - Catchall phrase; lots of types: papillomatosis, sclerosing adenosis, apocrine metaplasia, duct adenosis, epithelial hyperplasia, ductal hyperplasia, and lobular hyperplasia
  - **Symptoms:** breast pain, nipple discharge (uncommon, can be yellow to brown), masses, lumpy breast tissue that varies with hormonal cycle
  - **Only cancer risk is in atypical ductal or lobular hyperplasia (an unusual finding)**
    - Do not need to get negative margins with atypical hyperplasia; just remove all suspicious areas (i.e., calcifications) that appear on mammogram
  - **Sclerosing adenosis** can manifest as a cluster of calcifications on mammogram without a mass or pain → can look like breast CA
    - Is differentiated from breast CA by regularity of nuclei and absence of mitoses
  - Risk factors for benign breast disease – early menarche, late menopause, small breast size, normal or low body weight, history of cyclic breast discomfort, irregular menses, history of spontaneous abortions, premenopausal status
- **Intraductal papilloma**
  - **Most common cause of bloody discharge from nipple**
  - Are usually small, nonpalpable, and close to the nipple
  - These lesions are <u>not</u> premalignant → can get contrast ductogram to find papilloma
  - Tx: resection (subareolar resection usually curative)

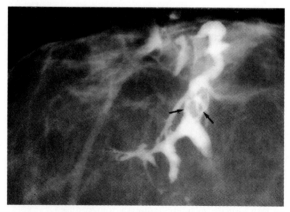

Ductogram. A large defect *(arrow)* represents an intraductal papilloma.

- **Fibroadenoma**
  - Most common breast lesion in adolescents and young women; 10% multiple
  - Usually painless, slow growing, well circumscribed, firm, and rubbery
  - Often grows to several cm in size and then stop
  - Can change in size with menstrual cycle and can enlarge in pregnancy
  - Giant fibromas can be >5 cm (treatment is the same)
  - Prominent fibrous tissue compressing epithelial cells on pathology
  - Can have large, coarse calcifications (popcorn lesions) on mammography from degeneration

- **In patients < 30 years**
  - Mass needs to feel clinically benign (firm, rubbery, rolls, not fixed)
  - Ultrasound or mammogram needs to be consistent with fibroadenoma
  - Need fine-needle aspiration (FNA) or core needle biopsy showing the lesion (not just normal breast tissue)
- **In patients > 30 years** → excisional biopsy to ensure diagnosis
- Avoid resection of breast tissue in teenagers and younger children → can affect breast development

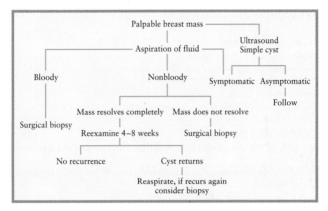

Diagnosis and management of cystic lesions. Bloody fluid on aspiration, failure of the mass to resolve completely, and prompt refilling of the same cyst are indications for surgical biopsy.

Classification of Benign Breast Disease

Nonproliferative: No Increase in Risk
Cysts: micro or macro
Ductal ectasia
Simple fibroadenoma
Mastitis
Fibrosis
Metaplasia: squamous or apocrine
Mild hyperplasia

Proliferative: RR 1.5–2.0
Complex fibroadenoma
Papilloma
Sclerosing adenosis
Hyperplasia; moderate or severe

Proliferative With Atypia: RR 4.5–5.0
Atypical ductal hyperplasia
Atypical lobular hyperplasia

RR, relative risk.

NIPPLE DISCHARGE
- **Most nipple discharge is benign**
- All of these patients need H and P and bilateral mammogram
- Try to find the trigger point or mass on exam
- **Green discharge** – usually due to fibrocystic disease
  - Tx: if cyclical and nonspontaneous, reassure patient
- **Bloody discharge** – most commonly intraductal papilloma; occasionally ductal CA
  - Tx: need galactogram and excision of that ductal area

- **Serous discharge** – worrisome for cancer, especially if coming from only 1 duct or spontaneous
  - Tx: excisional biopsy of that ductal area
- **Spontaneous discharge** – no matter what the color or consistency is worrisome for cancer
  - All these patients need some sort of biopsy in the area of the duct causing the discharge
- **Nonspontaneous discharge** (occurs only with pressure, tight garments, exercise, etc.) – not as worrisome but may still need excisional biopsy (i.e., if bloody)

- May have to do a complete subareolar resection if the area above cannot be properly identified (no trigger point or mass felt)

DIFFUSE PAPILLOMATOSIS
- Affects multiple ducts of both breasts
- Papillomas are larger than when they occur solitarily
- Usually have serous discharge
- Mammogram shows Swiss cheese appearance
- ↑ risk of breast CA with diffuse papillomatosis (40% get breast CA)

DUCTAL CARCINOMA IN SITU
- **Malignant cells of the ductal epithelium without invasion of the basement membrane**
- 50%–60% get cancer if not resected (ipsilateral breast); 5%–10% get cancer in contralateral breast
- Considered a **premalignant lesion**
- Usually not palpable and presents as a cluster of calcifications on mammography
- Need a 2–3-mm margin with excision
- Can have solid, cribriform, papillary, and comedo patterns
  - **Comedo pattern** – most aggressive subtype; has necrotic areas
    - High risk for multicentricity, microinvasion, and recurrence
    - Tx: simple mastectomy
- ↑ **recurrence risk with comedo type and lesions > 2.5 cm**

- Tx: **lumpectomy and XRT; possibly tamoxifen**
  - **Simple mastectomy** if high grade (i.e., comedo type, multicentric, multifocal), if a large tumor not amenable to lumpectomy, or if not able to get good margins; **no ALND**

- Ductal carcinoma in situ (DCIS) with a small focus (<10%) of microinvasive disease can be treated with lumpectomy and XRT or simple mastectomy; need negative margins, **no ALND**

LOBULAR CARCINOMA IN SITU
- 40% get cancer (either breast)
- Considered a marker for the development of breast CA, **not premalignant itself**
- Has no calcifications; is not palpable
- Primarily found in premenopausal women
- Patients who develop breast CA are more likely to develop a **ductal CA (70%)**
- Usually an incidental finding; multifocal disease is common
- 5% risk of having a synchronous breast CA at the time of diagnosis of lobular carcinoma in situ (LCIS; most likely ductal)
- **Do not** need negative margins
- Tx: nothing, tamoxifen, or bilateral subcutaneous mastectomy (no ALND)

BREAST CANCER
- Breast CA decreased in economically poor areas
- Japan has lowest rate of breast CA worldwide

- Breast CA risk – **1 in 8 women (12%)**; 4%–5% in women with no risk factors
- **Screening** decreases mortality by 25%
- Untreated breast cancer – median survival 2–3 years
- 10% of breast CAs have negative mammogram and negative ultrasound
- **Clinical features of breast CA** – distortion of normal architecture, skin/nipple distortion or retraction, hard, tethered, indistinct borders
- **Symptomatic breast mass workup**
  - **<30 years old** – ultrasound
    - **If solid → FNA; excisional biopsy** if FNA is nondiagnostic
    - These patients most commonly have fibroadenomas that can be left alone if FNA is diagnostic. However, if the fibroadenoma enlarges, need excisional biopsy
  - **30–50 years** – bilateral mammograms and FNA; excisional biopsy if FNA nondiagnostic
  - **>50 years** – bilateral mammograms and excisional or core needle biopsy
  - **Core needle biopsy** – gives architecture
  - **FNA** – gives cytology (just the cells)
  - **Cyst fluid** – if bloody, need cyst excisional biopsy; if clear and recurs, need cyst excisional biopsy
    - If complex cyst, need cyst excisional biopsy

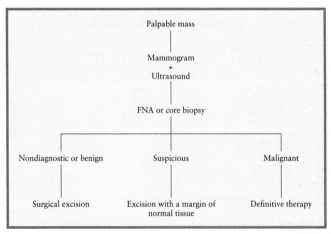

Diagnosis and management of the patient with a clinically indeterminate or suspect solid breast mass. In this circumstance, imaging studies are insufficient to exclude malignancy, and tissue sampling is required.

Management of Breast Masses Based on Fine-Needle Aspiration (FNA) Diagnosis	
FNA Diagnosis	**Treatment**
Malignant	Definitive therapy
Suspicious	Surgical biopsy
Atypia	Surgical biopsy
Benign	Possible observation[a]
Nondiagnostic	Repeated FNA or surgical biopsy

[a]See discussion in text on clinical approach to the patient with a solid breast mass.

- **Mammography**
  - Has 90% sensitivity/specificity
  - Sensitivity increases with age as the dense parenchymal tissue is replaced with fat
  - Mass needs to be ≥5 mm to be detected

- Irregular borders; spiculated; multiple clustered, small, thin, linear, and/or branching calcifications; can have crushed appearance; asymmetric density, ductal asymmetry, distortion of architecture
- 5% of cancers have sharp margin
- Suspicious lesion on mammogram → needle localization and excisional biopsy (core needle biopsy also an option)

■ Screening
- **Mammogram every 2–3 years after age 40, yearly after 50**
- **High-risk screening** – mammogram 10 years before the youngest age of diagnosis of breast CA in first-degree relative
- **No mammography in patients < 30** unless high risk → hard to interpret because of dense parenchyma
  - ↓ radiation dose in young patients
- **Suspicious calcifications or architecture on mammography** → perform localized stereotactic needle excisional biopsy
- **Indeterminate calcifications or architecture on mammography** → can perform core needle biopsy; if indeterminate, perform localized stereotactic needle excisional biopsy

BI-RADS Classification of Mammographic Abnormalities

Category	Assessment	Recommendation
1	Negative	Routine screening
2	Benign finding	Routine screening
3	Probably benign finding	Short-interval follow-up
4	Suspicious abnormality consider biopsy	Definite probability of malignancy;
5	Highly suggestive of malignancy	High probability of cancer; appropriate action should be taken.

BI-RADS, breast imaging, reporting, and data system.

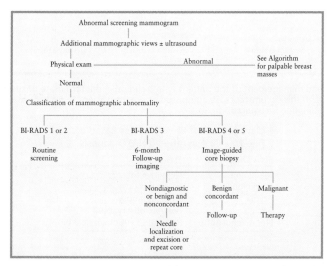

Diagnosis and management of mammographically detected breast lesions. A careful physical examination and a diagnostic imaging workup must be performed before a decision is made about the need for biopsy. BI-RADS, breast imaging, reporting, and data system.

▧ **Node levels**
- **I** – lateral to pectoralis minor muscle
- **II** – beneath pectoralis minor muscle
- **III** – medial to pectoralis minor muscle
- Rotter's nodes – between the pectoralis major and pectoralis minor muscles

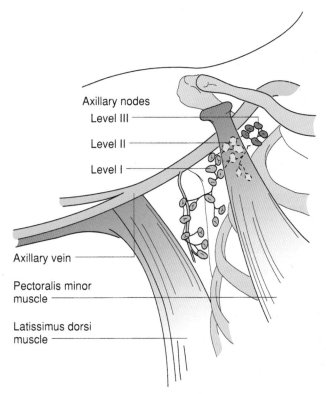

The axillary lymph nodes are divided into three levels by the pectoralis minor muscle. The level I nodes are inferior and lateral to the pectoralis minor, the level II nodes are below the axillary vein and behind the pectoralis minor, and the level III nodes are medial to the muscle against the chest wall.

- Need to sample only level I nodes

- **Nodes are the most important prognostic staging factor. Other factors include tumor size, tumor grade, progesterone, and estrogen receptor status**
  - Survival is directly related to the number of positive nodes
  - Larger tumors are more likely to have positive nodes
  - 30% of nonpalpable nodes are positive at surgery
    - 0 nodes positive   75% 5-year survival
    - 1–3 nodes positive   60% 5-year survival
    - 4–10 nodes positive   40% 5-year survival
▧ **Bone** – most common distant metastasis (can also go to lung, liver, brain)
▧ Takes approximately 5–7 years to go from single malignant cell to 1-cm tumor
▧ **Central and subareolar tumors** have increased risk of multicentricity

TNM STAGING SYSTEM FOR BREAST CANCER

T1: <2 cm. **T2:** 2–5 cm. **T3:** >5 cm. **T4:** skin or chest wall involvement (does <u>not</u> include pectoral muscles), peau d'orange, inflammatory cancer

N1: ipsilateral axillary nodes. **N2:** fixed ipsilateral axillary nodes. **N3:** ipsilateral internal mammary nodes

M1: distant metastasis (includes ipsilateral supraclavicular nodes)

Stage	TNM Status
I	T1,N0,M0
IIa	T0–1,N1,M0 or T2,N0,M0
IIb	T2,N1,M0 or T3,N0,M0
IIIa	T0–3,N2,M0 or T3,N1–2,M0
IIIb	Any T4 or N3 tumors
IV	M1

AJCC. *Cancer Staging Handbook.* 6th ed. New York: Springer-Verlag; 2002:265–266.

- **Breast cancer risk**
  - **Greatly increased risk**
    - BRCA gene in patient with family history of breast CA
    - ≥2 primary relatives with bilateral or premenopausal breast CA
    - DCIS (ipsilateral breast at risk) and LCIS (both breasts have same high risk)
    - Fibrocystic disease with atypical hyperplasia
  - **Moderately increased risk**
    - Family history of breast cancer other than above
    - Early menarche (<12 years), late menopause (>55 years)
    - Nulliparity or first birth after age 30
    - Radiation
    - Previous breast CA
    - Environmental risk factor – **high-fat diet (obesity)**

Magnitude of Known Breast Cancer Risk Factors
RELATIVE RISK < 2
Early menarche
Late menopause
Nulliparity
Proliferative benign disease
Obesity
Alcohol use
Hormone replacement therapy
RELATIVE RISK 2–4
Age > 35 first birth
First-degree relative with breast cancer
Radiation exposure
Prior breast cancer
RELATIVE RISK > 4
Gene mutation
Lobular carcinoma in situ
Atypical hyperplasia

	General	*BRCA1*	*BRCA2*
Estimated Lifetime Cancer Risks for *BRCA1* and *BRCA2* Mutations (to Age 70)			
Type of Cancer	Population (%)	Carrier (%)	Carrier (%)
Breast cancer	8.0	40–85	40–85
Contralateral breast cancer	0.5–1/yr	40–65	40–65
Male breast cancer	0.1	1–5	5–10
Ovarian cancer	1.4	30–45	10–20

Modified from Isaacs C, Peshkin BN, Lerman C. Evaluation and management of women with a strong family history of breast cancer. In: Harris JR, Lippman ME, Morrow M, et al., eds. *Diseases of the Breast.* 3rd ed. Philadelphia: Lippincott Williams & Wilkins; 2004:316.

- **First-degree relative with bilateral, premenopausal breast cancer** increases breast CA risk to 50%
  - BRCA I – associated with ovarian (50%), endometrial CA
  - BRCA II – associated with male breast CA
  - **Consider TAH and bilateral oophorectomies in BRCA I families**
- **Considerations for prophylactic mastectomy**
  - Family history + BRCA gene
  - LCIS
  - **Also need one of the following**: high patient anxiety, poor patient access for follow-up exams and mammograms, difficult lesion to follow on exam or with mammograms, or patient preference for mastectomy

■ **Receptors**
- **Positive receptors** – better response to hormones, chemotherapy, surgery, and better overall prognosis
  - Receptor-positive tumors are more common in **postmenopausal women**
- **Progesterone receptor–positive tumors** have better prognosis than estrogen receptor–positive tumors
- Tumor that is both progesterone receptor– and estrogen receptor–positive has best prognosis
- 10% of breast CAs negative for both receptors

■ **Male breast cancer**
- <1% of all breast CAs; usually ductal
- Poorer prognosis because of late presentation
- Have ↑ pectoral muscle involvement
- Associated with steroid use, previous XRT, family history, Klinefelter's syndrome, prolonged hyperestrogenic state
- Tx: modified radical mastectomy (MRM)

■ **Ductal CA**
- 85% of all breast CAs
- Can have various subtypes
  - **Medullary breast CA** – smooth borders, ↑ lymphocytes, ductal type cancer with bizarre cells
    - Vast majority are estrogen- and progesterone receptor–positive
    - More favorable prognosis
  - **Tubular CA** – small tubule formations
    - Nodes positive in 10%
    - More favorable prognosis
  - **Mucinous CA (colloid)** – produces an abundance of mucin
    - More favorable prognosis
  - **Scirrhotic CA** – worse prognosis
- Tx: MRM or lumpectomy with ALND (or SLNB); postop XRT

- **Lobular cancer**
  - 10% of all breast CAs
  - Does not form calcifications; extensively infiltrative; ↑ bilateral, multifocal, and multicentric disease
  - **Signet ring cells** confer worse prognosis
  - Tx: MRM or lumpectomy with ALND (or SLNB); postop XRT

- **Inflammatory cancer**
  - May need chemotherapy and XRT 1st, then mastectomy
  - Considered T4 disease
  - Very aggressive → median survival of 36 months
  - Has **dermal lymphatic invasion,** which causes <u>peau d'orange lymphedema</u> appearance; erythematous and warm

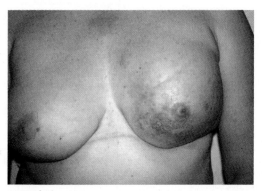

Locally advanced breast cancer. The breast is lifted and the upper half is bulging because of the large tumor. Distortion in the inferolateral contour is evident. The medial skin changes are caused by dermal tumor satellites.

- **Other histologic types**
  - Metaplastic adenocarcinoma – takes on the appearance of nonglandular cells
    - Most common types → squamous and pseudosarcomatous
    - Prognosis is the same as the tumor cell line from which it was derived
  - Adenoid cystic carcinoma
    - Large, well-circumscribed lesions
    - Better prognosis than ductal CAs

- **Preoperative studies**
  - CXR, bilateral mammograms, CBC, LFTs
  - Abdominal CT if LFTs elevated
  - Head CT if patient reports headaches
  - Bone scan if patient has bone pain or abnormal alkaline phosphatase
  - For patients with more advanced local primary, consider more extensive preop evaluations (head and abdominal CT, bone scan)

- **Surgical options**
  - **Subcutaneous (simple) mastectomy**
    - Leaves 1%–2% of breast tissue, preserves the nipple
    - <u>Not</u> indicated for breast CA treatment
    - Used for DCIS and LCIS
  - **Lumpectomy and SLNB (or ALND), postop XRT** – need 1-cm margin

Contraindications to Breast-Conserving Therapy in Invasive Carcinoma

ABSOLUTE CONTRAINDICATIONS
- Two or more primary tumors in separate quadrants of the breast
- Persistent positive margins after reasonable surgical attempts
- Pregnancy is an absolute contraindication to the use of breast irradiation. When cancer is diagnosed in the third trimester; it may be possible to perform breast-conserving surgery and treat the patient with irradiation after delivery
- A history of prior therapeutic irradiation to the breast region that would result in retreatment to an excessively high radiation dose
- Diffuse malignant-appearing microcalcifications

RELATIVE CONTRAINDICATIONS
- A history of scleroderma or active systemic lupus erythematosus
- Extensive gross, multifocal disease in the same quadrant. Studies in this area are not definitive
- Large tumor in a small breast that would result in cosmesis unacceptable to the patient
- Very large or pendulous breasts if reproducibility of patient setup and adequate dose homogeneity cannot be ensured

- **SLNB**
- Fewer complications than ALND
- Indicated only for malignant tumors >1 cm
- <u>Not</u> indicated in patients with clinically positive nodes; they need ALND
- Accuracy best when primary tumor is present (finds the right lymphatic channels)
- Well suited for small tumors with low risk of axillary metastases
- Radioactive material or blue dye can be used
- Dye or radiotracer is injected directly into the tumor area
- Type I hypersensitivity reactions have been reported with Lymphazurin blue dye
- Usually find 1–3 nodes; 95% of the time, the sentinel node is found
- During **SLND** – if no radiotracer or dye is found, need to do a formal ALND

  - **Contraindications** – pregnancy, multicentric disease, neoadjuvant, clinically positive nodes, prior axillary surgery, inflammatory or locally advanced disease

- **Modified radical mastectomy**
  - Removes all breast tissue including the nipple areolar complex
  - Includes axillary node dissection (level I nodes)

- **Radical mastectomy**
  - Includes MRM and overlying skin, pectoralis major and minor muscles, and level I, II, and III lymph nodes
  - Rarely performed anymore

- **Complications of mastectomy** – infection, flap necrosis, seromas

- **Complications of axillary lymph node dissection**
  - Infection, lymphedema, lymphangiosarcoma
  - **Axillary vein thrombosis** – sudden, early, postop swelling
  - **Lymphatic fibrosis** – slow swelling over 18 months
  - **Intercostal brachiocutaneous nerve** – hyperesthesia of inner arm and lateral chest wall; most commonly injured nerve after mastectomy; no significant sequelae
  - **Drains** – leave in until drainage < 40 cc/day

- ▣ Radiotherapy
  - **Usually consists of 5,000 rad for lumpectomy and XRT**
  - **Complications of XRT** – edema, erythema, rib fractures, pneumonitis, ulceration, sarcoma, contralateral breast CA
  - **Contraindications to XRT** – scleroderma (results in severe fibrosis and necrosis), previous XRT, SLE (relative), active rheumatoid arthritis (relative)
  - **Indications for XRT after <u>mastectomy</u>**
    - >4 nodes
    - Skin or chest wall involvement
    - Positive margins
    - Tumor > 5 cm (T3)
    - Extracapsular nodal invasion
    - Inflammatory CA
    - Fixed axillary nodes (N2) or internal mammary nodes (N3)
  - **Lumpectomy with XRT**
    - 10% chance of local recurrence, usually occurs within 2 years of 1st operation
    - These patients often also have distant disease
    - Need salvage MRM for local recurrence
    - Need to have negative margins following lumpectomy before starting XRT

- ▣ Chemotherapy
  - TAC for 6–12 weeks
  - **Positive nodes** – everyone gets chemo except <u>postmenopausal women with positive estrogen receptors</u> → tamoxifen
  - **>1 cm and negative nodes** – everyone gets chemo except patients with <u>positive estrogen receptors</u> → tamoxifen
  - **<1 cm and negative nodes** – no further treatment

Recommendations for Adjuvant Therapy

Patient Group	Recommended Treatment
NODE-NEGATIVE, LOW RISK	
Tumor < 1 cm	No treatment or endocrine therapy if ER+
Special histologic types 1–2 cm, grade 1, ER+	
NODE-NEGATIVE, HIGHER RISK	
ER+	Endocrine therapy OR chemotherapy + endocrine therapy
ER−	Chemotherapy
NODE-POSITIVE	
ER+	
Premenopausal	Chemotherapy + endocrine therapy
Postmenopausal	Chemotherapy + endocrine therapy or endocrine therapy alone
ER−	Chemotherapy

ER+ estrogen receptor–positive; ER−, estrogen receptor–negative.

- **Alternative hormonal/chemotherapy options** – androgenic steroid, aminoglutethimide, bilateral oophorectomy, Megace, aromatase inhibitors (anastrozole, letrozole)
- Both chemotherapy and hormonal therapy have been shown to decrease recurrence and improve survival
- **Tamoxifen** – decreases short-term risk of breast CA by 50%–60%
  - 1% risk of blood clots; 0.1% risk of endometrial CA

- ▣ **Almost all women with recurrence die of disease**

▣ Increased recurrences and metastases occur with **positive nodes, large tumors, negative receptors, unfavorable subtype**

▣ **Metastatic flare** – pain, swelling, erythema in metastatic areas; XRT can help
- XRT is good for bone metastases

▣ **Occult breast CA** – breast CA that presents as axillary metastases with unknown primary
- 70% are found to have breast CA at mastectomy

▣ **Benign conditions that mimic breast CA**
- Radial scar – can present as a stellate, irregular, spiculated mass lesion
- Fibromatosis – locally invasive spindle cells; can have skin retraction/dimpling
- Granular cell tumors (skin retraction/dimpling)
- Fat necrosis – poorly defined borders, skin retraction; accompanying fibrosis causes these findings; thought to be related to trauma
- Pathology shows macrophages laden with fat or foreign body giant cells (FNA or core needle biopsy)

▣ **Malignant tumors with a benign appearance (smooth, rounded masses)** – mucinous CA, medullary CA, cystosarcoma phyllodes

▣ **Most masses that contain fat are benign** – nodes, posttraumatic oil cyst, hamartomas, fibrolipoadenomas

▣ **Paget's disease**
- Scaly skin lesion on nipple; biopsy shows Paget's cells
- Patients have DCIS or ductal CA in breast
- Tx: need MRM if cancer present; otherwise simple mastectomy

▣ **Cystosarcoma phyllodes**
- 10% malignant, based on mitoses per high-power field (>5–10)
- <u>No</u> nodal metastases, hematogenous spread in any (rare)
- Resembles giant fibroadenoma; has stromal and epithelial elements (mesenchymal tissue)
- Can often be large tumors
- Tx: WLE with negative margins; **<u>no</u> ALND**

▣ **Stewart–Treves syndrome**
- Lymphangiosarcoma from chronic lymphedema following axillary dissection (MRM)
- Patients present with dark purple nodule or lesion on arm 5–10 years after surgery

▣ **Pregnancy with mass**
- Tends to present late, leading to worse prognosis
- Mammography and ultrasound do not work as well during pregnancy
- Try to use ultrasound to avoid radiation
- If **cyst**, drain it and send FNA for cytology
- If **solid**, perform core needle biopsy or FNA
- If core needle and FNA equivocal, need to go to excisional biopsy
- If breast CA
  - 1st trimester – MRM
  - 2nd trimester – MRM
  - 3rd trimester – MRM or if late can perform lumpectomy with ALND and postpartum XRT
  - May be able to wait until delivery for treatment
  - No chemotherapy or XRT while pregnant; no breast-feeding after delivery

CHAPTER 25. THORACIC

ANATOMY AND PHYSIOLOGY
- **Azygos vein** runs along the right side and dumps into superior vena cava
- **Thoracic duct** runs along the right side, crosses midline, and dumps into left subclavian vein at junction with internal jugular vein. Crosses at T4–5

THORACIC DUCT

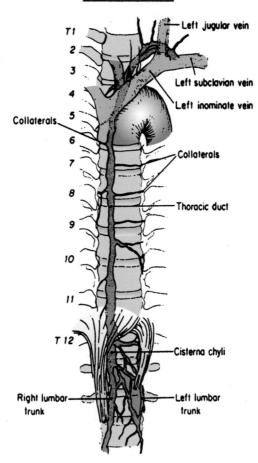

Schematic drawing of the most usual pattern and course of the thoracic duct. The single duct that enters the chest through the aortic hiatus between T12 and T10 is a relatively consistent finding and the usual site for surgical ligation.

- Left mainstem bronchi longer than right
- Right pulmonary artery longer than left before 1st branch
- **Phrenic nerve** – runs anterior to hilum
- **Vagus nerve** – runs posterior to hilum

- Right lung volume 55% (3 lobes: RUL, RML, and RLL), left lung volume 45% (2 lobes: LUL and LLL and lingula)
- Quiet inspiration – diaphragm 80%, intercostals 20%
- Greatest change in dimension superior/inferior
- Accessory muscles – sternocleidomastoid muscle (SCM), levators, serratus posterior, scalenes

- **Type I pneumocytes** – gas exchange
- **Type II pneumocytes** – surfactant production

- **Pores of Kahn** – direct air exchange between alveoli
- **Pleural fluid** – 1–2 L/day; parietal pleura produces pleural fluid cleared by **lymphatics** in the visceral pleura

PULMONARY FUNCTION TESTS
- Need predicted postop **FEV₁ > 0.8** (or at least 40% of the predicted value)
  - If it is close → get qualitative V/Q scan to see contribution of that portion of lung to overall FEV_1 → if low, may still be able to resect
- Need predicted postop **DLCO > 11–12** mL/min/mm Hg CO (at least 50% of the predicted value)
  - Represents carbon monoxide diffusion capacity
  - This value is based on pulmonary capillary surface area, hemoglobin content, and alveolar architecture
- **Need predicted postop FVC > 1.5 L**
- No resection if preop **pCO_2 > 45 or pO_2 <50** at rest
- No resection if preop **VO_2 max <10 mL/min/kg**

- **Persistent air leak** – most common after segmentectomy/wedge
- **Atelectasis and arrhythmias** – common problems after lobectomy or pneumonectomy

LUNG CANCER

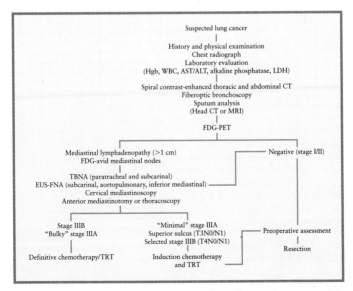

Decision making in patients who present with a solitary pulmonary nodule.

- Symptoms: patients can be asymptomatic with finding on routine CXR or present with atelectasis, PNA, pain, or weight loss
- **Most common cause of cancer-related death in the United States**
- **Nodal involvement** has strongest influence on survival
- **Brain** – single most common site of metastasis
  - Can also go to supraclavicular nodes, other lung, bone, liver, and adrenals
- **Recurrence** most commonly appears as disseminated metastases (brain most common)
  - 80% of recurrences are within the 1st 3 years

- Lung CA overall 5-year survival rate 10%; 30% with resection
- Stage I and II disease resectable; T3,N1,M0 (stage IIIa) possibly resectable
- Lobectomy or pneumonectomy most common; need to sample suspicious nodes
- Adenocarcinoma most common lung CA (<u>not</u> squamous)

- **Non–small cell carcinoma**
  - **80% of lung CA**
  - Squamous cell carcinoma usually more central
  - Adenocarcinoma usually more peripheral
  - **Local recurrence** increased with squamous cell CA
  - **Distant metastases** increased with adenocarcinoma
  - Other types of non–small cell CA – undifferentiated large cell and mixed tumors

---

TNM STAGING SYSTEM FOR LUNG CANCER

- **T1:** <3 cm. **T2:** >3 cm but >2 cm away from carina. **T3:** invasion of chest wall, pericardium, diaphragm or <2 cm from carina. **T4:** mediastinum, esophagus, trachea, vertebra, heart, great vessels, malignant effusion (all indicate unresectability)
- **N1:** ipsilateral hilum nodes. **N2:** ipsilateral mediastinal nodes (unresectable). **N3:** contralateral mediastinal or supraclavicular nodes (unresectable)
- **M1:** distant metastasis

Stage	TNM Status
I	T1–2,N0,M0
II	T1–2,N1,M0 or T3,N0,M0
IIIa	T1–3,N2,M0 or T3,N1,M0
IIIb	Any T4 or N3
IV	M1

Modified from AJCC. *Cancer Staging Handbook*. 6th ed. New York, NY: Springer-Verlag; 2002:197–198.

- **Small cell carcinoma**
  - **20% of lung CA neuroendocrine in origin**
  - Usually unresectable at time of diagnosis (< 5% candidates for surgery)
  - Overall 5-year survival rate; very poor prognosis
  - Stage T1,N0,M0 5-year survival rate – 50%
  - Most get just chemotherapy and XRT

- **Paraneoplastic syndromes**
  - **Squamous cell CA** – <u>PTH-related peptide</u>
  - **Small cell CA** – <u>ACTH, ADH</u>
  - **Small cell ACTH** – most common paraneoplastic syndrome

- **Mesothelioma**
  - Most malignant lung tumor

- Aggressive local invasion, nodal invasion, and distant metastases common at the time of diagnosis
- Asbestos exposure

▓ **Non–small cell CA chemotherapy (stage II or higher)** – carboplatin, Taxol
▓ **Small cell lung CA chemotherapy** – cisplatin, etoposide
▓ XRT can be used as well

▓ **Mediastinoscopy**
  - Use for **centrally located tumors** and patients with **suspicious adenopathy** > (0.8 cm or subcarinal > 1.0 cm) on chest CT
  - Does <u>not</u> assess aortopulmonary (AP) window nodes (left lung drainage)
  - Assesses **ipsilateral (N2) and contralateral (N3) mediastinal nodes**
  - <u>If positive, tumor unresectable</u>
  - Looking into **middle mediastinum with mediastinoscopy**
    - Left-sided structures – RLN, esophagus, aorta, main PA
    - Right-sided structures – azygous and SVC
    - Anterior structures – innominate vein, innominate artery, right PA
▓ **Chamberlain procedure** – assesses aortopulmonary window nodes; go through left 2nd rib cartilage
▓ **Bronchoscopy** – needed for centrally located tumors

▓ **Pancoast tumor** – tumor invades apex of chest wall and patients have Horner's syndrome (invasion of sympathetic chain → ptosis, miosis, anhidrosis) or **ulnar** nerve symptoms
▓ **Coin lesion**
  - Overall 5%-10% are malignant
  - Age <50 → <5% malignant; age > 50 → >50% malignant
  - No growth in 2 years, smooth contour suggests benign disease
  - Core needle biopsy frequently nondiagnostic

▓ **Asbestos exposure** increases lung CA risk 90×
▓ **Bronchioalveolar CA** – can look like pneumonia; grows along alveolar walls; multifocal
▓ **Metastases to the lung** – if isolated and <u>not</u> associated with any other systemic disease, may be resected for colon, renal cell CA, sarcoma, melanoma, ovarian, or endometrial CA

CARCINOIDS
▓ Neuroendocrine tumor, usually central
  - 5% have metastases at time of diagnosis; 50% have symptoms
▓ Typical carcinoid – 90% 5-year survival rate; atypical carcinoid – 60% 5-year survival
▓ Tx: resection; treat like cancer
▓ Outcome closely linked to histology; recurrence increased with positive nodes or tumors >3 cm

BRONCHIAL ADENOMAS
▓ **Malignant tumors** → adenoid cystic adenoma, mucoepidermoid adenoma, mucous gland adenoma
  - Slow growth, <u>no</u> metastases
  - Tx: resection
▓ **Adenoid cystic adenoma**
  - Submucosal glands; spread along perineural lymphatics, well beyond endoluminal component; XRT sensitive
  - Slow growing; can get 10-year survival with incomplete resection
  - Tx: resection; if unresectable, XRT can provide good palliation

HAMARTOMAS
- Most common benign adult lung tumor
- Have calcifications and can appear as a **popcorn lesion on chest CT**
- Diagnosis can be made with CT
- **Do not require resection**
- Repeat chest CT in 6 months to confirm diagnosis

MEDIASTINAL TUMORS IN ADULTS
- Most are asymptomatic; can present with chest pain, cough, dyspnea
- **Neurogenic tumors** – most common mediastinal tumor in adults and children, usually in posterior mediastinum
- **Location**
  - **Anterior** (thymus) – most common site for mediastinal tumor
    - **T's → T**hymoma (#1 anterior mediastinal mass in adults)
    - **T**hyroid CA and goiters
    - **T**-cell lymphoma
    - **T**eratoma (and other germ cell tumors)
    - Parathyroid adenomas
  - **Middle** (heart, trachea, ascending aorta)
    - Bronchiogenic cysts
    - Pericardial cysts
    - Enteric cysts
    - Lymphoma
  - **Posterior** (esophagus, descending aorta)
    - Enteric cysts
    - Neurogenic tumors
    - Lymphoma
- **Thymoma**
  - All thymomas require resection
  - Thymus too big or associated with refractory myasthenia gravis → resection
  - 50% of thymomas are malignant
  - 50% of patients with thymomas have symptoms
  - 50% of patients with thymomas have myasthenia gravis
  - 10% of patients with myasthenia gravis have thymomas
  - Myasthenia gravis – fatigue, weakness, diplopia, ptosis; antibodies to acetylcholine receptors
  - Tx: anticholinesterase medications, plasmapheresis, steroids
  - 80% get improvement with thymectomy, including patients who do not have thymomas

- **Lymphoma**
  - T-cell most common (non-Hodgkin's lymphoma) – lymphoblastic variant most common
  - Hodgkin's lymphoma – nodular sclerosing most common
  - Tx: chemotherapy and XRT

- **Germ cell tumors**
  - **Need to biopsy (usually done w/mediastinoscopy)**
  - **Teratoma** – most common germ cell tumor in mediastinum
    - Tx: resection and chemotherapy
  - **Seminoma** – most common malignant germ cell tumor in mediastinum
    - Tx: XRT (extremely sensitive); chemotherapy for positive nodes or residual disease; surgery for residual disease after that
  - **Nonseminoma** – 90% have elevated beta-HCG and alpha-fetoprotein
    - Tx: cisplatin-based chemotherapy and XRT; surgery for residual disease

- ■ Cysts
  - **Bronchiogenic** – posterior to carina. Tx: resection
  - **Pericardial** – at right costophrenic angle. Tx: resection

  - **Neurogenic tumors** – have pain, neurologic deficit. Tx: resection
    - 10% have intraspinal involvement that requires simultaneous spinal surgery
    - **Neurolemmoma** – most common
    - **Paraganglioma** – produce catecholamines
  - **Nerve sheath** – associated with von Recklinghausen's disease
  - **Can also get neuroblastomas and neurofibromas**

  - 50% of symptomatic mediastinal masses are malignant
  - 90% of asymptomatic mediastinal masses are benign

TRACHEA
- ■ Benign tumors – adults: **papilloma**; children: **hemangioma**
- ■ Malignant – **squamous cell carcinoma**

- ■ Most common late complication after tracheal surgery – granulation tissue formation
- ■ Most common early complication after tracheal surgery – laryngeal edema
  - Tx: reintubation, racemic epinephrine, steroids
- ■ Postintubation stenosis – at stoma site with tracheostomy, at cuff site with ET tube
  - May be able to treat with serial dilatation or with laser
- ■ May need resection with end-to-end anastomosis if severe
- ■ **Tracheoinnominate fistula**
  - Tracheostomy – needs to be between the 1st and 2nd tracheal rings not >3 rings → risk tracheoinnominate fistula
  - Tx: overinflate balloon to plug hole or stick your finger in hole and depress innominate artery. Resect innominate and place graft. Leave trachea alone. Use new tracheostomy site
- ■ **Tracheoesophageal fistula** (see also Chap. 43)
  - Use large-volume cuff below fistula
  - May need decompressing gastrostomy
  - Tx: tracheal resection, reanastomosis, sternohyoid flap

LUNG ABSCESS
- ■ Necrotic area; most commonly associated with aspiration
- ■ Most commonly in posterior segment of RUL and superior segment of RLL
- ■ Tx: antibiotics 95% successful; CT guided drainage if that fails
  - Surgery if this fails or cannot rule out cancer (>6 cm, failure to resolve after 6 weeks)
- ■ Chest CT can help differentiate empyema from lung abscess

EMPYEMA
- ■ Usually secondary to **pneumonia and subsequent parapneumonic effusion** (staph, strep)
- ■ Can also be due to esophageal, pulmonary, or mediastinal surgery
- ■ Symptoms: pleuritic chest pain, fever, cough, SOB
- ■ Pleural fluid often has WBCs > 500 cells/cc, bacteria, positive Gram stain
- ■ **Exudative phase** (1st week) – Tx: chest tube, antibiotics
- ■ **Fibroproliferative phase** (2nd week) – Tx: chest tube, antibiotics
- ■ **Organized phase** (3rd week) – Tx: likely need decortication; fibrous peel occurs around lung

- May need Eloesser flap (direct opening to external environment) for chronic unresolving empyema
- Can also place a chronic chest tube that is gradually pulled out

CHYLOTHORAX
- Fluid milky white; has ↑ lymphocytes and TAGs (>110 mL/μL); Sudan red stains fat
- **Fluid resistant to infection**
- 50% secondary to trauma or iatrogenic injury
- 50% secondary to tumor (lymphoma most common, due to tumor burden in the lymphatics)
- Injury above T5–6 results in left-sided chylothorax
- Injury below T5–6 results in right-sided chylothorax
- 3–4 weeks of conservative therapy (chest tube, octreotide, low-fat diet or TPN)
  - If that fails, surgery with ligation of thoracic duct on right side low in mediastinum (80% successful) if chylothorax secondary to trauma or iatrogenic injury
  - For malignant causes of chylothorax, can perform mechanical or talc pleurodesis (less successful than above)

MASSIVE HEMOPTYSIS
- **>600 cc/24 h**; bleeding is from high-pressure **bronchial arteries**
- Most commonly secondary to infection, **mycetoma** most common; death due to asphyxiation
- Tx: Place bleeding side down if known; rigid bronchoscopy to identify site; mainstem intubation to side opposite of bleeding to prevent drowning in blood; to OR for lobectomy or pneumonectomy; bronchial artery embolization if not suitable for surgery

SPONTANEOUS PNEUMOTHORAX
- Tall, healthy, thin, young males
- Recurrence risk after 1st pneumothorax 20%, after 2nd pneumothorax 60%, after 3rd pneumothorax 80%
- Results from rupture of a bleb in the apex of the upper lobe of the lung; can occur in the superior segment of the lower lobe
- More common on the right
- Tx: **chest tube**
- Surgery for recurrence, large blebs on CT scan, air leak > 7 days, nonreexpansion
- Also need surgery for high-risk profession (airline pilot, diver, mountain climber) or patients who live in remote areas
- Surgery consists of thoracoscopy, apical blebectomy, and mechanical pleurodesis

OTHER CONDITIONS
- **Bronchiogenic cysts** (see also Chap. 43)
  - Most common cysts of the mediastinum
  - Abnormal lung tissue outside lung; did not get connected to bronchial system
  - Usually posterior to the carina
  - Tx: remove cyst

- **Sequestration** (see also Chap. 43)
  - Lung tissue in lung not connected to bronchial tree
  - Receives blood supply from anomalous systemic arteries → usually off thoracic aorta
    - Can also come from the abdominal aorta through the inferior pulmonary ligament
  - Venous blood supply is either the pulmonary vein or systemic veins
  - **Extralobar** – more common in children; more likely to have systemic venous drainage
  - **Intralobar** – more common in adults; more likely to have pulmonary vein drainage
  - Tx: lobectomy

- **Solitary pulmonary nodule with history of previous cancer**
  - **Sarcoma/melanoma** → nodule more likely metastases
  - **Head/neck/breast** → nodule more likely primary lung CA
  - **GI/GU** → metastases or primary
  - In case of primary cancer with a resectable lung metastasis, take out primary 1st, then metastasis
- **Tension pneumothorax** – most likely to cause arrest after blunt trauma; impaired venous return
- **Catamenial pneumothorax** – occurs in temporal relation to menstruation
  - Caused by **endometrial implants** in the visceral lung pleura
- **Residual hemothorax despite 2 good chest tubes** → OR for thoracoscopic drainage
- **Clotted hemothorax** – surgical drainage if >25% of lung, air–fluid levels, or signs of infection (fever, ↑WBCs); surgery in 1st week to avoid peel
- **Broncholiths** – usually secondary to infection
- **Mediastinitis** – usually after cardiac surgery
- **Whiteout on chest x-ray**
  - Midline shift toward whiteout – most likely collapse → need bronchoscopy to remove plug
  - No shift – CT scan to figure it out
  - Midline shift away from whiteout – most likely effusion → place chest tube
- **Bronchiectasis** – acquired from infection, tumor, **cystic fibrosis**
  - Diffuse nature prevents surgery in most patients
- **Tuberculosis** – lung apices; get calcifications, caseating granulomas
  - Ghon complex → parenchymal lesion + enlarged hilar nodes
  - Tx: INH, rifampin, pyrazinamide
- **Sarcoidosis** – has noncaseating granulomas
- **Effusions – exudative**: protein >3, specific gravity >1.016, LDH ratio (pleural fluid:serum) >0.6, ↓glucose

Evaluation of Pleural Fluid

Test	Transudate	Exudate	Empyema
WBC	<1,000	>1,000	>1,000 >50,000 most specific
pH	7.45–7.55	≤7.45	<7.30
Pleural fluid protein to serum ratio	<0.5	>0.5	>0.5
Pleural fluid LDH to serum ratio	<0.6	>0.6	>0.6

From Knight C, Paauw D. Respiratory tract infections. In: Shah SS, Hu KK, Crane HM, eds. *Blueprints Infectious Diseases*. Philadelphia: Lippincott Williams & Wilkins; 2006, with permission.

- **Recurrent pleural effusions** can be treated with mechanical pleurodesis
  - Talc pleurodesis for malignant pleural effusions
- **Airway fires** – usually associated with the laser
  - Tx: stop gas flow, remove ET tube, reintubate for 24 hours; bronchoscopy
- **AVMs** – connections between the pulmonary arteries and pulmonary veins; usually in lower lobes; can occur with Osler–Weber–Rendu disease
  - Symptoms: hemoptysis, SOB, neurologic events
  - Tx: embolization
- **Chest wall tumors**
  - **Benign** – **osteochondroma** most common
  - **Malignant** – **chondrosarcoma** most common

CHAPTER 26. **CARDIAC**

CONGENITAL HEART DISEASE

- **R → L shunts cause cyanosis**
  - Children squat to ↑ SVRI and ↓ R → L shunts
  - **Cyanosis** – can lead to polycythemia, strokes, brain abscess, endocarditis, hypertrophic osteoarthropathy
  - **Eisenmenger's syndrome – shift from L → R shunt to R → L**
    - Sign of increasing pulmonary vascular resistance and pulmonary HTN
    - This condition is generally irreversible

- **L → R shunts cause CHF** – can manifest as failure to thrive, ↑ HR, tachypnea, hepatomegaly
  - **CHF in children** – hepatomegaly 1st sign

- **L → R shunts (patients get symptoms of CHF)** – VSD, ASD, PDA
- **R → L shunts (patients have cyanosis)** – tetralogy of Fallot, transposition of the great vessels, truncus arteriosus

- **Ductus arteriosus** – connection between descending aorta and left pulmonary artery (PA); blood shunted away from lungs in utero
- **Ductus venosum** – connection between portal vein and IVC; blood shunted away from liver
- **Fetal circulation to placenta** – 2 umbilical arteries
- **Fetal circulation from placenta** – 1 umbilical vein

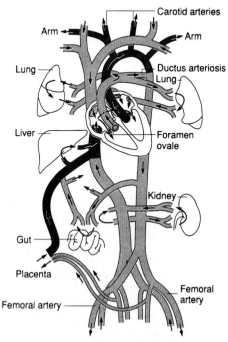

Persistent fetal circulation.

■ **Ventricular septal defect (VSD)**
- **Most common congenital heart defect**
- **L → R shunt** – most close spontaneously by age 6 months
- Large VSDs – usually cause symptoms after 4–6 weeks of life, as PVR ↓ and shunt ↑
- Get CHF, failure to thrive, tachypnea, tachycardia
- Medical Tx: diuretics and digoxin
- Timing of repair
  - **CHF resulting in failure to thrive** – most common reason for repair
  - **Before school age if does not close spontaneously**
  - **PVR > 4–6 Woods units** also indication for repair
  - PVR > 10-2 Woods units contraindication for repair → use vasodilators to see if it is reversible; if so, can repair

■ **Atrial septal defect (ASD)**
- **L → R shunt**
- **Ostium secundum** – most common; centrally located, patent foramen ovale (80%)
  - Can have anomalous pulmonary venous return (to right atrium or IVC)
  - IVC can connect to left atrium
- **Ostium primum** (or atrioventricular septal defects or endocardial cushion defects)
  - Defect more inferior
  - Can get mitral valve and coronary sinus defects
  - Caused by deficiency in remnant of left horn of sinus venosus
- Usually symptomatic when Qp/Qs > 2 → CHF (fatigue, SOB, recurrent infections)
- Rare for ASD to cause increase in PVR before adulthood
- Can get paradoxical emboli and arrhythmias in adulthood
- Medical Tx: diuretics and digoxin
- Timing of repair
  - **Volume overload** (occurs with Qp/Qs > 1.5)
  - **Before school age if does not close spontaneously**
  - PVR > 10–12 Woods units contraindication for repair
  - All ostium primum atrioventricular septal defects (ASDs) need repair

■ **Tetralogy of Fallot**
- VSD, pulmonic stenosis, overriding aorta, right ventricular (RV) hypertrophy
- **R → L shunt**
- **Most common congenital heart defect that results in cyanosis**
- Morphologic abnormality – anterior and superior displacement of the infundibular septum
- Medical Tx: β-blocker
- Timing of operation: ↑ cyanosis
- Repair: Blalock–Taussig (BT) shunt can be used for palliation to delay repair

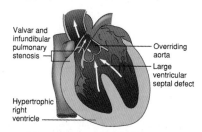

Valvar and infundibular pulmonary stenosis

Overriding aorta

Large ventricular septal defect

Hypertrophic right ventricle

The four anatomic features of the tetralogy of Fallot. The primary morphologic abnormality, anterior and superior displacement of the infundibular septum, results in a malalignment ventricular septal defect, overriding of the aortic valve, and obstruction of the right ventricular outflow. Right ventricular hypertrophy is a secondary occurrence.

- Definitive repair: RV outflow tract obstruction division, patch enlargement of outflow tract, and VSD repair

■ **Transposition of the great vessels**
- Most common cyanotic disorder presenting in the 1st week of life
- **R → L shunt**
- Mixing most often occurs through ASD; VSD or PDA can serve as additional mixing conduit
- Medical Tx: atrial septostomy, PGE_1
- In patients with large VSDs, significant CHF and pulmonary hypertension may occur by 3 months of age
- Repair: optimal – early switch with coronary reimplantation posteriorly (first 2–3 weeks of life) while LV is still getting high resistance
- Patients with LVOT obstruction not candidates for early switch
  - Most also have large VSDs
  - Palliation with systemic to PA shunting preferred early on (BT shunt)
  - Definitive repair at 3–5 years of age

■ **Truncus arteriosus**
- Usually has associated VSD
- **R → L shunt**
- Mixing causes arterial saturations of 85%–90%
- Neonates present with CHF; 80% die in 1st year due to CHF
- CXR shows cardiomegaly
- Medical Tx: diuretics, digoxin, fluid restriction, afterload reduction
- Timing of repair: onset of tachypnea is sign of ↓ PVR
- Tx: repair VSD, remove PAs from aorta, and repair aorta; restore RV outflow tract with Dacron graft to PAs

■ **Patent ductus arteriosus (PDA)**
- **L → R shunt**
- Indomethacin – causes the PDA to close; rarely successful beyond the neonatal period
- Usually requires surgical repair through left thoracotomy if persists
- PGE_1 – keeps PDA open

■ **Coarctation of the aorta**
- Usually occurs just distal to the left subclavian artery
- Associated with Turner's syndrome
- Rib notching from the IMA and intercostal collaterals
- Can present with profound CHF
- All patients should undergo repair to prevent heart failure
- Try to perform end-to-end repair

■ **Univentricular heart**
- Need Fontan procedure to direct all vena cava blood to the PA
- Best approach is to attach the right atrium and SVC to the PA directly
- Prerequisites – normal PA pressure (<20 mm Hg) and normal PVR (<2 Woods units)

■ **Hypoplastic left heart**
- Need Norwood procedure
- Main PA becomes outlet tract for aorta for what is to become single-ventricle physiology
- Tx: aorta is augmented with large piece of allograft artery and attached to main PA trunk
  - Distal PAs are separated and supplied through systemic-PA shunt (BT shunt)
  - Many patients eventually need heart TXP

■ **Anomalous pulmonary venous return** – goes to SVC instead of left atrium
  • Most often seen in patients with ASDs

■ **Vascular rings** – double aortic arch most common
  • May manifest as recurrent pulmonary infections or dysphagia
  • Trachea most commonly affected
  • Tx: divide smaller arch through left thoracotomy

ADULT CARDIAC DISEASE
■ **Coronary artery disease**
  • Most common cause of death in the United States
  • Risk factors – smoking, HTN, male gender, family history, hyperlipidemia, diabetes
  • Medical Tx: nitrates, smoking cessation, weight loss, statin drugs, ASA

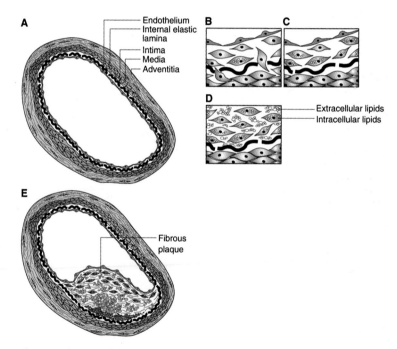

Developmental stages of the lesions of atherosclerosis. *(A)* The normal muscular artery consists of an internal intima with endothelium and internal elastic lamina. The smooth muscle of the vessel wall is in the media, and the thin adventitial layer contains connective tissue and the vasa vasorum. With age, the thickness and smooth-muscle cell content of the thin and sparsely muscled intima increase. *(B)* The first phase of an atherosclerotic lesion consists of focal thickening of the intima with smooth-muscle cells and extracellular matrix and an initial accumulation of intercellular lipid deposits. *(C)* Extracellular lipid may also develop. *(D)* Intercellular and extracellular lipid in the earliest phase is referred to as a *fatty streak*. *(E)* A fibrous plaque results as fibroblasts that cover the proliferating smooth-muscle cells laden with lipids and cell debris continue to accumulate. The lesion becomes more complex as continuing cell degeneration leads to an ingress of blood constituents and calcification. (After Glomset JA, Ross R. Atherosclerosis and the arterial smooth-muscle cells. *Science* 1973;180:1332, with permission.)

- **Right dominant circulation** (most common) – posterior descending artery comes off the right coronary artery
- **Left dominant circulation** – posterior descending artery comes off the circumflex coronary artery
- Left main coronary artery branches into left anterior descending and circumflex
- Most atherosclerotic lesions are **proximal**
- Complications of myocardial infarction
  - **VSD (pansystolic murmur), papillary muscle rupture, and free wall rupture.** Most likely to occur at 3–7 days post-MI
  - **Post-MI VSD** (pansystolic murmur) – **transesophageal echo** best test
    - Usually occurs **5–7 days after MI**
    - **Step-up in oxygen content** between right atrium and pulmonary artery secondary to L → R shunt
  - **LV aneurysm** – most commonly occurs after large, transmural, anterior MI
    - **Symptoms**: CHF, arrhythmias, angina
    - **Indications for surgery**: refractory symptoms, arrhythmias
- **PTCA** – restenosis in 20%–30% in <1 year
- **Saphenous vein graft** – 80%–90% 5-year patency
- **Internal mammary artery** – off subclavian arteries
  - Best conduit for CABG – >90% 10-year graft patency rate
  - Collateralizes with superior epigastric **artery**
- **CABG procedure**
  - **Potassium and cold solution cardioplegia** – causes arrest of the heart in diastole; keeps the heart protected and still while grafts are placed
  - **Indications**[1]
  - Left main disease
  - Left main equivalent disease (LAD > 70% and proximal left complications)
  - 3-vessel disease
  - 2-vessel disease with:
    - Proximal LAD stenosis and either LVEF < 50% or extensive ischemia on noninvasive imaging study
  - 1- or 2-vessel disease with:
    - Stable angina, large area of viable myocardium, and high-risk criteria on non-invasive testing *or*
    - Disease causing life-threatening arrhythmias *or*
    - Disabling stable angina despite medications when patient has acceptable risk
  - Unstable angina – patients with ongoing ischemia despite maximal nonsurgical therapy
  - **High mortality risk factors**: emergency operations (#1 risk factor), age, reoperation, and low EF

VALVE DISEASE
- **Aortic stenosis** – most common valve lesion

- **Calcification** – produces stenosis

- **Rheumatic heart disease** – most common cause of valve dysfunction
  - **Mitral** most commonly involved valve

- **Stenosis** predominates; see regurgitation with progressive valve degeneration (volcano orifice, sticks open)

---

[1]Eagle KA, et al. ACC/AHA guidelines for coronary artery bypass graft surgery: a report of the American College of Cardiology/American Heart Association Task Force on Practice Guidelines. *J Am Coll Cardiol.* 1999;34:1262–1347.

■ **Degenerative processes** – 3rd or 4th decade of life; **mitral** most commonly affected; **insufficiency** predominates

■ **Tissue valves** (do not require anticoagulation)
- For patients who want pregnancy, have contraindication to anticoagulation, are older and unlikely to require another valve in their lifetime, or have frequent falls
- Not as durable as mechanical valves
- Because of rapid calcification in children and young patients, use of tissue valves is contraindicated in these populations
- Chronic renal dialysis is also a contraindication

■ **Mitral stenosis**
- Leads to signs of pulmonary congestion
- Can develop mural thrombi – 50% go to cerebral circulation
- Indications for operation – when symptomatic (usually have valve area $<$1 cm^2)

■ **Mitral regurgitation**
- LV becomes dilated, wall tension ↑
- **Ventricular function** – key index of disease progression in patients with MR
- In end-stage disease, left atrium becomes less compliant → pulmonary congestion ensues and can lead to right-sided heart failure. Atrial fibrillation is common
- Indications for operation – symptoms may not develop until after irreversible heart dysfunction has occurred
  - Repair indicated for any functional class II heart failure (SOB on exertion)

■ **Aortic stenosis**
- Adequate CO and normal systemic pressures are maintained until late in the disease
- Eventually, LV hypertrophy leads to ↓ ventricular compliance and pulmonary congestion. LV failure ultimately develops
- Cardinal symptoms
  - Angina – develops in 65%; mean survival is 5 years
  - Syncope – develops in 25%, mean survival is 3 years
  - Heart failure – mean survival is 2 years (strongest prognostic indicator)
- Indications for operation – when symptomatic (usually have a peak gradient of 50 mm Hg and a valve area $<$ 1.0 cm^2)

■ **Aortic insufficiency**
- Produces volume loading strain on the LV
- LV becomes more dilated, wall tension ↑ (law of Laplace)
- Cardiac output can increase to 30 L/min
- Indications for operation – symptoms may not develop until after irreversible heart dysfunction has occurred
  - Repair indicated for any functional class II heart failure (SOB with exertion)

ENDOCARDITIS
■ Fever, chills, sweats
■ **Aortic valve** – most common site of prosthetic valve infections
■ **Mitral valve** – most common site of native valve infections
■ Most commonly left-sided except in drug abusers
■ *Staphylococcus aureus* responsible for 50% of cases
■ Medical therapy first – successful in 75%; sterilizes valve in 50%
■ Indications for surgery – **failure of antimicrobial therapy, valve failure, perivalvular abscesses, pericarditis**

■ **Periprocedural endocarditis prophylaxis indicated for patients**
  • Prosthetic valves
  • Rheumatic heart disease
  • Congenital cardiac malformations
  • Mitral valve prolapse with mitral regurgitation
  • Previous history of bacterial endocarditis
  • 1st-generation cephalosporins usually used → need to start oral antibiotics 1 day prior

Modified Duke Criteria for Diagnosis of Infective Endocarditis

Major Criteria
  Typical organism (e.g., *S. aureus*, streptococci) from 2 BCs
  Any organism grown persistently positive BC
  Positive serologic test or single BC for *C. burnetii* (Q fever)
  Echocardiogram showing oscillating intracardiac mass, abscess, or new dehiscence of prosthetic valve
  Physical exam showing new valvular regurgitation (change in preexisting murmur not sufficient)

Minor Criteria
  Predisposing heart condition or injection drug use
  Fever (temperature over 100.4°F [38.0°C])
  Vasculare phenomena (e.g., major arterial emboli, septic pulmonary infarcts, mycotic aneurysm, intracranial hemorrhage, conjunctival hemorrhages, Janeway lesions [petechiae or splinter hemorrhages not sufficient])
  Immunologic phenomena (e.g., glomerulonephritis, Osler's nodes, Roth's spots, positive rheumatoid factor)
  Serologic evidence or positive BC not meeting a major criterion

Diagnosis
  Definite endocarditis: either 2 major, 1 major + 3 minor, or 5 minor criteria
  Possible endocarditis: either 1 major + 1 minor, or 3 minor criteria

Abbreviation: BC, blood culture.
From Hagman, MM. Cardiac infections. In: Shah SS, Hu KK, Crane HM, eds. *Blueprints Infectious Diseases*. Philadelphia, PA: Lippincott Williams & Wilkins; 2006, with permission.

OTHER CARDIAC CONDITIONS
■ **Most common tumors of heart**
  • Most common benign tumor – **myxoma**; 75% in LA, mitral valve stenosis-type symptoms
  • Most common malignant tumor – **angiosarcoma**
  • Most common metastatic tumor to the heart – **lung CA**

■ Coming off cardiopulmonary bypass and aortic root vent blood is dark and aortic perfusion cannula blood is red
  • Tx: **ventilate the lungs**
■ **Coronary veins** have the lowest oxygen tension of any tissue in the body due to high oxygen extraction by myocardium
■ **Superior vena cava (SVC) syndrome** – swelling of the upper extremities and face
  • Most cases secondary to lung CA invading the SVC
  • These tumors are unresectable since the tumor has invaded the mediastinum
  • Tx: XRT
■ **Idiopathic hypertrophic subaortic stenosis**
  • Too much volume can cause pulmonary edema due to stenosis region
  • Not enough afterload will cause the aortic outflow tract to collapse, also resulting in pulmonary edema
  • Very tricky management

- **Intra-aortic balloon pump (IABP)** – see Chap. 16
- **Mediastinal bleeding** – >500 cc for 1st hour or >250 cc/h for 4 hours → ↑
  re-explore after cardiac procedure
- **Risk factors for mediastinitis** – obesity, use of bilateral internal mammary arteri↓
  diabetes
  - Tx: debridement with pectoralis flaps; can also use omentum
- **Postpericardiotomy syndrome** – pericardial friction rub, fever, chest pain, SOB
  - EKG – diffuse ST segment elevation in multiple leads
  - **Tx: NSAIDs, steroids**
- **1st sign of cardiac tamponade on echocardiogram** – ↓ right atrial diastolic filling

ASCULAR

hypercoagulable disorder – resistance to activated protein C

hypercoagulability disorder – smoking

ATHEROSCLEROSIS STAGES

- **1st** – **foam cells** → macrophages that have absorbed fat and lipids in the vessel wall
- **2nd** – **smooth muscle cell proliferation** → caused by growth factors released from macrophages; results in wall injury
- **3rd** – **intimal disruption** (from smooth muscle cell proliferation) → leads to exposure of collagen in vessel wall and eventual **thrombus formation** → fibrous plaques then form in these areas with underlying atheromas
- Risk factors: smoking, HTN, hypercholesterolemia, DM, hereditary factors
- **Atherosclerosis** – disease of intima
- **Hypertension** – disease of media

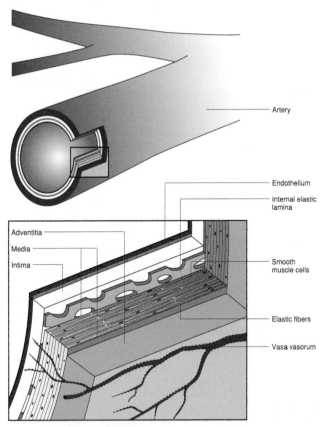

The artery wall is made of multiple layers (intima, media, and adventitia) that vary in composition depending on the artery.

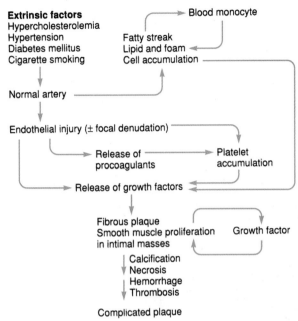

Atherogenesis and progression of atherosclerosis is probably the consequence of multiple factors acting on the arterial wall.

CEREBROVASCULAR DISEASE

▇ Stroke 3rd most common case of death in the United States

▇ **HTN** – most important risk factor for stroke in asymptomatic patients
▇ Carotids supply 85% of blood flow to brain
  • **Bifurcation** – most common site of stenosis
▇ Normal internal carotid artery has **continuous forward flow**
▇ Normal external carotid artery has **triphasic flow**
  • 1st branch of external carotid artery – **superior thyroid artery**
  • Communication between internal carotid artery and external carotid artery with **ophthalmic artery** (1st branch of ICA) and **internal maxillary artery (off ECA)**

▇ **Middle cerebral artery** – most commonly diseased <u>intracranial artery</u>
▇ **Cerebral ischemic events** – most commonly from **arterial embolization** (not thrombosis) from the ICA
  • Can also occur from a **low-flow state** through a severely stenotic lesion
  • **Heart** 2nd most common source of emboli
▇ **Anterior cerebral artery events** – mental status changes, release, slowing
▇ **Middle cerebral artery events** – contralateral motor and speech (if dominant side); contralateral facial droop
▇ **Amaurosis fugax** – occlusion of the ophthalmic branch of the ICA (visual changes → shade coming down over eyes); visual changes are transient
  • See **Hollenhorst plaques** on ophthalmologic exam
▇ **Carotid traumatic injury with major fixed deficit**
  • If occluded do <u>not</u> repair → can exacerbate injury with bleeding
  • If not occluded – repair

■ **Carotid endarterectomy (CEA)**
  • Should be considered in any patient <u>with >70% stenosis</u> and symptoms
  • Asymptomatic patients with 70%–80% stenosis more controversial
  • Any patient <u>with >80%–90% stenosis</u> should have CEA if technically possible
  • **Recent completed stroke** → wait 4-6 weeks and then perform CEA if it meets criteria (bleeding risk if performed earlier)
  • **Emergent CEA** may be of benefit with <u>fluctuating neurologic symptoms or crescendo/evolving TIAs</u>

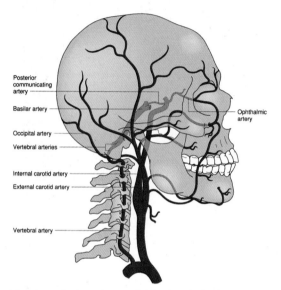

The paired carotid and vertebral arteries supply blood to the brain. Extensive extracranial collaterals between the external carotid and vertebral systems allow for antegrade perfusion when a proximal occlusion develops in either vessel. Likewise, periorbital collaterals allow for retrograde flow through the ophthalmic artery to the internal carotid artery in the presence of a cervical internal carotid artery occlusion. Extensive side-to-side collaterals are found between the right and left external carotid arteries and right and left vertebral arteries.

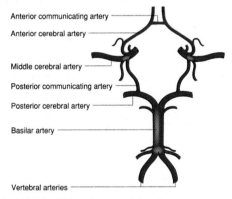

The circle of Willis is a highly efficient intracranial collateral network; however, multiple important variations occur, and an incomplete circle producing an isolated hemisphere is not uncommon.

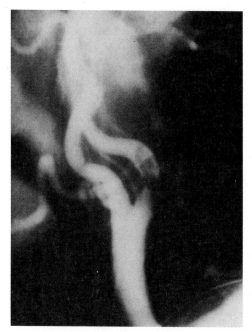

An isolated atherosclerotic lesion at the origin of the internal carotid artery. Free-floating intraluminal thrombus can be seen distal to the atherosclerotic plaque in this patient with crescendo transient ischemic attacks.

- **Shunt during CEA for stump pressures < 50**
- **Repair the tightest side first if the patient has bilateral stenosis** (symptomatic side)
- **Repair the dominant side first if the patient has equally tight carotid stenosis bilaterally**

Carotid Sheath: common carotid artery, vagus nerve, int. jugular

- **Complications**
  - **Vagus nerve** – <u>most common cranial nerve injury with CEA</u> → secondary to vascular clamping during endarterectomy; patients get hoarseness
  - **Hypoglossal nerve** – tongue deviation to the side of injury → speech and mastication difficulty
  - **Glossopharyngeal nerve** – unlikely injury; could occur with really high carotid lesion → causes difficulty swallowing
  - **Ansa cervicalis** – strap muscles; no serious deficits
  - **Mandibular branch of facial nerve** – affects corner of mouth (smile)
  - **Acute event immediately after CEA** → back to OR to check for flap or thrombosis
  - **Pseudoaneurysm** – pulsatile, bleeding mass after CEA
  - Tx: drape and prep before intubation, intubate, then repair
  - **20% have hypertension following CEA** – caused by injury to carotid body
  - Tx: Nipride to avoid bleeding
  - **Myocardial infarction** – most common nonstroke morbidity and mortality following CEA
  - **15% restenosis** rate after CEA

- **Carotid stenting is another option compared with CEA** – this new technology seems most beneficial for high-risk patients (e.g., patients w/ previous CEA, medical disease that makes them too high risk for surgery, etc.)

Terminal branches of external carotid: Maxillary, superficial temporal artery

High-Risk Patients to be Considered for Carotid Artery Stenting

Medical Comorbidity	Local Factors
Age > 80	Carotid restenosis after carotid endarterectomy
Coronary artery disease	Anatomically high lesion (above second cervical vertebrae)
Acute myocardial infarction in prior 4 weeks	
CABG within prior 6 months	Contralateral internal carotid artery occlusion
Congestive heart failure – (class III/IV)	Contralateral laryngeal nerve palsy
Ejection fraction – 30%	Radiation-induced internal carotid artery stenosis
Dialysis-dependent renal failure	Prior neck dissection
Severe chronic obstructive pulmonary disease	Permanent tracheal stoma
$FEV_1 < 1.01$	Cervical scarring

CABG, coronary artery bypass graft.

- ▥ **Vertebral disease**
  - Usually bilateral, at origins; usually need bilateral disease to have symptoms
  - Caused by spurs, bands, trauma; get vertebrobasilar insufficiency
  - Symptoms: diplopia, dysarthria, vertigo, tinnitus, drop attacks, incoordination, binocular vision loss
  - Tx: PTA, vertebral artery transposition to subclavian, transsubclavian endarterectomy, osteophyte resection, unroofing of transverse process foramina, and resection of musculotendinous bands all options

- ▥ **Carotid body tumors** – present as a painless neck mass, usually near bifurcation, neural crest cells
  - Tx: resection

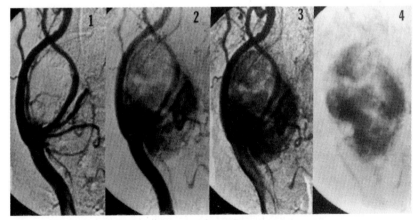

Typical angiographic appearance of a carotid body tumor. Initial injection view (1) demonstrates the characteristic "splaying" of the carotid bifurcation. Subsequent delayed views (2–4) show the anatomic extent of lesion and the degree of vascularity. (From Moore WS. Carotid body tumors. In: Fischer JE, Bland KI, et al., eds. *Mastery of Surgery*. 5th ed. Philadelphia, PA: Lippincott Williams & Wilkins; 2007, with permission).

THORACIC AORTIC DISEASE
- ▥ **Thoracic aortic transection** (see also Chap. 15)
  - From trauma, usually a deceleration injury

- Address other life-threatening injuries first (severe solid organ laceration, pelvic fracture with hemorrhage, etc. → then repair aorta)
- Get **mediastinal widening** from bridging veins and arteries, <u>not</u> leaking from aorta itself
- Usually tears at the **ligamentum arteriosum**, just distal to the left subclavian
- Use left heart bypass with repair (TEUAR better than open)
- 90% of these patients die at the scene

■ **Ascending aortic aneurysms**
- Usually caused by connective tissue disorders; **cystic medial necrosis** most common abnormality – Marfan's syndrome
- Dx: chest CT or aortography
- Can get aortic insufficiency
- Often asymptomatic and picked up on routine CXR
- Can also get compression of vertebra (back pain), RLN (voice changes), bronchi (dyspnea or PNA), or esophagus (swallowing trouble)
- Symptomatic patients usually have CHF secondary to aortic insufficiency
- Indications for repair: acutely symptomatic, ≥5.5 cm; with Marfan's > 5.0 cm, diameter 2× normal, or rapid ↑ in size (> 1 cm/year)

■ **Transverse aortic arch aneurysms**
- From atherosclerosis
- Repair indications same as for ascending aortic aneurysms
- Patients will likely need to be cooled down and have circulatory arrest to perform repair

■ **Descending aortic aneurysms (or thoracoabdominal aneurysms)**
- From atherosclerosis; can become quite large before symptoms occur
- Risk of paraplegia 5%–10%
- Repair indications same as for ascending aortic aneurysms
- Reimplant intercostal vessels below T8 to help prevent paraplegia

■ **Dissections**
- **Stanford classification** – based on the presence or absence of involvement of ascending aorta
  - **Class A** – any ascending aortic involvement
  - **Class B** – descending aortic involvement only
- **DeBakey classification** – based on the site of tear and extent of dissection
  - **Type I** – ascending and descending
  - **Type II** – ascending only
  - **Type III** – descending only

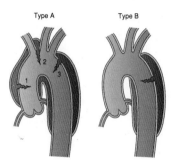

Stanford classification of aortic dissections based on the presence or absence of involvement of the ascending aorta. Numbers indicate the locations of the site of primary intimal tear.

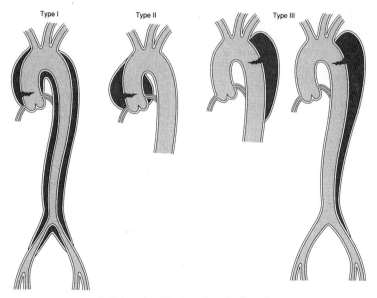

DeBakey classification of aortic dissection.

- Most dissections start in **ascending aorta**
- Can mimic myocardial infarction
- Symptoms: searing-like chest pain; can have unequal pulses or BP in upper extremities
- 95% of patients have **severe HTN**
- **Other risk factors**: Marfan's syndrome, previous coarctation repair, atherosclerosis, infection (syphilis)
- CXR – usually normal; may have wide mediastinum
- Dx: chest CT with contrast
- Dissection occurs in **media layer of blood vessel wall**
- **Aortic insufficiency** occurs in 70% with acute disease, caused by annular dilatation or when aortic valve cusp is sheared off
- Can also have occlusion of the coronaries and major aortic branches
- Death with ascending aortic dissections usually secondary to **cardiac failure from aortic insufficiency or tamponade**; can also have **rupture**
- Medical Tx if possible → control BP with hydralazine and β-blockers
- Surgery aims at obliterating the false lumen and placing graft
  - **Operate on all ascending aortic dissections**
  - **Operate on descending aortic dissections with visceral, renal, or leg ischemia; persistent pain; large size** (from aortic dilatation after dissection)
  - Need to follow these patients with lifetime serial CT scans; 30% will eventually get aneurysm formation requiring surgery
- **Postop complications for thoracic aortic surgery** – MI, renal failure, paraplegia (especially descending thoracic aortic surgery)
- Paraplegia caused by ischemia due to occlusion of the intercostal arteries and artery of Adamkiewicz during repair

ABDOMINAL AORTIC DISEASE
■ **Abdominal aortic aneurysms (AAAs)**
  - **Normal aorta 2–3 cm**

- Aneurysms form from **degeneration of the medial layer**
- **Most commonly due to atherosclerosis**
- Usually found incidentally
- Risk factors: HTN, male gender, smoking, elderly age

Independent Risk Factors for Detecting an Unknown ≥ 4 cm Diameter AAA During Ultrasound Screening		
Risk Factor	**Odds Ratio**	**95% CI**
Increased risk		
Smoking history	5.1	4.1–6.2
Family history of AAA	1.9	1.6–2.3
Older age (per 7-year interval)	1.7	1.6–1.8
Coronary artery disease	1.5	1.4–1.7
High cholesterol	1.4	1.3–1.6
COPD	1.2	1.1–1.4
Height (per 7-cm interval)	1.2	1.1–1.3
Decreased risk		
Abdominal imaging within 5 years	0.8	0.7–0.9
Deep vein thrombosis	0.7	0.5–0.8
Diabetes mellitus	0.5	0.5–0.8
Black race	0.5	0.4–0.7
Female gender	0.2	0.1–0.5

Odds ratio indicates relative risk compared with patients without that risk factor.
CI, confidence interval; COPD, chronic obstructive pulmonary disease; AAA, abdominal aortic aneurysm.
From Schermerhorn ML, Simosa HF. Type IV thoracoabdominal, infrarenal and pararenal aortic aneurysms. In: Fischer JE, Bland KI, et al., eds. *Mastery of Surgery*. 5th ed. Philadelphia, PA: Lippincott Williams & Wilkins, 2007, with permission.

- Can present with rupture, distal embolization (can cause lower extremity ischemic symptoms, compression of adjacent organs)

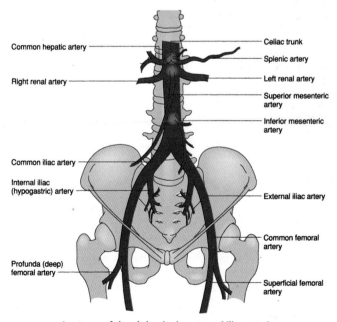

Anatomy of the abdominal aorta and iliac arteries.

- **Rupture**
  - Leading cause of death without an operation
  - Patients often have back or abdominal pain; can have profound hypotension
  - Dx: ultrasound or abdominal CT
  - **AAA rupture risk** – starts to rise in AAAs > 5 cm (5-cm AAA has 15%–20% 5-year risk of rupture); >**8 cm** → 100% rupture risk within 5 years
  - CT shows **fluid** in retroperitoneal space, **extraluminal contrast** with rupture

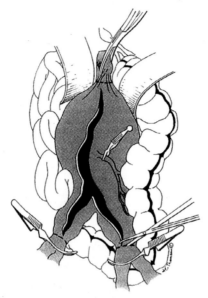

Typical appearance of a ruptured infrarenal aortic aneurysm (AAA) on a contrast-enhanced CT scan. Note the large hematoma to the right of the aorta, obscuring the right psoas muscle and displacing the bowl anteriorly. (From Pomposelli F, Bojovic B. Ruptured abdominal aortic aneurysm. In: Fischer JE, Bland KI, et al., eds. *Mastery of Surgery*. 5th ed. Philadelphia, PA: Lippincott Williams & Wilkins; 2007, with permission.)

  - Most likely to rupture on **left posterolateral wall, 2–4 cm below renals**
  - More likely to rupture in presence of **diastolic HTN or COPD** (thought to be predictors of expansion)
  - **50% mortality with rupture** if patient reaches hospital alive

- **Tx: repair if symptomatic, >5 cm, or growth > 0.5 cm/yr**

  - **Reimplant IMA if backpressure < 40 mm Hg** (poor backbleeding), previous colonic surgery, stenosis at SMA, or flow to left colon appears inadequate
  - **Ligate bleeding lumbar arteries**
  - Maintain flow to at least **one internal iliac artery** (hypogastric) to avoid **vasculogenic impotence**

  - **Complications**
  - **Major vein injury with proximal cross-clamp** – retroaortic renal vein
  - **Impotence** in ⅓ secondary to disruption of autonomic nerves and blood flow to the pelvis
  - 5% mortality with elective repair

- **#1 cause of acute death after surgery** – MI
- **#1 cause of late death after surgery** – renal failure
- **Graft infection rate** – 1%
- **Pseudoaneurysm after graft placement** – 1%
- **Atherosclerotic occlusion** – most common late complication after aortic graft placement
- **Diarrhea (especially bloody)** after AAA worrisome for **ischemic colitis**
- **Inferior mesenteric artery** often sacrificed with AAA repair and can cause ischemia of left colon
  - Dx: endoscopy or abdominal CT; rectum spared from ischemia
  - If patient has peritoneal signs → take to OR for colectomy and colostomy placement
  - Can follow closely if no peritoneal signs

- **Endovascular repair of AAAs** – perioperative complication rates seem to be lower after endovascular repair; however, the long-term outcome of endovascular repair is unknown

Ideal Criteria for Abdominal Aortic Aneurysm (AAA) Endovascular Repair

AAA Morphology	Criteria
Neck length	>15 mm
Neck diameter	<30 mm
Neck angulation	<60 degrees
Common iliac artery length	>35 mm
Common iliac artery diameter	<22 mm
Other	Nontortuous, noncalcified iliac arteries
	Lack of neck thrombus

From Schermerhorn ML, Simosa HF. Type IV thoracoabdominal, infrarenal, and pararenal aortic aneurysms. In: Fischer JE, Bland KI, et al., eds. *Mastery of Surgery*. 5th ed. Philadelphia, PA: Lippincott Williams & Wilkins; 2007, with permission.

Classification of Endoleaks

Classification	Failure Site	Treatment
Type I	Proximal or distal attachment zones	Proximal or distal extension cuffs
	Stent migration	
Type II	Retrograde endoleaks	Percutaneous coil embolization
	Patent lumbar, IMA, intercostals, accessory renal, etc.	Observe (may spontaneously close)
Type III	Midgraft component disconnection	Secondary endograft
	Fabric tear	
Type IV	Graft wall porosity or suture holes	Secondary stenting (nonporous stent)
		Observe
Type V (Endotension)	High intrasac pressure without endoleaks shown	Secondary repair
		Open repair

IMA, inferior mesenteric artery.
From Schermerhorn ML, Simosa HF. Type IV thoracoabdominal, infrarenal, and pararenal aortic aneurysms. In: Fischer JE, Bland KI, et al., eds. *Mastery of Surgery*. 5th ed. Philadelphia, PA: Lippincott Williams & Wilkins; 2007, with permission.

■ **Inflammatory aneurysms**
  - Occurs in 10% of patients with AAA; males
  - Adhesions to the **3rd and 4th portions of the duodenum**
  - **Ureteral entrapment** in 25%
  - <u>Not</u> secondary to infection
  - Weight loss, ↑ ESR, thickened rim above calcifications on CT scan

- May need to place preoperative ureteral stents
- Inflammatory process resolves after aortic graft placement

▪ **Mycotic aneurysms**
- ***Salmonella #1***, *Staphylococcus* #2
- Pain, fevers, positive blood cultures in 50%
- Periaortic fluid, gas, retroperitoneal soft tissue edema, lymphadenopathy
- Usually need extra-anatomic bypass (axillary–femoral w/ femoral to femoral crossover) and resection of infrarenal abdominal aorta to clear infection
- Bacteria infect atherosclerotic plaque, cause aneurysm

▪ **Aortic graft infections**
- ***Staphylococcus #1***, *E. coli* #2
- See fluid, gas, thickening around graft
- Blood cultures negative in many patients
- Treatment of choice is to resect the graft and bypass through noncontaminated field
- More common with grafts going to groin (aortobifemoral grafts)

▪ **Aortoenteric fistula**
- Usually occurs >6 months after surgery
- **Herald bleed with hematemesis**, then blood per rectum
- In 3rd or 4th portion of duodenum near proximal suture line
- Tx: bypass through noncontaminated field; resection of graft with aortic stump closure

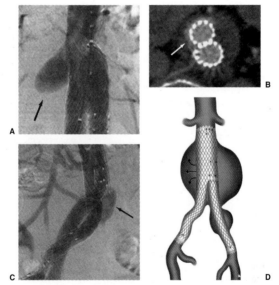

The various endoleaks are demonstrated. *(A)* Type 1 leaks originate at either the proximal or distal attachment sites. Note the large blush of contrast outside of the graft lumen at the proximal fixation site. *(B)* Type 2 leaks are from the collateral circulation originating in the lumbar or inferior mesenteric arteries. Note the contrast filled limbs of the graft and the rim of contrast outside the limbs of the graft but within the lumen of the aorta. The other CT images demonstrated that the leak originated from the inferior mesenteric artery. *(C)* Type 3 leaks are caused by fabric tears or problems at the graft interfaces of the modular devices. Note the contrast blush outside of the lumen of the graft at the modular interface. *(D)* Type 4 leaks are usually transient (<24 hours) transgraft extravasations and can result from the porosity of the graft and needle holes.

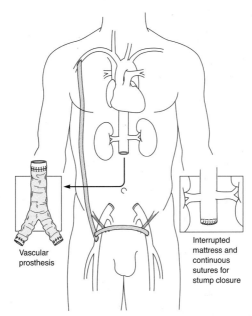

Vascular
prosthesis

Interrupted
mattress and
continuous
sutures for
stump closure

Standard treatment for an infected aortic vascular prosthesis. An axillobifemoral bypass is performed first. This is followed a few days later by removal of the infected aortic prosthesis and careful oversewing of the aortic stump as illustrated. This operation has its greatest usefulness in patients with infected aortoiliac prostheses and who have femoral areas free of infection and good runoff.

PERIPHERAL VASCULAR DISEASE

◼ **Leg compartments**
- **Anterior** – deep peroneal nerve (dorsiflexion, sensation between 1st and 2nd toes), anterior tibial artery
- **Lateral** – superficial peroneal nerve (eversion, lateral foot sensation)
- **Deep posterior** – tibial nerve (plantarflexion), posterior tibial artery, peroneal artery
- **Superficial posterior** – sural nerve

◼ **Signs of PVD** – pallor, hair loss, dependent rubor, abnormal nail growth, slow capillary refill
- Most commonly due to **atherosclerosis**

◼ **Statin drugs (lovastatin)** – #1 preventive agent for atherosclerosis

◼ **Homocystinuria** can ↑ risk of atherosclerosis. Tx: folate, B_6, B_{12}

◼ **Claudication** – medical therapy first → ASA, smoking cessation, exercise until pain occurs to improve collaterals
- 2%/yr **gangrene risk** and 1%/yr **amputation risk** with claudication

◼ **Symptoms occur one level below occlusion**
- **Buttock claudication** – aortoiliac disease
- **Midthigh claudication** – external iliac
- **Calf claudication** – common femoral artery or proximal superficial femoral artery disease
- **Foot claudication** – distal superficial femoral artery or popliteal disease

◼ **Lumbar stenosis** can mimic claudication

◼ **Diabetic neuropathy** can mimic rest pain

◼ **Leriche syndrome**
- No femoral pulses
- Buttock or thigh claudication

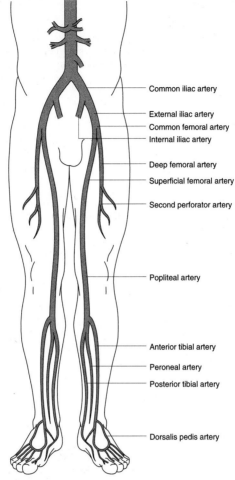

Anatomy of the arterial circulation to the lower extremity.

- Impotence (from hypogastric obstruction and ↓ flow in the internal iliacs)
- Lesion at aortic bifurcation or above

▓ **Most common atherosclerotic occlusion in lower extremities** – Hunter's canal (distal superficial femoral artery exits here). Sartorius muscle covers Hunter's canal

▓ **Collateral circulation** – forms from abnormal pressure gradients
  - Circumflex iliacs to subcostals
  - Circumflex femoral arteries to gluteal arteries
  - Geniculate arteries around the knee

▓ **Postnatal angiogenesis** – budding from preexisting vessels; angiogenin involved

▓ **Ankle–brachial index (ABI)**
  - <0.9 – start to get claudication (typically occurs at same distance each time)

- <0.5 – start to get rest pain (usually across the distal arch and foot)
- <0.4 – ulcers (usually starts in toes)
- <0.3 – gangrene
- ABIs can be very **inaccurate in patients with diabetes** secondary to incompressibility of vessels; often have to go off Doppler waveforms in these patients
- In patients with claudication, the ABI in the extremity drops with walking (i.e., resting ABI may be 0.9 but can drop to <0.6 with exercise resulting in pain)
- ■ **Pulse volume recordings** (PVRs) – to find significant occlusion and at what level
- ■ **Arteriogram** if PVRs suggest significant disease – can also at times treat the patient with angiographic intervention; gold standard for vascular imaging

- ■ **Surgical indications for PVD** – rest pain, ulceration or gangrene, lifestyle limitation, atheromatous embolization
  - **PTFE (Gortex)** – decreases patency when crosses knee
  - **Dacron** – good for aorta and large vessels

  - **Aortoiliac occlusive disease** – most get aortobifemoral repair
    - In high-risk patients can perform bilateral axillary–femoral bypasses or an axillary–femoral bypass with a femoral–femoral crossover (keeps you out of the abdomen)
  - **Isolated iliac lesions** – angioplasty with stent 1st choice; if that fails can perform aortobifemoral repair or femoral-to-femoral crossover
  - **Femoropopliteal grafts**
    - 75% 5-year patency
    - Improved patency rate in patients with surgery for claudication as opposed to limb salvage

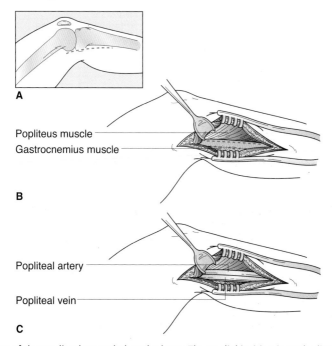

A

Popliteus muscle
Gastrocnemius muscle

B

Popliteal artery

Popliteal vein

C

Exposure of the popliteal artery below the knee. The medial incision is made directly overlying the course of the greater saphenous vein.

- Femoral-distal grafts (peroneal, anterior tibial, or posterior tibial artery)
  - 50% 5-year patency; patency not influenced by level of distal anastomosis
  - Distal lesions more limb threatening because of lack of collaterals
  - **Bypasses distal to knee; usually used only for limb salvage**

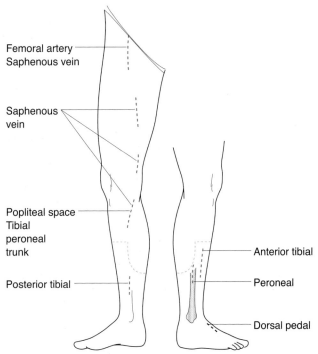

Femoral artery
Saphenous vein

Saphenous
vein

Popliteal space
Tibial
peroneal
trunk

Posterior tibial

Anterior tibial

Peroneal

Dorsal pedal

Placement of incisions for femoropopliteal and femorotibial bypass and for greater saphenous vein harvest. These should avoid the incision lines for a below-knee amputation.

- **Synthetic grafts have decreased patency below the knee** → need to use saphenous vein
- **Extra-anatomic grafts** to avoid hostile conditions in the abdomen (aortic graft infections, multiple previous operations)
- **Femoral-to-femoral crossover graft** – doubles blood flow to donor artery; can get vascular steal in donor leg

- Swelling following lower extremity bypass
  - Get lower extremity duplex to check for DVT
  - 2nd most common cause - **edema from reperfusion injury**
- Complications of reperfusion of ischemic tissue - **lactic acidosis, hyperkalemia, myoglobinuria, compartment syndrome**
- **Atherosclerosis** – #1 cause of late failure of reversed saphenous vein grafts
- **Technical problem** – #1 cause of early failure of reversed saphenous vein grafts

- **Patients with heel ulceration to bone** → amputation

■ **Dry gangrene** – noninfectious; can allow to autoamputate if just toes
  • Larger lesions should probably be amputated
  • See if patient has correctable vascular lesion
■ **Wet gangrene** – infectious; amputation to remove infected necrotic material, antibiotics, surgical emergency
■ **Malperforans ulcer**
  • At metatarsal heads – 2nd MTP most common
  • Diabetics; can have osteomyelitis
  • Tx: nonweightbearing, debridement of metatarsal head (need to remove cartilage), antibiotics; assess need for revascularization

■ **Percutaneous transluminal angioplasty**
  • Excellent for common iliac lesions
  • Best for short stenoses (<15cm)
  • Intima usually ruptured and media stretched, pushes the plaque out
  • Requires passage of wire first
  • **Pseudoaneurysm after arteriography** – thrombin injection with ultrasound guidance
    • Ultrasound duplex best 1st test for this

■ **Compartment syndrome**
  • Most likely to occur in the **anterior compartment of leg (get footdrop)**
  • Pressure > 20–30 mm Hg abnormal; consider fasciotomies → leave open 5–10 days
  • Dx: based on clinical suspicion

■ **Popliteal entrapment syndrome**
  • Most present with mild intermittent claudication
  • Men, 40s; loss of pulses with plantarflexion
  • Usually have medial deviation of artery around medial head of gastrocnemius muscle
  • Tx: **resection of medial head of gastrocnemius muscle**; may need arterial reconstruction

■ **Adventitial cystic disease**
  • Men, 40s; **popliteal most common area**
  • Often bilateral – ganglia originate from adjacent joint capsule or tendon sheath
  • Symptoms: intermittent claudication; changes in symptoms with knee flexion/extension
  • Dx: angiogram
  • Tx: vein graft if vessel occluded; otherwise just resection of cyst

■ **Arterial autografts** – internal iliac artery for children needing renal artery repair, radial grafts for CABG, IMA for CABG

AMPUTATIONS
■ For gangrene, nonhealing ulcers, or unrelenting rest pain not amenable to surgery
■ 50% mortality within 3 years of above-knee amputation (AKA) or below-knee amputation (BKA)
■ **BKA** – 80% heal, 70% walk again, 5% mortality
■ **AKA** – 90% heal, 30% walk again, 10% mortality
■ Emergency amputation for systemic complications, extensive infection, failure of antibiotics

ACUTE ARTERIAL EMBOLI
■ Usually do not have collaterals with emboli (do have collaterals with thrombosis)
■ Usually do not have signs of chronic limb ischemia

- **Contralateral leg** usually has no chronic signs of ischemia and pulses are usually normal
- Usually have no history of claudication
  - 1st pallor → cyanosis → marbling
- Symptoms: pain, pallor, pulselessness, paresthesia, poikilothermia, paralysis
- **Most common cause** – atrial fibrillation
  - Other causes – LV aneurysm with thrombus, prosthetic heart valve, cardiac tumors (myxoma), paradoxical embolus from patent foramen ovale, peripheral arterial or aortic atherosclerotic plaque embolism, aortic or arterial aneurysms with embolism
- **Common femoral artery** most common site of peripheral obstruction from emboli
- Tx: **embolectomy usual**; need to get pulses back; postop angiogram
  - Consider fasciotomy if ischemia >4–6 hours → permanent muscle and nerve damage begins at 4–6 hours
  - Aortoiliac emboli (loss of pulses to both feet) can be treated with bilateral femoral artery cutdowns and bilateral embolectomies

- **Atheroma embolism** – renals most commonly involved; cholesterol clefts in small arteries
  - **Blue toe syndrome** – flaking atherosclerotic emboli off abdominal aorta or branches
    - Patients typically have good distal pulses
    - Aortoiliac disease most common source
  - Dx: need chest/abdomen/pelvis CT scan to look for aneurysmal source, ECHO, angiogram to rule out atherosclerotic disease
  - TX: may need aneurysm repair, endarterectomy, arterial exclusion with bypass

Clinical Distinctions Between Acute Arterial Embolism and Acute Arterial Thrombosis

Embolism	Thrombosis
Arrhythmia	No arrhythmia
No prior claudication or rest pain	History of claudication or rest pain
Normal contralateral pulses	Contralateral pulses absent
No physical findings of chronic limb ischemia	Physical findings of chronic limb ischemia

ACUTE ARTERIAL THROMBOSIS

- These patients usually do <u>not</u> have arrhythmias
- Do have a history of claudication and have signs of chronic limb ischemia and poor pulses in the contralateral leg
- Tx: threatened limb → give heparin and go to OR for thrombectomy; if limb not threatened can go to angiography for thrombolytics
- **Thrombosis of PTFE graft** → thrombolytics and anticoagulation; if limb threatened → OR

Limb threatening ischemia / Critical Limb Ischemia / chronic Limb ischemia:
(1) rest pain or (2) tissue loss —(a) gangrene (b) non-healing ulcers

RENAL VASCULAR DISEASE – RENOVASCULAR HYPERTENSION

- Right renal artery runs posterior to IVC
- Accessory renal arteries in 25%
- **Most renal emboli from heart**
- **Renal atherosclerosis** – left side, proximal ⅓, men
  - Tx: PTA with stent
- **Fibromuscular dysplasia** – right side, distal ⅓, women
  - Tx: PTA with stent
- **Suggestive of renovascular HTN** – bruits, diastolic blood pressure > 115, worsening HTN, children, premenopausal women, rapid onset after age 50, HTN resistant to drug therapy

- ■ Need to rule out other sources of HTN (pheochromocytoma, etc.)
- ■ **Dx of renal artery stenosis**: angiogram
- ■ Tx: PTA with stent
- ■ **Indications for nephrectomy with renal HTN** → atrophic kidney < 6 cm and minimal collaterals with persistently ↑ renin levels

UPPER EXTREMITY

- ■ **Occlusive disease** – proximal lesions usually asymptomatic secondary to ↑ collaterals
  - Subclavian most common site of stenosis
  - Tx: PTA with stent; can also perform common carotid to subclavian bypass

- ■ **Subclavian steal syndrome** – proximal subclavian artery stenosis resulting in reversal of flow through ipsilateral vertebral artery into subclavian
  - Operate with limb or neurologic (usually vertebrobasilar) symptoms
  - Tx: carotid to subclavian bypass or PTA

- ■ **Thoracic outlet syndrome**
  - **Normal anatomy**
    - **Subclavian vein** – passes over the 1st rib anterior to the anterior scalene muscle, then behind clavicle
    - **Brachial plexus and subclavian artery** – pass over the 1st rib posterior to the anterior scalene muscle, and anterior to the middle scalene muscle
  - Dx: CXR, cervical spine x-ray, angiography if thought to be vascular etiology; EMG
  - Can get back and neck symptoms
  - **Adson's test** – ↓ radial pulse with head turned ipsilateral side (subclavian artery compression)
  - **Tinsel's test** – tapping reproduces symptoms

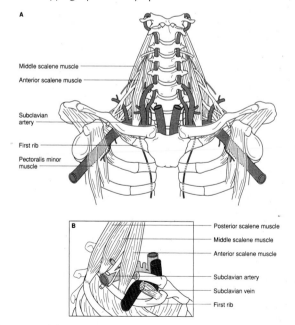

The normal anatomy of the thoracic outlet in anteroposterior *(A)* and oblique *(B)* views. The brachial plexus and subclavian artery traverse the narrow triangle formed by the anterior and middle scalene muscles and the first rib. The subclavian vein lies anteriorly.

- **Neurologic involvement** – much more common than vascular
- **#1 anatomic abnormality** – cervical rib
- **#1 cause of pain** – brachial plexus irritation

- **Brachial plexus irritation**
  - Usually have normal neurologic exam
  - ↑ back and neck symptoms
  - Palpation/manipulation – can ↑ symptoms
  - **Ulnar nerve** distribution (C8–T1) most common
  - Triceps weakness and atrophy, weakness of intrinsic muscles of hand, weak wrist flexion
  - Located on inferior portion of brachial plexus
  - **Radial nerve** – located on superior portion of brachial plexus
  - Finger extensors, wrist extension
  - Tx: resection of cervical ribs, divide **anterior scalenes** and middle scalenes, +/− 1st rib resection

- **Subclavian artery**
  - Compression usually secondary to **anterior scalene hypertrophy** (pitchers)
  - Absent radial pulse with maximal arm abduction
  - Tx: **surgery** → cervical rib and 1st rib resection, divide anterior scalene muscle, bypass graft

- **Subclavian vein**
  - Usually presents as effort-induced thrombosis of subclavian vein (Paget–von Schrötter disease)
  - Venous thrombosis – much more common than arterial
  - Venography – gold standard for diagnosis
  - Male gender; pain and swelling ↑ with activity, ↓ with rest
  - 80% have associated thoracic outlet problem
  - Tx: **thrombolytics, heparin, warfarin** initial treatment; repair at that admission

■ **Motor function can remain in digits** after prolonged ischemia because motor groups are in proximal forearm

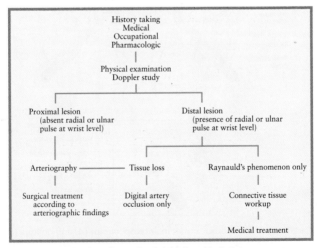

Workup for patients with hand ischemia.

MESENTERIC ISCHEMIA

■ Overall mortality 50%–70%
■ Findings on abdominal CT that suggest intestinal ischemia – bowel wall thickening, intramural gas, portal venous gas, vascular occlusion
■ Most common causes of visceral ischemia
  • **Acute embolic occlusion** – 50%
  • **Thrombotic occlusion** – 25%
  • **Low-flow state** – 15%
  • **Venous thrombosis** – 5%

■ **Superior mesenteric artery embolism**
  • Most commonly occurs near origin of SMA – heart #1 source
  • Pain out of proportion to exam; pain usually of sudden onset; hematochezia; peritoneal signs late finding
  • May have a history of atrial fibrillation, endocarditis, recent MI, recent angiography
  • Dx: angiogram or abdominal CT with IV contrast
  • Tx: volume resuscitation, antibiotics, **embolectomy**, resect infarcted bowel, heparin

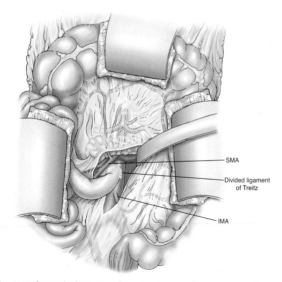

Exposure of the SMA for embolectomy. The omentum and transverse colon are lifted cephalad. All small bowel is retracted to the right, and the sigmoid colon packed to the left. The ligament of Treitz and the superior attachments of the duodenum are sharply divided, with the goal of mobilizing the last portion of the duodenum to the right. Then, with four fingers behind the small bowel mesentry and with the thumb anteriorly, the SMA should be palpable near the base of the transverse colon mesentery. (From Ozaki CK. Superior mesenteric artery embolectomy. In: Fischer JE, Bland KI, et al., eds. *Mastery of Surgery*. 5th ed. Philadelphia, PA: Lippincott Williams & Wilkins; 2007, with permission.)

■ **Superior mesenteric artery thrombosis**
  • Usually have history of chronic problems (food fear from mesenteric angina), weight loss
  • May have a history of vasculitis or hypercoagulable state
  • Symptoms: similar to embolism; may have developed some collaterals

- Dx: angiogram or abdominal CT with IV contrast
- Tx: **thrombectomy**, usually need **SMA bypass**, resection of infarcted bowel, heparin

■ **Mesenteric vein thrombosis**
- Usually short segments of intestine involved; bloody diarrhea, crampy abdominal pain
- May have a history of vasculitis, hypercoagulable state, portal HTN
- Dx: abdominal CT scan or angiogram
- Tx: **heparin**, thrombolytics; can try mesenteric vein thrombectomy if diagnosed early; resection of infarcted bowel

■ **Nonocclusive mesenteric ischemia**
- Spasm, low-flow states, hypovolemia, hemoconcentration, digoxin → final common pathway is low cardiac output state to visceral vessels
- Risk factors: prolonged shock, CHF, prolonged cardiopulmonary bypass
- Bloody diarrhea, pain
- Watershed areas (Griffith's and Sudak's points) most vulnerable
- Tx: volume resuscitation, glucagon, papaverine, nitrates can ↑ visceral blood flow; also need to ↑ cardiac output; resection of infarcted bowel

■ **Median arcuate ligament syndrome**
- Causes celiac compression
- **Bruit near epigastrium**, chronic pain, weight loss, diarrhea
- Tx: transect median arcuate ligament; may need arterial reconstruction

■ **Chronic mesenteric angina**
- Weight loss secondary to food fear
- Visceral angina occurs 30 minutes after meals (food fear)
- May need PTA, bypass, or endarterectomy
- Get lateral visceral vessel aortography to see origins of celiac and SMA

■ Arc of Riolan is an important collateral between the SMA and celiac

ANEURYSMS
■ **Rupture** – most common complication of aneurysms above inguinal ligament
■ **Thrombosis and emboli** – most common complications of aneurysm below inguinal ligament
■ **Visceral**
- **Repair all splanchnic aneurysms when diagnosed (50% risk for rupture) except splenic**
- **Splenic artery aneurysm** – most common visceral aneurysm (more common in women, 2% risk of rupture)
  - Repair splenic artery aneurysms if **symptomatic, if patient is pregnant, or if occurs in women of childbearing age**
  - High rate of pregnancy-related rupture – usually occurs in **3rd trimester**
- **Diameters > 2 cm considered aneurysmal**
- Most visceral aneurysms are treated with exclusion and bypass graft
- **Splenic and proximal common hepatic** can just be excluded (have good collaterals)
- Risk factors: medial fibrodysplasia, portal HTN, arterial disruption secondary to inflammatory disease (i.e., pancreatitis)

■ **Iliac**
- Surgical indications: symptomatic (thrombosis, emboli, or compression), >3.0 cm, mycotic
- Tx: bypass with exclusion

- ▨ **Femoral**
  - Surgical indications: symptomatic (thrombosis, emboli, or compression), >2.5 cm, mycotic
  - Tx: bypass with exclusion
- ▨ **Popliteal**
  - Most common peripheral aneurysm
  - Leg exam reveals prominent popliteal pulses
  - ½ are **bilateral**
  - ½ have **another aneurysm elsewhere** (AAA, femoral, etc.)
  - Most likely to get **thrombosis or emboli with limb ischemia**
  - Can also get leg pain from compression of adjacent structures
  - Surgical indications: symptomatic, >2 cm, mycotic
  - Dx: ultrasound
  - Tx: exclusion and bypass of all popliteal aneurysms; 25% have complication that requires amputation if not treated
- ▨ **Femoral pseudoaneurysm**
  - Collection of blood in continuity with the arterial system but unenclosed by all 3 layers of the arterial wall
  - Can result from disruption of a suture line between graft and artery or from percutaneous interventions
  - Tx: if occurs after percutaneous intervention, need ultrasound-guided compression with thrombin injection → if flow remains in the pseudoaneurysm or if pseudoaneurysm is at a suture site, need surgical repair
- ▨ **Renal**
  - Surgical indications: symptomatic, expansion, >1.5 cm; women who want pregnancy
  - Tx: reconstruction with vein patch; nephrectomy if rupture occurs

Percutaneous stents mat be an option for many of the above

OTHER VASCULAR DISEASES
- ▨ **Fibromuscular dysplasia**
  - Young women; HTN if renal involved
  - Renal (right side) most commonly involved vessel, followed by carotid and iliac
  - String of beads
  - Medial fibrodysplasia most common variant (80%–90%)
  - Tx: PTA (1st choice) or bypass

- ▨ **Buerger's disease**
  - Young men, smokers, corkscrew collateral on angiogram and severe distal disease
  - Severe rest pain with bilateral ulceration
  - Gangrene of the digits, especially the fingers
  - Normal arterial tree proximal to popliteal and brachial vessels (small vessel disease)
  - Tx: stop smoking or will require continued amputations

- ▨ **Cystic medial necrosis syndromes**
  - **Marfan's disease**
    - Type I collagen defect; Marfanoid habitus, retinal detachment, aortic root dilatation
  - **Ehlers–Danlos syndrome**
    - Many types of collagen defects identified
    - Easy bruising, hypermobile joints, tendency for **arterial rupture**, especially abdominal vessels

- Get aneurysms and dissections
- <u>No</u> angiograms → risk of laceration to vessel
- Often too difficult to repair and need ligation of vessels to control hemorrhage

■ **Immune arteritis**
- **Large arteries**
  - **Temporal arteritis**
    - Giant cell arteritis, granulomatous disease
    - Involves inflammation of large vessels
    - Long segments of smooth stenosis alternating with segments of larger diameter
    - Women, age > 55; visual changes (risk of blindness)
    - Symptoms: fever, arthralgia, myalgia, anorexia
    - Can affect branches of aorta and aorta itself and pulmonary artery
    - Tx: **steroids**, bypass of large vessels if needed; <u>no</u> endarterectomy
  - **Takayasu's arteritis** – same pathology, symptoms, and treatment as temporal arteritis; affects women < 35 years
- **Medium arteries**
  - **Polyarteritis nodosa**
    - Get aneurysms that thrombose or rupture
    - Renals most commonly involved
    - Tx: **steroids**
  - **Kawasaki's disease**
    - Children; get dilated coronaries and brachiocephalic vessels
    - Die from arrhythmias
    - Tx: **steroids, possible CABG**
- **Small arteries**
  - **Hypersensitivity angiitis**
  - Often secondary to drug/tumor antigens
  - Symptoms: rash, fever, symptoms of end-organ dysfunction
  - Tx: **calcium channel blockers, pentoxifylline,** stop offending agent

■ **Radiation arteritis**
- **Early** – sloughing and thrombosis (obliterative endarteritis)
- **Late** (1–10 years) – fibrosis, scar, stenosis
- **Late late** (3–30 years) – advanced atherosclerosis

■ **Raynaud's disease** – young women; pallor → cyanosis → rubor
- **Tx: calcium channel blockers, warmth**

VENOUS DISEASE
■ **Greater saphenous vein** – joins femoral vein near groin; runs medially
■ **Lesser saphenous vein** – joins popliteal vein in lower leg; runs lateral at first
■ <u>No</u> clamps on IVC → will tear
■ **Left renal vein** can be ligated safely because of increased collaterals → left gonadal vein, left adrenal vein
■ **Access grafts**
- Most common failure of A-V grafts for dialysis – **venous obstruction secondary to intimal hyperplasia**
- **Cimino** – radial artery to cephalic vein; wait 6 weeks to use → allows vein to mature
- **Interposition graft** – wait 6 weeks to allow fibrous scar to form

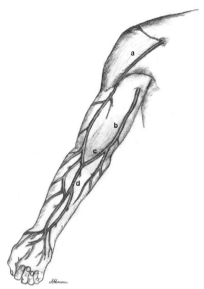

Veins of the arm. *a.* Cephalic vein. *b.* Basilic vein. *c.* Median cubital vein. *d.* Median ante-brachial vein. (From Hamdan AD, Evenson AR, Grunwaldt L. Use of arm vein conduit for lower extremity revascularization. In: Fischer JE, Bland KI, et al., eds. *Mastery of Surgery.* 5th ed. Philadelphia, PA: Lippincott Williams & Wilkins; 2007, with permission.)

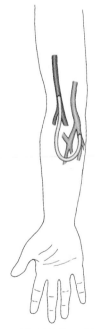

Brachiobasilic loop graft. (From Hayashi MS, Wilson SE. Prosthetic bridge grafts. In: Fischer JE, Bland KI, et al., eds. *Mastery of Surgery.* 5th ed. Philadelphia, PA: Lippincott Williams & Wilkins; 2007, with permission.)

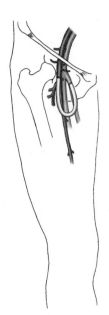

Femoro-saphenous loop graft. (From Hayashi MS, Wilson SE. Prosthetic bridge grafts. In: Fischer JE, Bland KI, et al., eds. *Mastery of Surgery*. 5th ed. Philadelphia, PA: Lippincott Williams & Wilkins; 2007, with permission.)

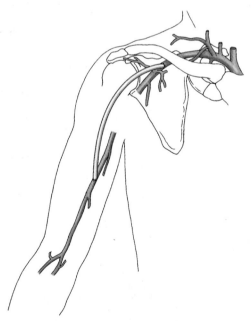

Brachioaxillary straight graft. (From Hayashi MS, Wilson SE. Prosthetic bridge grafts. In: Fischer JE, Bland KI, et al., eds. *Mastery of Surgery*. 5th ed. Philadelphia, PA: Lippincott Williams & Wilkins; 2007, with permission.)

■ **Acquired A-V fistula** – usually secondary to trauma; can get peripheral arterial insufficiency, CHF, aneurysm, limb-length discrepancy
■ Most need repair → lateral venous suture; arterial side may need bypass graft

■ **Varicose veins**
- Smoking, obesity, low activity
- Tx: stockings, elevation, exercise, sclerotherapy → most do <u>not</u> need surgery
- Surgery for severe symptoms, recurrent ulcers, severe varicosities
- DVT contraindication to sclerotherapy and vein stripping

■ **Venous ulcers**
- Secondary to venous valve incompetence (90%)
- Unna boot compression cures 90%
- May need to ligate perforators or have vein stripping of greater saphenous vein

■ **Venous insufficiency**
- Aching, swelling, night cramps, brawny edema
- Ulceration occurs above and posterior to malleoli
- Edema – secondary to incompetent perforators
- Elevation brings relief
- **Trendelenburg test**
  - 1st part – elevate leg, occlude greater saphenofemoral vein junction, lower leg → rapid filling of greater saphenous vein suggests incompetent perforators
  - 2nd part – if 1st part did not fill greater saphenous vein, release pressure on saphenofemoral junction → rapid filling of greater saphenous vein suggests incompetent valves in greater saphenous
- Tx: leg wraps, ambulation with avoidance of long standing; ulcers < 3 cm often heal without surgery
  - Greater saphenous vein stripping with moderate to severe symptoms, recurrent ulceration despite medical Tx

■ **Superficial thrombophlebitis** – nonbacterial inflammation
- Tx: NSAIDs, warm packs, ambulation
■ **Suppurative thrombophlebitis** – fever, ↑ WBCs, erythema, fluctuance
- Tx: resect vein
■ **Migrating thrombophlebitis** – pancreatic CA
■ **Mondor's disease** – self-limiting thrombophlebitis of the breast

■ **Normal venous Doppler ultrasound** – augmentation of flow with distal compression or release of proximal compression

■ **Sequential compression devices (SCDs)** – help prevent blood clots by ↓ venous stasis, ↑ AT-III, tPA, and ↑ fibrinolysin

■ **Deep venous thrombosis (DVT)**
- Most common in calf
- Pain, tenderness, calf swelling
- **Left leg 2×** more involved than right (longer left iliac vein compressed by right iliac artery)
- **Risk factors: Virchow's triad** → venous stasis, hypercoagulability, venous wall injury
- **Calf DVT** – minimal swelling
- **Femoral DVT** – ankle and calf swelling
- **Iliofemoral DVT** – severe leg swelling
- **Phlegmasia alba dolens** – tenderness, pallor (whiteness), edema
  - Tx: heparin

- **Phlegmasia cerulea dolens** – tenderness, cyanosis (blueness), massive edema
  - Tx: heparin; rarely need surgery
- **Long-term Tx**
  - 1st – Coumadin 6 months
  - 2nd – Coumadin 1 year
  - 3rd or pulmonary embolism – Coumadin lifetime
- **Filter** – contraindication to anticoagulation; PE while on Coumadin, free-floating ileofemoral thrombi; after pulmonary embolectomy
- **Pulmonary embolism with filter in place** – comes from ovarian veins, inferior vena cava superior to filter, or from upper extremity

■ **Pulmonary embolism**
  - Get ↓ pO_2 and ↓ pCO_2, ↑ RR, respiratory alkalosis, shock if massive
  - Most PEs arise from above the knee
  - Tx: heparin if symptomatic; lifetime Coumadin
    - Some say all of these patients should get a filter
    - If patient is in shock, go to OR for emergency pulmonary artery thrombectomy

■ **Venous thrombosis with central line** – pull out if not needed; can try to treat with systemic heparin or TPA down line

LYMPHATICS
■ **Do not contain a basement membrane**
■ **Not found in bone, muscle, tendon, cartilage, brain, or cornea**

■ **Lymphedema**
  - Occurs when lymphatics are obstructed, too few in number, or nonfunctional
  - Leads to woody edema secondary to fibrous tissue in subcutaneous tissue – toes, feet, ankle, leg
  - Cellulitis and lymphangitis secondary to minor trauma – big problem
  - Strep most common infection
  - Deep lymphatics have valves
  - **Congenital lymphedema L > R**
  - Tx: leg elevation, compression, antibiotics for infection

■ **Lymphangiosarcoma**
  - Raised blue/red coloring; early metastases to lung
  - Stewart–Treves syndrome – associated with breast axillary dissection

■ **Lymphangiectasia** – dilation of preexisting lymphatic channels
  - Dx: lymphangiography
  - Tx: resection

■ **Lymphocele** following surgery
  - Usually after dissection in the groin (i.e., for femoral to popliteal bypass)
  - Leakage clear fluid; need to rule out an infectious source for the fluid (send cultures, get CT scan of area)
  - Small lymphoceles can be observed (may resorb spontaneously)
  - Large or symptomatic or lying close to graft material – need early excision
  - Tx: inject **isosulfan blue dye** into foot to identify the lymphatic channels supplying the lymphocele
  - Resect the lymphocele and ligate the supplying lymphatic channel

Gastrin – produced by G cells in **antrum**
  Secretion stimulated by amino acids, vagal input (acetylcholine), calcium, ETOH, antral distention, pH > 3.0
  Secretion inhibited by pH < 3.0, somatostatin, secretin, CCK, vasoactive intestinal peptide, gastric inhibitory peptide
  Target cells – parietal cells and chief cells
  Response – ↑ HCl, intrinsic factor, and pepsinogen secretion
  Omeprazole blocks H/K ATPase of parietal cell **(final pathway for H$^+$ release)**

Somatostatin – produced by D (somatostatin) cells in **antrum**
  Secretion stimulated by acid in duodenum
  Target cells – many; is the great inhibitor
  Response – inhibits gastrin and HCl release; inhibits release of insulin, glucagons, secretin, GIP, motilin, neurotensin, enteroglucagon; ↓ pancreatic and biliary output
  Octreotide (somatostatin analogue) – can be used to ↓ pancreatic fistula output

Gastric inhibitory peptide – produced by K cells in **duodenum**
  Secretion stimulated by amino acids, glucose, long-chain fatty acids, ↓ pH
  Target cells – parietal cells of stomach and beta cells of pancreas
  Response – ↓ HCl secretion and pepsin; ↑ insulin release

CCK – produced by I cells of **duodenum** and jejunum
  Secretion stimulated by amino acids and fatty acid chains
  Response – gallbladder contraction, relaxation of sphincter of Oddi, ↑ pancreatic enzyme secretion, some ↑ in intestinal motility

Secretin – produced by S cells of **duodenum**
  Secretion stimulated by fat, bile, pH < 4.0
  Secretion inhibited by pH > 4.0, gastrin
  Response – ↑ pancreatic HCO$_3^-$ release, ↑ bile flow, inhibits gastrin release (this is reversed in patients with gastrinoma), and inhibits HCl release
    High pancreatic duct output – ↑ HCO$_3^-$, ↓ Cl$^-$
    Slow pancreatic duct output – ↑ Cl$^-$, ↓ HCO$_3^-$ (carbonic anhydrase in duct exchanges HCO$_3^-$ for Cl$^-$)

Vasoactive intestinal peptide – produced by cells in **gut and pancreas**
  Secretion stimulated by fat, acetylcholine
  Response – ↑ intestinal secretion (water and electrolytes) and motility
  Inhibits gastrin release

Insulin – released by beta cells of the **pancreas**
  Secretion stimulated by glucose, glucagons, CCK
  Secretion inhibited by somatostatin, pancreatostatin
  Response – cellular glucose uptake; promotes protein synthesis

Glucagon – released by alpha cells of the **pancreas** (also from alpha cells in stomach, intestine)
  Secretion stimulated by ↓ glucose, ↑ amino acids, acetylcholine, gastrin-releasing peptide
  Secretion inhibited by ↑ glucose, ↑ insulin, somatostatin

Response – glycogenolysis, gluconeogenesis, lipolysis, ketogenesis, ↓ gastric acid secretion, ↓ pancreatic secretion, ↓ intestinal motility, ↓ stomach motility, ↑ LES pressure, ↓ MMCs

Pancreatic polypeptide – secreted by islet cells in **pancreas**
Secretion stimulated by food, vagal stimulation, other GI hormones
Response – ↓ pancreatic and gallbladder secretion

Motilin – release by intestinal cells of gut
Secretion stimulated by duodenal acid, food, vagus input, gastrin-releasing peptide
Secretion inhibited by somatostatin, secretin, pancreatic polypeptide, duodenal fat
Response – ↑ intestinal (small bowel) motility → **erythromycin** acts on this receptor

Bombesin (gastrin-releasing peptide) – ↑ intestinal motor activity, ↑ pancreatic enzyme secretion, ↑ gastric acid secretion
Peptide YY – released from terminal ileum following a fatty meal → inhibits acid secretion and stomach contraction; inhibits gallbladder contraction and pancreatic secretion

Anorexia – mediated by hypothalamus

Bowel recovery
Small bowel 24 hours
Stomach 48 hours
Large bowel 3–5 days

ANATOMY AND PHYSIOLOGY

- Squamous epithelium, circular inner muscle layer, outer longitudinal muscle layer; no serosa

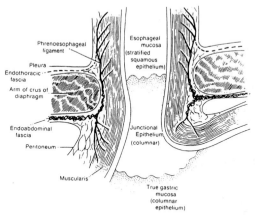

Coronal section through gastroesophageal junction and esophageal hiatus of diaphragm. (From Skandalakis LJ, Colborn GL, Skandalakis JE, et al. The stomach and duodenum. In: Fischer JE, Bland KI, et al., eds. *Mastery of Surgery*. 5th ed. Philadelphia, PA: Lippincott Williams & Wilkins; 2007, with permission.)

- Vessels directly off the aorta are the major blood supply to the esophagus

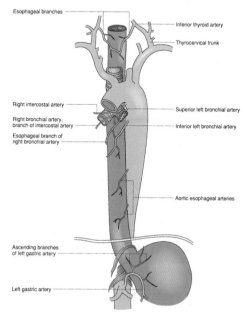

Arterial blood supply of the esophagus.

- Cervical esophagus – supplied by the inferior thyroid artery
- Abdominal esophagus – supplied by the left gastric artery and inferior phrenic arteries
- Lymphatics – upper ⅔ drains cephalad, lower ⅓ caudad
- Upper esophagus – **striated muscle**
- Lower esophagus – **smooth muscle**

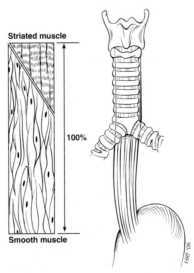

Graduation of striated to smooth muscle fibers. (From Lerut T, Stamenkovic S, Coosemans W, et al. The esophagus. In: Fischer JE, Bland KI, et al., eds. *Mastery of Surgery*. 5th ed. Philadelphia, PA: Lippincott Williams & Wilkins; 2007, with permission.)

- **Right vagus nerve** – travels on posterior portion of stomach as it exits chest; becomes **celiac plexus**; also has the criminal nerve of Grassi → can cause persistently high acid levels postoperatively if left undivided
- **Left vagus nerve** – travels on anterior portion of stomach; goes to **liver and biliary tree**
- **Thoracic duct** – travels from right to left in chest at upper ⅓ of mediastinum; inserts into left subclavian vein
- **Upper esophageal sphincter (15 cm from incisors)** – cricopharyngeus muscle (circular muscle, prevents air swallowing); has recurrent laryngeal nerve innervation
  - Normal UES pressure with food bolus – 12–14 mm Hg
  - Normal UES pressure at rest – 50–70 mm Hg
  - **Cricopharyngeus muscle** – most common site of esophageal perforation (usually occurs with EGD)
  - **Aspiration with brainstem stroke** – failure of UES (cricopharyngeus) to relax
- **Lower esophageal sphincter (40 cm from incisors)** – relaxation mediated by inhibitory neurons; muscle is normally contracted at resting state → prevents reflux
  - Normal LES pressure at rest 10–20 mm Hg

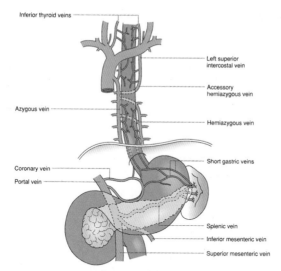

Venous drainage of the esophagus.

- ■ **Anatomic areas of narrowing**
  - Cricopharyngeus muscle
  - Compression by the left mainstem bronchus and aortic arch
  - Diaphragm
- ■ **Swallowing stages** – CNS initiates swallow
  - Normal esophageal pressures with food bolus – 70–120 mm Hg
  - **Primary peristalsis** – occurs with food bolus and swallow initiation
  - **Secondary peristalsis** – occurs with incomplete emptying and esophageal distention, propagating waves
  - **Tertiary peristalsis** – nonpropagating, nonperistalsing (dysfunctional)
  - UES and LES are normally contracted between meals
- ■ **Swallowing mechanism** – soft palate occludes nasopharynx, larynx rises and airway opening is blocked by epiglottis, cricopharyngeus relaxes, pharyngeal contraction moves food into esophagus. **LES relaxes** soon after initiation of swallow

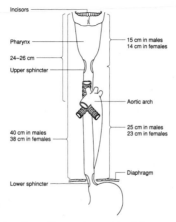

Important clinical endoscopic measurements of the esophagus in adults.

- **Surgical approach**
  - Cervical esophagus – **left**
  - Upper ⅔ thoracic – **right (avoids the aorta)**
  - Lower ⅓ thoracic – **left (left-sided course in this region)**

- **Hiccoughs**
  - Causes – gastric distention, temperature changes, ETOH, tobacco
  - Reflex arc – vagus, phrenic, sympathetic chain T6–12

- **Esophageal dysfunction**
  - <u>Primary</u> – unknown cause
  - <u>Secondary</u> – systemic disease, gastroesophageal reflux disease (GERD; most common), scleroderma, polymyositis

- **Endoscopy** – procedure of choice for **heartburn** → can visualize esophagitis, etc.
- Barium swallow – **procedure of choice for** dysphagia and odynophagia **(better at picking up masses)**
- **Meat impaction** – Dx and Tx: endoscopy

PHARYNGOESOPHAGEAL DISORDERS
- Trouble in transferring food from mouth to esophagus
- Most commonly neuromuscular disease – myasthenia gravis, Parkinson's disease, polymyositis, muscular dystrophy, Zenker's diverticulum, lye ingestion, stroke
- **Liquids worse than solids**
- **Cervical esophageal dysphagia** – Plummer–Vinson syndrome; usually due to web; Fe-deficient anemia. Tx: **dilation, Fe; need to screen for oral CA**

DIVERTICULA
- **Zenker's diverticulum** – caused by ↑ pressure during swallowing
- Is a **false diverticulum** – **posterior**
  - **Occurs between the cricopharyngeus and pharyngeal constrictors**
  - Symptoms: upper esophageal dysphagia, choking, halitosis
  - Dx: **barium swallow studies**, manometry; risk for perforation with EGD and Zenker's

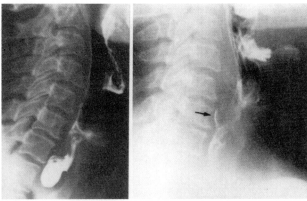

A   B

(A) Contrast study with preoperative appearance of Zenker diverticulum. *(B)* Same patient after extramucosal myotomy and diverticulopexy; with free passage of the contrast material. The suspended diverticulum is visible as a small contrast line *(arrow)*. (From Lerut ALR, Coosemans W, Decker G, et al. Pathophysiology and treatment of Zenker diverticulum. In: Fischer JE, Bland KI, et al., eds. *Mastery of Surgery*. 5th ed. Philadelphia, PA: Lippincott Williams & Wilkins; 2007, with permission.)

- Tx: <u>**cricopharyngeal myotomy**</u> (key point); Zenker's itself can either be resected or suspended (removal of diverticula not necessary)
  - Left cervical incision; leave drains in; esophagogram POD #1

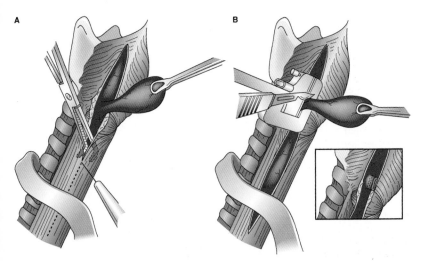

Cervical esophagomyotomy and concomitant resection of a pharyngoesophageal diverticulum. *(A)* An esophagomyotomy is performed for several centimeters in either vertical direction from the base of the mobilized diverticulum. *(B)* After completion of the esophagomyotomy, the base of the pouch is crossed with a TA-30 stapler and amputated.

- **Traction diverticulum**
  - Is a **true diverticulum** – usually lies **lateral**
  - Due to inflammation, granulomatous disease, tumor
  - Usually found in the mid-esophagus
  - Symptoms: regurgitation of undigested food, dysphagia
  - Tx: excision and primary closure, may need palliative therapy (i.e., XRT) if due to invasive CA

- **Epiphrenic diverticulum**
  - Rare; associated with esophageal motility disorders
  - Most common in the distal 10 cm of the esophagus
  - Most are asymptomatic; can have dysphagia and regurgitation
  - Dx: esophagram and esophageal manometry
  - Tx: diverticulectomy and long esophageal myotomy on the side opposite the diverticulectomy

ACHALASIA
- Dysphagia, regurgitation, weight loss, respiratory symptoms
- Caused by **failure of peristalsis and lack of LES relaxation** after food bolus
- Secondary to **neuronal degeneration** in muscle wall
- Manometry – ↑ **LES pressure, incomplete LES relaxation, no peristalsis**
- Can get tortuous dilated esophagus and epiphrenic diverticula; birdbeak appearance

- Tx: calcium channel blocker, LES dilation → effective in 60%; nitrates
  - If medical Tx and dilation fail → Heller myotomy – left thoracotomy, transect circular layer of muscle <u>lower</u> esophagus; also need partial Nissen fundoplication
- *T. cruzi* can produce similar symptoms

DIFFUSE ESOPHAGEAL SPASM
- Chest pain; other symptoms can be similar to achalasia. May have psychiatric history
- Manometry – frequent strong body contractions of ↑ amplitude and duration, **normal LES tone, strong unorganized contractions**
- Surgery better at resolving dysphagia than pain
- Nutcracker esophagus has similar symptoms
- Tx: calcium channel blocker, nitrates, antispasmodics, Heller myotomy (transect circular layer of <u>upper</u> and <u>lower</u> esophagus)
- Treatment usually less effective for diffuse esophageal spasm than for achalasia

SCLERODERMA
- Causes dysphagia, loss of LES tone; most have strictures, fibrous replacement of smooth muscle
- Tx: esophagectomy; Nissen may be effective in some

GASTROESOPHAGEAL REFLUX DISEASE
- **Normal anatomic protection from GERD** – need LES competence, normal esophageal body, normal gastric reservoir
- ↑ acid exposure to esophagus from loss of the normal gastroesophageal barrier
- Get heartburn symptoms 30–60 minutes after meals
- Can also have asthma symptoms (cough), choking, PNA
- Symptoms worse lying down
- Need to make sure patient does not have another cause for the pain
  - **Dysphagia/odynophagia** – need to worry about tumors
  - **Bloating** – suggests aerophagia and delayed gastric emptying (Dx gastric emptying study)
  - **Epigastric pain** – suggests peptic ulcer, tumor
- Dx: endoscopy, pH probe (best test), manometry (resting LES < 6 mm Hg), histology
- **Medical therapy 1st**: omeprazole for 12 weeks
- **Surgical indications**: GERD on pH monitoring, failure of medical Tx, complications of GERD (stricture, Barrett's esophagus, cancer)
- Tx: **Nissen** → divide short gastrics, pull esophagus into abdomen, repair defect in phrenoesophageal membrane; 270- (partial) or 360-degree gastric fundus wrap
  - Phrenoesophageal membrane is an extension of the transversalis fascia
  - Key maneuver is identification of the **left crura**
  - Complications – injury to spleen, diaphragm, esophagus, or pneumothorax
  - **Belsey** – approach is through the chest
  - **Collis gastroplasty** – when not enough esophagus exists to pull down into abdomen, can staple along stomach and create a "new" esophagus
  - Most common cause of dysphagia following Nissen – **wrap is too tight**

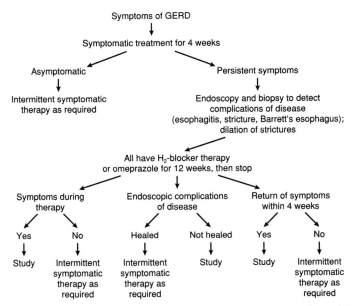

Algorithm for selecting patients with symptoms suggestive of GERD for further study.

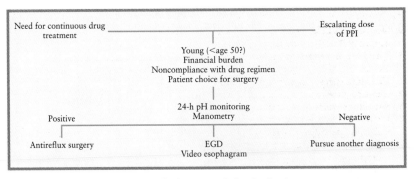

Indications for laparoscopic fundoplication.

HIATAL HERNIA (ALSO SEE GERD, ABOVE)
- Type I – sliding hernia from dilation of hiatus (most common); often associated with GERD
- Type II – paraesophageal; hole in the diaphragm alongside the esophagus, normal GE junction. Symptoms: chest pain, dysphagia, early satiety
- Type III – combined
- Type IV – entire stomach in the chest plus another organ (i.e., colon, spleen)
- With type II, still need **Nissen** as diaphragm repair can affect LES; also helps anchor stomach
- **Paraesophageal hernia (type II)** – all need repair → high risk of incarceration
- Most patients with type I hiatal hernia do not have reflux
- Most patients with significant reflux do have type I hiatal hernia

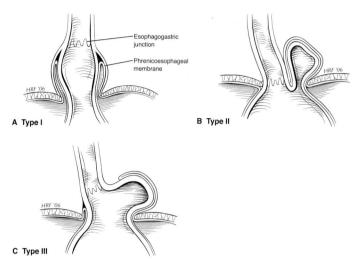

Classification of hiatal hernia. *(A)* Type 1, sliding. *(B)* Type II, pure paraesophageal. *(C)* Type III, mixed hernia. (From Critchlow J. Paraesophageal herniation. In: Fischer JE, Bland KI, et al., eds. *Mastery of Surgery.* 5th ed. Philadelphia, PA: Lippincott Williams & Wilkins; 2007, with permission.)

SCHATZKI'S RING

- Almost all patients have an associated sliding hiatal hernia
- Symptoms: short episodes of dysphagia following rapid swallowing
- Tx: dilatation of the ring usually sufficient; may need antireflux procedure

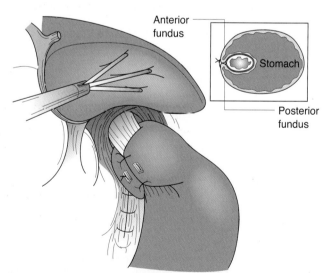

Fixation of the fundoplication. The fundoplication is sutured in place with a single U-stitch of 2-0 Prolene pledgeted on the outside. A 60-French mercury-weighted bougie is passed through the gastroesophageal junction prior to fixation of the wrap to assure a floppy fundoplication. Inset illustrates the proper orientation of the fundic wrap.

BARRETT'S ESOPHAGUS
- Squamous metaplasia to columnar epithelium
- Occurs with long-standing exposure to gastric reflux
- Cancer (adenocarcinoma) risk ↑ 50 times
- Severe Barrett's dysplasia is an indication for esophagectomy
- Uncomplicated Barrett's can be treated like GERD (i.e., PPI or Nissen) – surgery will ↓ esophagitis and further metaplasia but will <u>not</u> prevent malignancy or cause regression of the columnar lining
  - Need careful follow-up with EGD for lifetime, even after Nissen

ESOPHAGEAL CANCER
- Esophageal tumors are almost always malignant, early invasion of nodes
- Spreads quickly along **submucosal lymphatic channels**
- Symptoms: difficulty swallowing solids, dysphagia, weight loss
- Risk factors: achalasia, caustic injury, ETOH, tobacco, nitrosamines
- Dx: esophagram diagnostic procedure of choice in patients with dysphagia, odynophagia, or suspected mass lesions
- **Unresectability** – hoarseness (RLN), Horner's syndrome, phrenic nerve involvement, malignant pleural effusion, malignant fistula, airway invasion, vertebral invasion
  - **Chest/abdominal CT best test for unresectability**
- **Adenocarcinoma #1 esophageal cancer** – <u>not</u> squamous
  - **Adenocarcinoma** – most often occurs in lower ⅓ of esophagus
  - **Squamous cell carcinoma** – most often occurs in upper ⅔ of esophagus
- **Supraclavicular nodes** – M1 disease; unresectable
- **Distant metastases** – most go to lung or liver; <u>contraindication to esophagectomy</u>
  - Survival < 12 months
- **Nodal disease outside the area of resection** (i.e., SMA or celiac nodes) – contraindication to esophagectomy
- Preoperative XRT and chemotherapy may downstage tumors and make them resectable
- **Esophagectomy** – 5% mortality from surgery; curative in 20%
  - **Right gastroepiploic artery** – primary blood supply to stomach after replacing esophagus (have to divide left gastric and short gastrics)
  - **Transhiatal approach** – abdominal and neck incisions; bluntly dissect intrathoracic esophagus; may have ↓ mortality from esophageal leaks with cervical anastomosis
  - **Ivor Lewis** – abdominal incision and right thoracotomy → exposes all of the esophagus; intrathoracic anastomosis
  - **3-Hole esophagectomy** – abdominal, thoracic, and cervical incisions
  - Need **pyloromyotomy** with these procedures
  - **Colonic interposition** – may be choice in young patients with benign disease when you want to preserve gastric function; 3 anastomoses required; blood supply depends on marginal vessels
  - After esophagectomy → need contrast study on postop day 7 to rule out leak
  - **Postoperative stricture** – most can be dilated
  - Palliative esophagectomy may be indicated in some circumstances
- **Chemotherapy** – 5FU and cisplatin (for node-positive disease or use preop to shrink tumors)
- **XRT** – has been shown to be effective as both preop and postop treatment
- **Malignant fistulas** – most die within 3 months due to aspiration

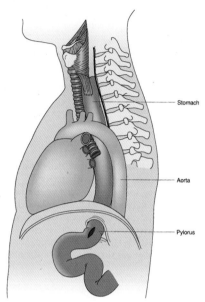

Final position of the mobilized stomach in the posterior mediastinum after transhiatal esophagectomy and cervical esophagogastric anastomosis. The gastric fundus has been suspended from the cervical prevertebral fascia, and an end-to-side cervical esophagogastrostomy has been performed. The pylorus is now located several centimeters below the level of the diaphragmatic hiatus.

LEIOMYOMA

- Most common benign tumor of the esophagus; submucosal
- Dx: esophagram, endoscopy needed to rule out cancer
- Symptoms: dysphagia, pain usually in lower ⅔ of esophagus
- **Do not biopsy** → can form scar and make subsequent resection difficult
- Tx: **>5 cm or symptomatic** → excision (enucleation) via thoracotomy

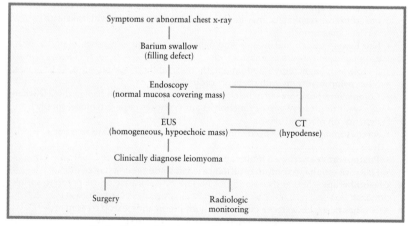

Evaluation and treatment of esophageal leiomyoma.

ESOPHAGEAL POLYPS
- Symptoms: dysphagia, hematemesis
- 2nd most common benign tumor of the esophagus; usually in the cervical esophagus
- Small lesions can be resected with endoscopy; larger lesions require cervical incision

CAUSTIC ESOPHAGEAL INJURY
- **No NG tube. Do <u>not</u> induce vomiting. Nothing to drink**
- **Alkali** – causes deep liquefaction necrosis, especially liquid (e.g., Drano)
  - Worse injury than acid; also more likely to cause cancer
- **Acid** – causes coagulation necrosis; mostly causes gastric injury
- **CXR and AXR to look for free air**
- **Endoscopy** to assess lesion
  - Do <u>not</u> use with suspected perforation and do <u>not</u> go past site of injury
- Serial exams and plain films required

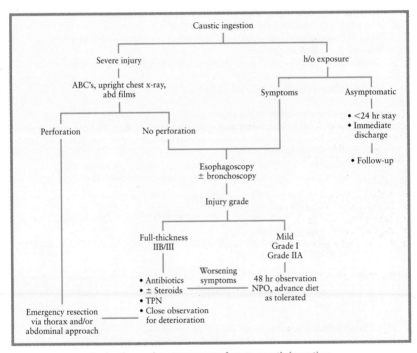

Evaluation and management of acute caustic ingestion.

- **Degree of injury**
  - **Primary burn** – hyperemia
    - Tx: observation and conservative therapy
    - **Conservative Tx**: IVFs, spitting, antibiotics, oral intake after 3–4 days; may need future serial dilation for strictures (usually cervical and near aortic indentation)
    - Can also get shortening of esophagus, requiring antireflux procedure
  - **Secondary burn** – ulcerations, exudates, and sloughing
    - Tx: prolonged observation and conservative therapy as above
    - Surgery with specific indications

- **Relative indications for surgery** – sepsis, peritonitis, persistent back and chest pain, metabolic acidosis, mediastinitis, free air, mediastinal air, crepitance, contrast extravasation, pneumothorax, effusion, air in stomach wall
- **Tertiary burn** – deep ulcers, charring, and lumen narrowing
  - Tx: as above; esophagectomy usually necessary
  - Alimentary tract not restored until after patient recovers from the caustic injury

- Need Gastrografin swallow followed by thin barium on HD 2–3 for 2nd- and 3rd-degree injuries

PERFORATIONS
- Usually the result of EGD
- Cervical esophagus near **cricopharyngeus muscle** most common site
- Symptoms: pain, dysphagia, respiratory distress, fever, tachycardia
- Dx: Gastrografin swallow followed by barium swallow
- **Criteria for nonsurgical management** – contained perforation by contrast, self-draining, no systemic effects
  - **Conservative Tx**: IVFs, NPO, spit (some say you can place NGT), broad-spectrum antibiotics
  - **No NG tube with caustic injuries** (see above)

- **Noncontained perforations in the chest**
  - **If free perforation has occurred and quick to diagnose it** (<24 hours) or if the area has minimal contamination → try **primary repair** with drains (chest tubes) and intercostal muscle pedicle flap
  - **For sick patients** → cervical esophagostomy for diversion, washout of the mediastinum, place chest tubes, and later placement of a feeding G or J tube
  - Later esophagectomy and gastric pull-up
  - **Esophagectomy** – may be needed in stable patients with intrinsic disease (burned out esophagus or malignancy)
    - Some will also go with esophagectomy and diversion in sick patients with intrinsic disease as the first procedure

- If in neck
  - primary repair and leave drains (if grossly contaminated, can just leave drains and will usually heal)

- **Need longitudinal myotomy** to see the full extent of injury
  - Consider **intercostal muscle flaps** to area of perforation to help the area heal

- **Proximal ⅔ of thoracic esophagus** – right thoracotomy (may have right effusion)
- **Distal ⅓ of thoracic esophagus** – left thoracotomy (may have left effusion)

- Use Gastrografin followed by barium swallow 10 days after repair to **rule out leak**
- Leave drains in until patient taking good oral intake without increase in drainage from drains

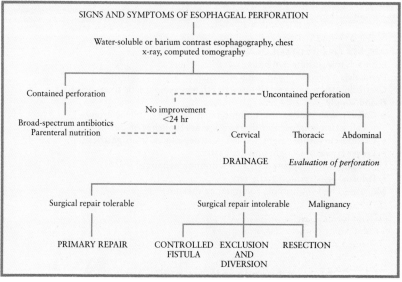

Evaluation and treatment of esophageal perforation.

- If patient has a leak without systemic effects, try to let it heal → give patient TPN or place distal feeding tube
- **Boerhaave's syndrome**
  - Forceful vomiting followed by chest pain – perforation most likely to occur in the left lateral wall of esophagus at level of T8, 3–5 cm above the GE junction
  - **Hartmann's sign** – mediastinal crunching on auscultation
  - **Early diagnosis and treatment improve survival**
  - **Dx:** Gastrografin swallow
  - **Tx:** left thoracotomy, longitudinal myotomy to see extent of injury, primary repair; leave chest tubes

ANATOMY AND PHYSIOLOGY
■ Stomach transit time 3–4 hours
■ **Peristalsis** – occurs only in distal stomach
■ Gastroduodenal pain sensed through afferent sympathetic fibers T5-10
■ **Blood supply**
  • **Celiac trunk** – left gastric, common hepatic artery, splenic artery
    • Left gastroepiploic and short gastric are branches of splenic artery
  • **Greater curvature** – right and left gastroepiploics, short gastrics
  • **Lesser curvature** – right and left gastrics
    • **Right gastric** is a branch of the common hepatic artery
  • **Pylorus** – gastroduodenal artery
■ Mucosa – lined with simple columnar epithelium

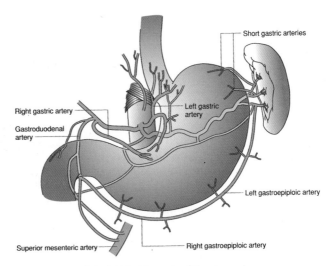

Arterial blood supply of the stomach.

■ **Cardia glands** – mucus secreting

■ **Fundus and body (oxyntic) glands**
  • **Chief cells** – pepsinogen (1st enzyme in proteolysis)
  • **Parietal cells** – release H^+ and intrinsic factor
    • **Acetylcholine, gastrin, and histamine** cause HCl release
    • **Acetylcholine (vagus) and gastrin** act on <u>phospholipase</u> → PIP → DAG + IP_3 to ↑ **Ca; activates phosphorylase kinase** →↑ HCl production
    • **Histamine** acts on <u>adenylate cyclase</u> → **cAMP** → **protein kinase A** to ↑ HCl
    • **Phosphorylase kinase and protein kinase C** phosphorylate <u>H/K ATPase</u> to ↑ acid production
    • **Omeprazole** blocks H/K ATPase in parietal cell membrane (**final pathway for** H^+ **release**)
    • **Inhibitors of parietal cells** – somatostatin, PGE_1, secretin, CCK
    • **Intrinsic factor** – binds B_{12} and the complex is reabsorbed in the terminal ileum

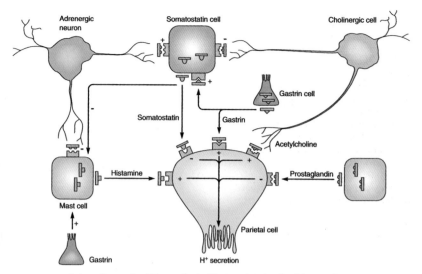

Interactions of cell types that affect parietal cell acid secretion.

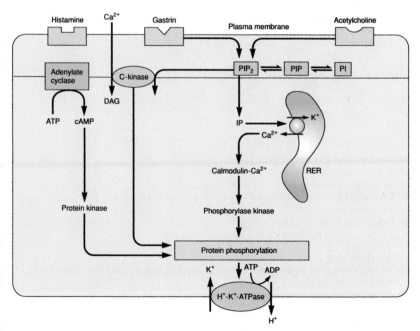

Cellular mechanisms controlling parietal cell acid secretion.

- **Antrum and pylorus glands**
  - Mucus and HCO_3^- secreting glands – protect stomach
  - **G cells** release **gastrin** – why antrectomy helpful
    - **Inhibited by H^+ in duodenum**
    - **Stimulated by amino acids, acetylcholine**
  - **D cells** – secrete **somatostatin**; inhibit gastrin and acid release
- **Brunner's glands** – in duodenum; secrete pepsinogen and alkaline mucus
- **Somatostatin, CCK, and secretin** – released with antral and duodenal acidification

- $\uparrow$ **acid and** $\uparrow$ **gastrin** – ZES, antral cell hyperplasia, retained antrum, renal failure, gastric outlet obstruction, short bowel syndrome
- $\uparrow$ **gastrin and normal/$\downarrow$ acid** – pernicious anemia, chronic gastritis, gastric CA, postvagotomy, medical acid suppression
- **Rapid gastric emptying** – previous surgery (#1), ZES, ulcers
- **Delayed gastric emptying** – opiates, anticholinergics, myxedema, hyperglycemia, diabetes

- **Billroth I** – antrectomy with gastroduodenal anastomosis
- **Billroth II** – antrectomy with gastrojejunal anastomosis

- **Trichobezoars (hair)** – hard to pull out
  - Tx: EGD generally inadequate; likely need gastrostomy and removal
- **Phytobezoars (fiber)** – often in diabetics with poor gastric emptying
  - Tx: enzymes, EGD, diet changes

- $\uparrow$ **marginal ulceration and diarrhea** with Billroth I and II versus Roux-en-Y gastrojejunostomy
- **Dieulafoy's ulcer** – vascular malformation
- **Ménétrièr's disease** – mucous cell hyperplasia, $\uparrow$ rugal folds

GASTRIC VOLVULUS
- Associated with type II (paraesophageal) hernia
- Nausea without vomiting; severe pain; usually organoaxial volvulus
- Tx: reduction and Nissen

MALLORY–WEISS TEAR
- Secondary to forceful vomiting
- Presents as hematemesis following severe retching
- Bleeding often stops spontaneously
- Dx/Tx: EGD; tear is usually near lesser curvature of the stomach (near GE junction), PPI, transfusion
- If continued bleeding, may need gastrostomy and oversewing of the vessel

VAGOTOMIES
- **Vagal denervation** – all forms $\uparrow$ liquid emptying → **vagally mediated receptive relaxation is removed**
  - Results in $\uparrow$ gastric pressure that accelerates liquid emptying
- **Truncal vagotomy** – divides vagal trunks at level of esophagus
- **Selective vagotomy** – divides nerves of Latarjet
- **Highly selective (proximal) vagotomy** – divides individual fibers, preserves "crow's foot"
  - **Complete vagotomy (truncal or selective)** – $\downarrow$ emptying of solids
  - **Highly selective vagotomy** – normal emptying of solids

- Addition of **pyloroplasty** to either of the above results in ↑ solid emptying
- **Other physiologic alterations caused by truncal vagotomy**
  - **Gastric effects** – ↓ acid output by 90%, ↑ gastrin, gastrin cell hyperplasia
  - **Nongastric effects** – ↓ exocrine pancreas function, ↓ postprandial bile flow, ↑ gall-bladder volumes, ↓ release of vagally mediated hormones
  - **Diarrhea (30%–50%)** – most common problem following vagotomy
    - Caused by sustained MMCs forcing bile acids into the colon

UPPER GASTROINTESTINAL BLEEDING

- **Risk factors**: previous UGI bleed, peptic ulcer disease, NSAID use, smoking, liver disease, esophageal varices, splenic vein thrombosis, sepsis, burn injuries, trauma, severe vomiting
- 1st **NGT and EGD to confirm bleeding is from ulcer**; can potentially treat the ulcer with EGD
  - EGD for bleeding duodenal ulcer – does not change mortality or operative rates; most important predictor of continued or recurrent bleeding is bleeding at the time of EGD

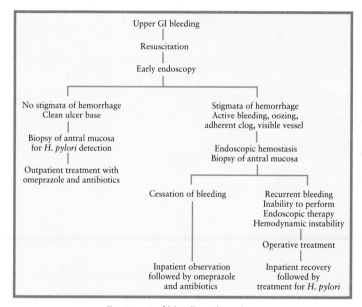

Treatment of bleeding ulceration.

- If patient hypotensive despite resuscitation and thought to be bleeding from ulcer → **go to OR**
- Having trouble localizing bleeding source → **tagged RBC scan**
- **Biggest risk factor for rebleeding at the time of EGD** – #1 spurting blood vessel (60% chance of rebleed), #2 visible blood vessel (40% chance of rebleed), #3 diffuse oozing (30% chance of rebleed)
- **Patient with liver failure** is likely bleeding from esophageal varices, <u>not</u> an ulcer
- Tx: EGD with sclerotherapy or TIPS, not OR

DUODENAL ULCERS
- ↑ acid production and ↓ defense

Pathogenesis of Peptic Ulcer

Helicobacter pylori infection

ENDOCRINE CONSEQUENCES
- Increased basal serum gastrin
- Increased gastrin response to a meal
- Increased responsiveness to gastrin-releasing peptide
- Production of Na-methylhistamine
- Decreased density of somatostatin cells
- Decreased mucosal somatostatin content

GASTRIC ACID SECRETION
- Increased acid secretory capacity
- Increased basal secretion
- Increased pentagastrin-stimulated output
- Increased meal response
- Abnormal gastric emptying

MUCOSAL DEFENSE
- Decreased duodenal bicarbonate production
- Decreased gastric mucosal prostaglandin production

ENVIRONMENT
- Cigarette smoking
- Nonsteroidal anti-inflammatory drugs

- Most frequent peptic ulcer; more common in men
- Usually in 1st part of the duodenum; **usually anterior**
  - **Anterior** ulcers <u>perforate</u>
  - **Posterior** ulcers <u>bleed from gastroduodenal artery</u>
- Symptoms: epigastric pain radiating to the back; abates with eating but recurs 30 minutes after
- Dx: endoscopy
- Tx: H$_2$ blockers (cimetidine, ranitidine), H-pump inhibitor (omeprazole), triple therapy for patients with *Helicobacter pylori* on biopsy → bismuth salts, amoxicillin, metronidazole/tetracycline (BAM or BAT)
- Surgery for ulcer rarely indicated since **introduction of proton pump inhibitors**
- **Surgical indications**
  - **Perforation**
  - **Protracted bleeding despite EGD therapy**
  - **Obstruction**
  - **Intractability** despite medical therapy
  - **Inability to rule out cancer** (ulcer remains despite treatment) → requires resection of ulcer
- If patient has been on **proton pump inhibitor therapy, acid-reducing surgical procedure is required in addition to surgery for the complication**
- Need to rule out gastrinoma in patients with complicated ulcer disease
- **Surgical options**
  - Truncal vagotomy and pyloroplasty
  - Truncal vagotomy and antrectomy with Billroth I or Billroth II – best surgery for prevention of recurrence

- Proximal or highly selective vagotomy – lowest rate of postoperative complications, 10% recurrence, no need for antral or pylorus procedure

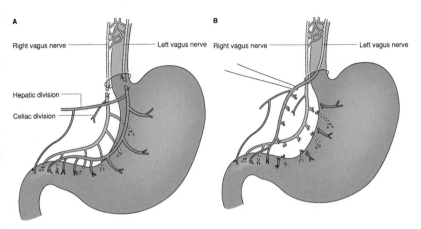

Truncal vagotomy and proximal gastric vagotomy. *(A)* With truncal vagotomy, both nerve trunks are divided at the level of the diaphragmatic hiatus. *(B)* Proximal gastric vagotomy involves division of the vagal fibers that supply the gastric fundus. Branches to the antropyloric region of the stomach are not transected, and the hepatic and celiac divisions of the vagus nerves remain intact.

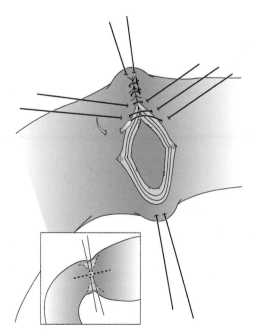

Pyloroplasty formation. A Heineke–Mikulicz pyloroplasty involves a longitudinal incision of the pyloric sphincter followed by a transverse closure.

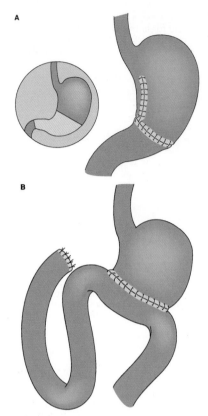

Antrectomy involves resection of the distal stomach *(pale pink area in inset).* Restoration of gastrointestinal continuity may be accomplished as a Billroth I gastroduodenostomy *(A)* or Billroth II gastrojejunostomy *(B)* reconstruction.

Clinical Results of Duodenal Ulcer Surgery

	PGV (%)	TV + P (%)	TV + A (%)
Mortality rate	0	0.5–1	1–2
Acid reduction			
Basal	80	70	85
Stimulated	50	50	85
Ulcer recurrence	10	12	1–2
Gastric emptying			
Liquids	Accelerated	Accelerated	Accelerated
Solids	No change	Accelerated	Slowed
Dumping			
Mild	<5	10	10–15
Disabling	0	1	1–2
Diarrhea			
Mild	<5	25	20
Disabling	0	2	1–2

PGV, proximal gastric vagotomy; TV + P, truncal vagotomy and pyloroplasty; TV + A, truncal vagotomy and antrectomy.

■ **Bleeding**
- Most frequent complication of duodenal ulcers
- Usually minor but can be life-threatening
- Major bleeding – >6 units of blood in 24 hours or patient remains hypotensive despite transfusion
- Tx: EGD 1st – sclerose, cauterize; vasopressin, omeprazole
- **Surgical options**
  ○ 1st duodenostomy and **gastroduodenal artery (GDA) ligation**
  ○ Avoid hitting common bile duct with GDA ligation
  ○ If patient has been on H-pump inhibitor therapy, need surgical ulcer procedure as well → **truncal vagotomy and pyloroplasty probably best option** (does not get rid of ulcer)
  ○ Can consider highly selective vagotomy as an alternative

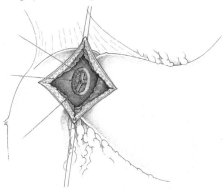

Proper suture ligation of a bleeding ulcer arising from the gastroduodenal artery requires a 3-suture ligation. The proximal and distal branches of the gastroduodenal artery are transfixed. A third suture, U type in configuration, is necessary to transfix the transverse pancreatic branch of the artery. (From Bailey RW, Martinez JM. Laparoscopic highly selective vagotomy. In: Fischer JE, Bland KI, et al., eds. *Mastery of Surgery*. 5th ed. Philadelphia, PA: Lippincott Williams & Wilkins; 2007, with permission.)

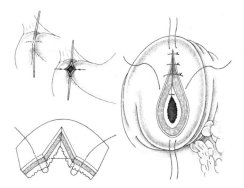

A standard Heineke–Mikulicz pyloroplasty performed with a single layer of sutures (Weinberg). The longitudinally oriented incision **(upper left)** is closed transversely **(middle left)**, such that the former end points of the longitudinal incision *(arrows)* are apposed; this transverse closure of the incision prevents potential functional gastric outlet obstruction after vagotomy. Sutures are placed as shown in the **lower left**, creating a single inverting layer **(right)**. (From Bailey RW, Martinez JM. Laparoscopic highly selective vagotomy. In: Fischer JE, Bland KI, et al., eds. *Mastery of Surgery*. 5th ed. Philadelphia, PA: Lippincott Williams & Wilkins; 2007, with permission.)

- **Obstruction**
  - Serial dilation initial treatment of choice
  - **Surgical options**
    - If near ampulla of Vater or if removing ulcer would be very difficult → **gastrojejunostomy (Billroth II, bypasses obstruction), antrectomy, and truncal vagotomy** → probably best option for most patients
    - If proximal to ampulla of Vater → **antrectomy (with ulcer excision) with Billroth II and truncal vagotomy**

- **Perforation**
  - 80% will have free air
  - Patients usually have sudden sharp epigastric pain; can have generalized peritonitis
  - Pain can radiate to the pericolic gutters with dependent drainage of gastric content
  - Elderly – some believe that elderly, high-risk patients can be safely observed
    - Need to get UGI to make sure that the perforation has sealed
  - **Surgical options**
    - **Graham patch and highly selective vagotomy** – probably best option for most if patient has been on H-pump inhibitor; otherwise just do Graham patch and place on omeprazole
    - Truncal vagotomy and pyloroplasty – need to include ulcer in pyloroplasty
    - Truncal vagotomy and antrectomy with Billroth I or II – need to include ulcer

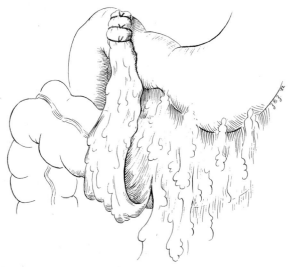

When the sutures are tied loosely enough so that the blood supply to the omentum is not compromised, the seal is complete, even with the larger perforations. (From Baker RJ. Perforated duodenal ulcer. In: Fischer JE, Bland KI, et al., eds. *Mastery of Surgery*. 5th ed. Philadelphia, PA: Lippincott Williams & Wilkins; 2007, with permission.)

- **Intractability**
  - >3 months without relief while on H-pump inhibitor therapy or recurrence <1 year after medical therapy
  - Based in EGD mucosal findings, not symptoms
  - **Surgical options**
    - **Highly selective vagotomy (does not get rid of ulcer)** – probably best option for most patients

- Truncal vagotomy and pyloroplasty (does not get rid of ulcer)
- Truncal vagotomy and antrectomy with Billroth I or Billroth II

ZOLLINGER–ELLISON SYNDROME
- Pancreatic tumors < 2 cm can be enucleated
- Secretin test results in high gastrin level
- Can often be multiple and metastatic
- Blind pancreatic resections are generally not indicated
- Resection and ablation of metastases are important for **palliation** and decreased need for drug treatment

GASTRIC ULCERS
- Older men; slow healing
- Risk factors: male, tobacco, ETOH, NSAIDs, *H. pylori*, uremia, stress (burns, sepsis, and trauma) steroids, chemotherapy
- **Most (type I and type IV) have normal acid secretion, due to abnormal mucosal defense**
- 70%–80% on lesser curvature of the stomach
- Hemorrhage is associated with higher mortality than duodenal ulcers
- Symptoms: epigastric pain radiating to the back; relieved with eating but recurs 30 minutes later; melena or guaiac-positive stools
- **CLO test** – test for *H. pylori* → detects urease released from *H. pylori*
- Biopsy for *H. pylori* needs to be from the **antrum**

- **Type A blood** – associated with type I ulcers
- **Type O blood** – associated with type II–IV ulcers

- **Surgical indications**
  - Perforation
  - Bleeding
  - Obstruction
  - Cannot exclude malignancy
  - Intractability – >3 months without relief or 2nd recurrence (based on mucosal findings)

- **Type I – lesser curve along body of stomach;** due to ↑ mucosal protection
  - Tx: distal gastrectomy including ulcer with Billroth I or Billroth II +/− vagotomy probably best option
    - Alternative → ulcer excision +/− highly selective vagotomy or truncal vagotomy and pyloroplasty
- **Type II – 2 ulcers (lesser curve and duodenal);** similar to duodenal ulcer with high acid secretion
  - Tx: Distal gastrectomy with Billroth I or Billroth II and truncal vagotomy probably best option
    - Alternative → truncal vagotomy and pyloroplasty (does not get rid of ulcers)
- **Type III – prepyloric ulcer;** similar to duodenal ulcer with high acid secretion; ↑ bleeding
  - Tx: distal gastrectomy with Billroth I or Billroth II and truncal vagotomy probably best option
    - Alternative → truncal vagotomy and pyloroplasty (does not get rid of ulcer)
- **Type IV – lesser curve high along cardia of stomach;** ↑ risk of bleeding due to ↓ mucosal protection
  - Tx: **ulcer excision** +/− highly selective vagotomy or truncal vagotomy and pyloroplasty
- **Type V – ulcer** associated with NSAIDs

STRESS GASTRITIS
- Occurs 3–10 days after event
- Lesions appear in fundus first
- Tx: proton pump inhibitor
- Selective angiography with vasopressin injection may help with bleeding
- EGD with cautery of specific bleeding point may be effective

CHRONIC GASTRITIS
- Type A (fundus) – associated with pernicious anemia, autoimmune disease
- Type B (antral) – associated with *H. pylori*

GASTRIC CANCER
- Pain unrelieved by eating, weight loss
- Antrum has 40% of gastric cancers
- 50% of cancer-related deaths in Japan
- Dx: EGD
- **Risk factors** – adenomatous polyps, tobacco, previous gastric operations, intestinal metaplasia, atrophic gastritis, pernicious anemia, type A blood, nitrosamines
- **Adenomatous polyps** – 10%–20% risk of cancer. Tx: endoscopic resection
- **Krukenberg tumor** – metastases to ovaries
- **Virchow's nodes** – metastases to supraclavicular node
- **Intestinal gastric cancer** – ↑ in high-risk populations, older men; rare in the United States
  - Associated with chronic atrophy, dysplasia; has blood invasion; glands on histology
  - Stage I disease – 85% cure rate; overall 5-year survival rate 10%
  - Surgical Tx: Try to perform subtotal gastrectomy (need 5-cm margins)

- **Diffuse gastric cancer (linitis plastica)** – in low-risk populations, women
  - Lymphatic invasion; <u>no</u> glands
  - Less favorable prognosis than intestinal gastric cancer
    - Stage II disease – <50% 5-year survival rate
  - Surgical Tx: patients require total gastrectomy because of diffuse nature of linitis plastica
  - Chemotherapy (poor response to chemo): 5FU, doxorubicin, mitomycin C
- Metastatic disease outside the area of resection – contraindication to resection unless performing surgery for palliation

- **Palliation of gastric cancer**
  - Obstruction – proximal lesions can be stented; distal lesion bypasses with gastrojejunostomy
  - Low to moderate bleeding or pain – XRT
  - If these fail, consider palliative gastrectomy for obstruction or bleeding

GASTRIC LEIOMYOMAS (ALSO CALLED GIST TUMORS)
- Most common benign gastric neoplasm
- Symptoms: usually asymptomatic but obstruction and bleeding can occur
- Hypoechoic on ultrasound; smooth edges
- Dx: biopsy
- Tx: resection
- Consider chemotherapy if >5 cm or >5–10 mitoses/HPF
- Need 1-cm margins
- Most are **C-KIT**-positive
- Chemotherapy → Gleevec (tyrosine kinase inhibitor)

Malignant Potential and Progress of Gastrointestinal Stromal Tumors			
Risk Classification	Size	Mitotic Rate	10-Year Survival (%)
High	Any size	>10/50 HPF	30
	>10 cm	Any rate	
	>5 mm	>5/50 HPF	
Intermediate	5–10 cm	<5/50 HPF	60
	<5 cm	6–10/50 HPF	
Low	2–5 cm	<5/50 HPF	75
Very low	<2 cm	<5/50 HPF	80
Normal population	—	—	80

HPF, high power field.

GASTRIC LEIOMYOSARCOMAS
- Need en bloc resection
- Cancer diagnosis based on mitoses/HPF (>5–10 associated with ↑ risk of metastases)
- **Hematogenous** spread

GASTRIC LYMPHOMAS
- Have ulcer symptoms; organ most commonly involved in extranodal lymphoma
- Usually non-Hodgkin's lymphoma
- Dx: EGD
- Chemotherapy and XRT are primary treatment modalities; surgery for complications
- Surgery possibly indicated only for stage I disease (tumor confined to stomach mucosa) and then only partial resection is indicated
- Overall 5-year survival rate >50%

MUCOSA-ASSOCIATED LYMPHOID TISSUE LYMPHOMA (MALT LYMPHOMA)
- Related to *H. pylori* infection
- Usually regresses after treatment for *H. pylori*
- Usually in GI tract; can also occur in lung and Waldeyer's ring
- Tx: triple-therapy antibiotics for *H. pylori* and surveillance; if MALT does not regress, need chemotherapy (CHOP)

MORBID OBESITY
- Central obesity – worse prognosis
- Surgical eligibility: BMI > 40 or BMI > 35 with comorbidities
- NIDDM, HTN, and sleep apnea often resolve after surgery

Criteria for Patient Selection for Bariatric Surgery
■ Body mass index >40 kg/m^2
■ Body mass index >35 kg/m^2 with coexisting comorbidities
■ Failure of nonsurgical methods of weight reduction
■ Psychological stability
■ Absence of drug and alcohol abuse

Resolution of Comorbidities Following Gastric Bypass

Comorbidity	Resolution Rate (%)
Diabetes	73
Obstructive sleep apnea (mild/moderate)	100
Obstructive sleep apnea (severe)	75
Hypertension (high blood pressure)	56
Urinary stress incontinence	91
Gastroesophageal reflux disease	90
Venous stasis ulcers	94
Pseudotumor cerebri	100
Joint pain	71

▥ Operative mortality is approximately 1%

▥ **Roux-en-Y gastric bypass**
  - Better weight loss than just stapling
  - Risk of marginal ulcers, leak, necrosis, B_{12} deficiency (intrinsic factor needs acidic environment to bind B_{12}), iron-deficiency anemia (bypasses duodenum, where Fe absorbed), gallstones (from rapid weight loss)
  - Perform **cholecystectomy** during operation if stones present
  - **UGI** on postop day 2
  - **10%–15% failure rate** due to high carbohydrate snacking
  - **Ischemia** – most common cause of leak
    - Signs of leak – ↑ RR, ↑ HR, pain, fever, elevated WBCs
  - **Marginal ulcers** – develop in 10%. Tx: omeprazole
  - **Stenosis** – usually responds to serial dilation
  - **Signs of obstruction following surgery** – hiccoughs, large stomach bubble

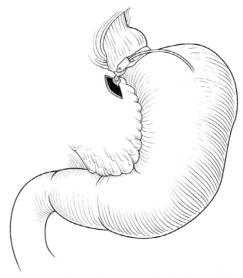

Laparoscopic adjustable gastric band. (From Jones DB, Schneider BE. Surgical management of morbid obesity. In: Fischer JE, Bland KI, et al., eds. *Mastery of Surgery*. 5th ed. Philadelphia, PA: Lippincott Williams & Wilkins; 2007, with permission.)

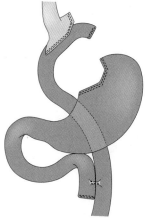

Laparoscopic proximal Roux-en-Y gastric bypass (retrocolic, retrogastric).

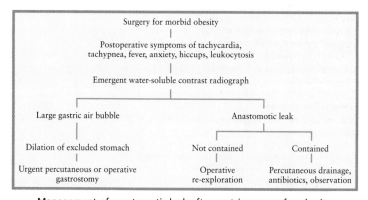

Management of anastomotic leak after gastric surgery for obesity.

Outcomes after Laparoscopic Roux-en-Y Gastric Bypass

Excess weight loss	65%–80%
Resolution of comorbidities	
Diabetes	82%–98%
Hypertension	52%–92%
Hypercholesterolemia	63%
NAFLD inflammation/fibrosis[a]	37%–20%
Gastroesophageal reflux	72%–98%
Sleep apnea	74%–98%
Degenerative joint disease	41%–76%
Migraines	57%
Pseudotumor cerebri	96%
Depression	55%
Venous stasis disease	95%
Polycystic ovarian syndrome	79%–100%
Urinary incontinence	44%–88%

NAFLD, nonalcoholic fatty liver disease.
[a]90% improvement in steatosis.

From Brethauer SA, Schauer PR. Laparoscopic gastric bypass. In: Fischer JE, Bland KI, et al., (eds.) *Mastery of Surgery*, 5th ed. Philadelphia, PA: Lippincott Williams & Wilkins; 2007, with permission.

- **Jejunoileal bypass**
  - These operations are no longer done
  - Associated with ↑ liver cirrhosis and kidney (stones) problems, osteoporosis (↓ Ca)
  - Need to correct these patients and perform Roux-en-Y gastric bypass if ileojejunal bypasses are encountered

POSTGASTRECTOMY COMPLICATIONS

- **Dumping syndrome**
  - Can occur after gastrectomy or after vagotomy and pyloroplasty
  - Occurs from rapid entering of carbohydrates into the small bowel
  - 90% of cases resolve with medical therapy
  - **2 phases**
    - Hyperosmotic load causes fluid shift into bowel (diarrhea, dizziness, hypotension)
    - Reactive ↑ in insulin and ↓ in glucose (2nd phase rarely occurs)
  - Can almost always be treated with medical and conservative (dietary changes) therapy
  - Tx: small, low-fat, low-carbohydrate, increased-protein meals; no liquids with meals, no lying down after meals
    - Octreotide may be effective
  - **Surgical options** (rarely needed)
    - Conversion of Billroth I or Billroth II to Roux-en-Y gastrojejunostomy
    - Operations to ↑ gastric reservoir (jejunal pouch) or ↑ emptying time (reversed jejunal loop)

- **Alkaline reflux gastritis**
  - Postprandial epigastric pain associated with N/V; pain not relieved with vomiting
  - Dx: evidence of bile reflux into stomach, histologic evidence of gastritis
  - Tx: H_2 blockers, cholestyramine, metoclopramide
  - Surgical option: conversion of Billroth I or Billroth II to Roux-en-Y gastrojejunostomy with afferent limb 60 cm distal to original gastrojejunostomy

- **Roux stasis**
  - Stasis of chyme in Roux limb due to loss of jejunal motility
  - Dx: EGD, emptying studies
  - Tx: metoclopramide, prokinetics
  - Surgical option: shorten Roux limb to 40 cm

- **Chronic gastric atony**
  - Delayed gastric emptying after vagotomy
  - Symptoms: nausea, vomiting, pain, early satiety
  - Dx: gastric emptying study
  - Tx: metoclopramide, prokinetics
  - Surgical option: near-total gastrectomy with Roux-en-Y

- **Small gastric remnant (early satiety)**
  - Actually want this for gastric bypass patients
  - Dx: EGD
  - Tx: small meals
  - Surgical option: jejunal pouch construction

- Duodenal stump blow-out – place duodenostomy and drains

■ **Blind-loop syndrome**
   • With Billroth II or Roux-en-Y
   • Symptoms: pain, diarrhea, malabsorption, B_{12} deficiency (bacteria use it up), steatorrhea (bacterial deconjugation of bile)
   • Caused by bacterial (*E. coli*, GNRs) overgrowth and stasis in afferent limb
   • Tx: tetracycline, Flagyl, metoclopramide
   • Surgical option: reanastomosis with shorter (40-cm) afferent limb

■ **Afferent-loop obstruction**
   • With Billroth II or Roux-en-Y
   • Nonbilious vomiting, pain relieved with bilious emesis
   • Symptoms: RUQ pain, steatorrhea
   • Caused by obstruction of afferent limb
   • Risk factors – long afferent limb with Billroth II or Roux-en-Y
   • Dx: CT scan
   • Tx: balloon dilation may be possible
   • Surgical option: reanastomosis with shorter (40-cm) afferent limb

■ **Efferent-loop obstruction**
   • Symptoms of obstruction
   • Dx: UGI, EGD
   • Tx: balloon dilation
   • Surgical option: find site of obstruction and relieve it

■ **Postvagotomy diarrhea**
   • Secondary to nonconjugated bile salts in the colon
   • Caused by sustained postprandial organized MMCs
   • Tx: cholestyramine, octreotide
   • Surgical option: reversed interposition jejunal graft

■ PEG complications – insertion into the liver or colon

ANATOMY AND PHYSIOLOGY

- **Hepatic artery variants**
- **Right hepatic artery off superior mesenteric artery** (#1 hepatic artery variant; 20%) courses behind pancreas, posterolateral to the common bile duct
- **Left hepatic artery off left gastric artery** (about 20%) – found in gastrohepatic ligament medially
- **Common hepatic artery** – most common variant is off SMA (2%)
- **Falciform ligament** – separates medial and lateral segments of the left lobe; attaches liver to anterior abdominal wall; extends to umbilicus and carries remnant of the umbilical vein
- **Ligamentum teres** – carries the obliterated umbilical vein to the undersurface of the liver; extends from the falciform ligament
- Line drawn from the middle of the **gallbladder fossa to IVC (portal fissure or Cantlie's line)** separates the right and left lobes

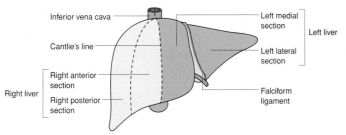

Anatomic division of the liver into right and left halves by a line extending from the gallbladder fossa posteriorly to the inferior vena cava.

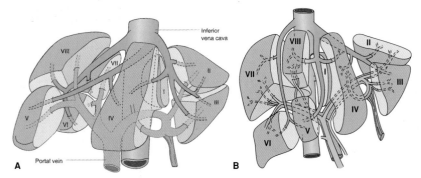

Functional divisions of the liver and liver segments according to Couinaud's nomenclature.

- **Segments**
  - I – caudate
  - II – superior left lateral segment
  - III – inferior left lateral segment
  - IV – left medial segment (quadrate lobe)
  - V – inferior right anteromedial segment
  - VI – inferior right posterolateral segment

- VII – superior right posterolateral segment
- VIII – superior right anteromedial segment
▦ Glisson's capsule – peritoneum that covers the liver
▦ Bare area – area on the posterior-superior surface of liver not covered by Glisson's capsule
▦ Triangular ligaments – lateral and medial extensions of the coronary ligament on the posterior surface of the liver; made up of peritoneum
▦ **Portal triad enters segments IV and V**
▦ **Gallbladder lies under segments IV and V**

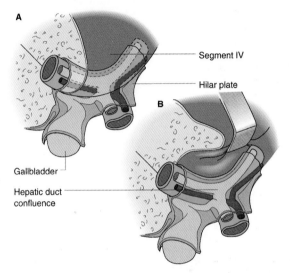

Lowering the hilar plate. *(A)* The inferior border of segment IV (quadrate lobe) overlies the hepatic duct confluence. *(B)* Division of the connective issue investment allows elevation of segment IV, which results in a "lower" hilar plate and surgical exposure to the hepatic duct confluence.

▦ **Kupffer cells – liver macrophages**
▦ **Hepatoduodenal ligament** – where bile duct, portal vein, and hepatic artery meet (portal triad)
▦ **Portal triad – portal vein** posteriorly, **common bile duct** laterally, **hepatic artery** medially
▦ **Pringle maneuver** – porta hepatis clamping; will not stop hepatic vein bleeding
▦ **Foramen of Winslow**
  - Anterior – portal triad
  - Posterior – IVC
  - Inferior – duodenum
  - Superior – liver

▦ **Portal vein**
  - Forms from superior mesenteric vein joining splenic vein (no valves)
  - **Inferior mesenteric vein** – enters splenic vein
  - **Portal veins** – 2 in liver; ⅔ of hepatic blood flow
    • <u>Left</u> – II, III, and IV
    • <u>Right</u> – V, VI, VII, and VIII
▦ **Arterial blood supply**
  - Right, left, and middle hepatic arteries (follows hepatic vein system)
  - Middle hepatic artery MC a branch off the left hepatic artery

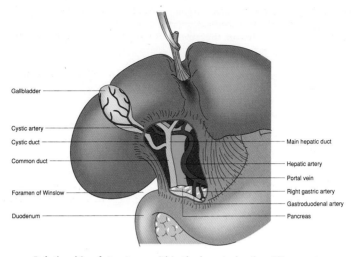

Gallbladder

Cystic artery

Cystic duct

Common duct

Foramen of Winslow

Duodenum

Main hepatic duct

Hepatic artery

Portal vein

Right gastric artery

Gastroduodenal artery

Pancreas

Relationship of structures within the hepatoduodenal ligament.

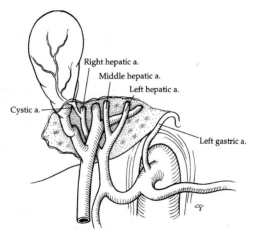

Right hepatic a.

Middle hepatic a.

Left hepatic a.

Cystic a.

Left gastric a.

The most common hepatic artery configuration. (From Trunkey D. Treatment of major hepatic trauma. In: Fischer JE, Bland KI, et al., eds. *Mastery of Surgery*. 5th ed. Philadelphia, PA: Lippincott Williams & Wilkins; 2007, with permission.)

- **Most primary and secondary tumors of the liver** are supplied by the <u>hepatic artery</u>
- **Hepatic veins**
  - 3 hepatic veins
- <u>Left</u> – II, III, and superior IV
- <u>Middle</u> – V and inferior IV
- <u>Right</u> – VI, VII, and VIII
- **Middle hepatic vein** joins left hepatic vein in 80% before going into IVC; other 20% go directly into IVC
- **Accessory right hepatic veins** – drain medial aspect of right lobe directly into the IVC
- **Inferior phrenic veins** – also drain directly into the IVC
- **Caudate lobe** – receives separate right and left portal and arterial blood flow; drains directly into IVC via separate hepatic veins

- **Alkaline phosphatase** – normally located in canalicular membrane
- **Nutrient uptake** – occurs in sinusoidal membrane
- **Ketones** – usual energy source for liver; glucose converted to glycogen and stored
  - Excess glucose converted to fat
- **Urea** – synthesized in the liver
- **Not made in the liver** – von Willebrand factor and factor VIII (endothelium)
- Liver stores large amount of **fat-soluble vitamins**
- **B$_{12}$** – the only water-soluble vitamin stored in the liver

- **Bleeding and bile leak** – most common problems with hepatic resection
- **Hepatocytes most sensitive to ischemia** – central lobular (acinar zone III)
- 75% of normal liver can be safely resected

BILIRUBIN
- Breakdown product of hemoglobin (Hgb → heme → biliverdin → bilirubin)
- Conjugated to **glucuronic acid (glucuronyl transferase)** in the liver → improves water solubility
- Conjugated bilirubin actively secreted into bile
- **Urobilinogen**
  - Breakdown of bilirubin by bacteria in the terminal ileum
  - Is reabsorbed in the blood, and released in the urine
  - Excess urobilinogen turns urine dark like cola

BILE
- Contains bile salts (85%), proteins, phospholipids (lecithin), cholesterol, and bilirubin
- Final bile composition determined by active (Na/K ATPase) reabsorption of water in gallbladder
- **Cholesterol** – used to make bile acids
- **Bile acids** conjugated to **taurine or glycine (improves water solubility)**
  - <u>Primary bile acids</u> – **cholic and chenodeoxycholic**
  - <u>Secondary bile acids</u> – **deoxycholic and lithocholic** (dehydroxylated primary bile acids by bacteria in gut)
- **Lecithin** – main biliary phospholipid; solubilizes cholesterol and emulsifies fats in the intestine

JAUNDICE
- Occurs when bilirubin >2.5; <u>1st evident under the tongue</u>
- Maximum bilirubin is 30 unless patient had underlying renal disease, hemolysis, or bile duct–hepatic vein fistula
- **Unconjugated bilirubin** – prehepatic causes (hemolysis); hepatic deficiencies of uptake or conjugation
- **Conjugated bilirubin** – secretion defects into bile ducts; excretion defects into GI tract (stones, strictures, tumor)
- **Syndromes**
  - **Gilbert's disease** – abnormal uptake; mildly high unconjugated bilirubin
  - **Crigler–Najjar disease** – inability to conjugate; deficiency of glucuronyl transferase; high unconjugated bilirubin → life-threatening disease
  - **Physiologic jaundice of newborn** – immature glucuronyl transferase; high unconjugated bilirubin
  - **Rotor's syndrome** – deficiency in storage ability; high conjugated bilirubin
  - **Dubin–Johnson syndrome** – deficiency in secretion ability; high conjugated bilirubin

VIRAL HEPATITIS
- All hepatitis viral agents can cause acute hepatitis and fulminant hepatic failure
- Hepatitis B, C, and D can cause chronic hepatitis and hepatoma

- ■ Hepatitis A (RNA) – serious consequences uncommon
- ■ Hepatitis B (DNA)
  - Infection IgM antibody dominates 1st 6 months
    - Anti-HBc rises 10–12 weeks after infection
    - Anti-HBe rises 12–14 weeks after infection
    - Anti-HBs rises 14–16 weeks after infection
  - Anti-HBc-IgM (c = core) is elevated in the first 6 months; IgG then takes over
  - Vaccination – have ↑ anti-HBs (s = surface) antibodies only
  - ↑ anti-HBc and ↑ anti-HBs antibodies and <u>no</u> HBs antigens (HBsAg) → patient had infection with recovery and subsequent immunity
- ■ Hepatitis C (RNA) – can have long incubation period; currently most common viral hepatitis leading to liver TXP
- ■ Hepatitis D (RNA) – cofactor for hepatitis B
- ■ Hepatitis E (RNA) – fulminant hepatic failure in pregnancy, most often in 3rd trimester

LIVER FAILURE
- ■ **Most common cause of liver failure** – cirrhosis
- ■ Best indicator of synthetic function in patient with cirrhosis - **prothrombin time (PT)**
- ■ **Acute fulminant hepatic failure** – 80% mortality
  - Outcome determined by the course of encephalopathy
- ■ **Hepatic encephalopathy**
  - Liver failure leads to inability to metabolize – buildup of ammonia, mercantanes, methane thiols, and false neurotransmitters
  - Causes other than liver failure for encephalopathy – GI bleeding, infection (spontaneous bacterial peritonitis [SBP]), electrolyte imbalances, drugs
  - May need to embolize previous therapeutic shunts or embolize other major collaterals
  - Tx: **lactulose** – cathartic that gets rid of bacteria in the gut and acidifies colon (preventing NH_3 uptake by converting it to ammonium), titrate to 2–3 stools/day
    - **Limit protein intake** (<70 g/day)
    - **Branched-chain amino acids** – metabolized by skeletal muscle, may be of some value
    - <u>No</u> antibiotics unless for a specific infection
    - Neomycin may help
    - **Dopamine receptor agonists** (L-dopa and bromocriptine) may help
    - **Tap ascites to rule out SBP**
    - **Guaiac stools and place NGT to R/O bleed**
- ■ **Cirrhosis mechanism** – hepatocyte destruction → fibrosis and scarring of liver → ↑ hepatic pressure → portal venous congestion → lymphatic overload → leakage of splanchnic and hepatic lymph into peritoneum → ascites
- ■ **Paracentesis for ascites** – replace with albumin (1 g for every 100 cc removed)
- ■ **Ascites** – from **hepatic/splanchnic** lymph
  - Tx: ↓ NaCl, diuretics (spironolactone counteracts hyperaldosteronism often seen with liver failure), paracentesis, TIPS, peritoneovenous shunts (Denver, LeVeen shunt → complications include DIC); prophylactic antibiotics to prevent SBP (ciprofloxacin 750 mg/week); water restriction
- ■ ↑ **aldosterone** – secondary to impaired hepatic metabolism and impaired GFR
- ■ **Hepatorenal syndrome** – same appearance as prerenal azotemia
  - Tx: stop diuretics, give volume
- ■ **Neurological changes** – asterixis; sign that liver failure is progressing
- ■ **Peritoneovenous shunts (Denver, LeVeen)** – shunt ascites into venous system; can get DIC complications

- ■ **Postpartum liver failure with ascites** – hepatic vein thrombosis
  - Dx: SMA arteriogram with venous phase contrast

Characteristics of Viruses

Virus	Genus	Genome	Genome Length (kb)	Mode of Transmission	Incubation[a](d) Mean	Range	Acute Hepatitis	Fulminant Hepatic Failure	Chronic Hepatitis	Hepatoma	Recipient to Allograft	New Acquisition
								Consequence of Infection			**Posttransplantation**	
Hepatitis A	Picornavirus	RNA	7.5	Fecal-oral	28	15–50	Yes	Yes	No	No	No	No
Hepatitis B	Hepadnavirus	DNA	3.2	Parenteral Venereal ? Fecal-oral	84	28–160	Yes	Yes	Yes	Yes	Yes	Yes
Hepatitis C	Flavivirus	RNA	10.2	Parenteral ? Venereal ? Fecal-oral	56	14–160	Yes	Probable	Yes	Yes	Yes	Yes
Hepatitis D	Viroid	RNA	1.67	Parenteral	—	—	Yes	Yes	Yes	No	Yes	Uncertain
Hepatitis E	Probably calicivirus	RNA	7.6	Fecal-oral	40	22–60	Yes	Yes[b]	No	No	Uncertain	No

[a] Time from exposure to clinical hepatitis.
[b] Especially in pregnant women in third trimester.

SPONTANEOUS BACTERIAL PERITONITIS
- Fever, abdominal pain, PMNs > 250 in fluid, positive cultures
- *E. coli* (#1), pneumococci, streptococci (see Chap. 5)
- Most commonly mono-organism; if not, need to worry about bowel perforation
- Risk factors – prior SBP, variceal hemorrhage, low-protein ascites, nephrotic syndrome, SLE in children
- Tx: 3rd-generation cephalosporins; patients usually respond within 48 hours

ESOPHAGEAL VARICES
- Bleed by rupture
- **Tx**: sclerotherapy (90% effective at treating)
  - vasopressin (splanchnic artery constriction)
  - octreotide (↓ portal pressure by ↓ blood flow)
  - Patients with history of CAD should receive NTG while on vasopressin
  - Sengstaken–Blakemore (S–B) tube – used to control variceal bleeding, risk of rupture of the esophagus (hardly used anymore)
  - Correct coags/blood transfusions
- Propranolol – may help prevent rebleeding; no good role acutely
- Can get later strictures from sclerotherapy; usually easily managed with dilatation
- TIPS needed for refractory variceal bleeding
- Bleeding varices have 33% mortality with 1st episode
- 50% will rebleed; 50% mortality with each subsequent bleeding episode

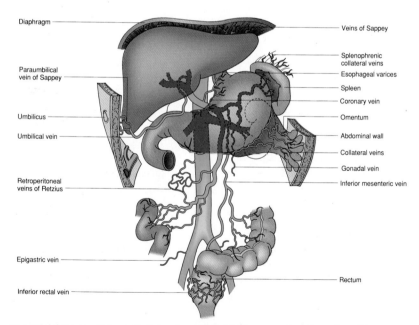

Potential venous collaterals that develop with portal hypertension. The veins of Sappey drain portal blood through the bare areas of the diaphragm and through paraumbilical vein collaterals to the umbilicus. The veins of Retzius form in the retroperitoneum and shunt portal blood from the bowel and other organs to the vena cava.

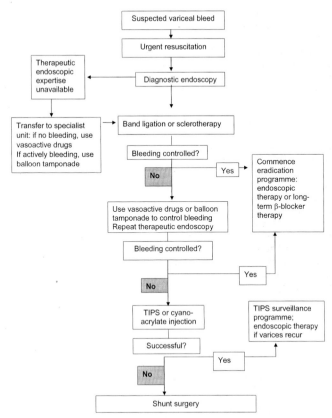

Algorithm for the management of acute variceal bleedings. TIPS, transjugular intrahepatic portosystemic shunt. (From Krige JEJ, Bornman PC. Endoscopic therapy in the management of esophageal varices: injection sclerotherapy and variceal ligation. In: Fischer JE, Bland KI, et al., eds. *Mastery of Surgery.* 5th ed. Philadelphia, PA: Lippincott Williams & Wilkins; 2007, with permission.)

PORTAL HYPERTENSION
- **Presinusoidal obstruction** – schistosomiasis, congenital hepatic fibrosis, portal vein thrombosis (50% of portal HTN in children)
- **Sinusoidal obstruction** – cirrhosis
- **Postsinusoidal obstruction** – Budd–Chiari syndrome (hepatic vein occlusive disease), constrictive pericarditis, CHF
- Normal portal vein pressure < 12 mm Hg
- **Coronary veins** act as collaterals between the portal vein and the systemic venous system of the lower esophagus
- Portal HTN leads to esophageal variceal hemorrhage, ascites, splenomegaly, and hepatic encephalopathy
- Shunts can decompress portal system

- **TIPS** – used for protracted bleeding, progression of coagulopathy, visceral hypoperfusion, refractory ascites
  - Allows antegrade flow
  - Risk – development of encephalopathy

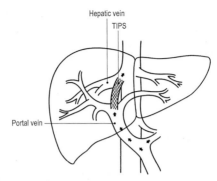

Transjugular intrahepatic portosystemic shunt (TIPS). A catheter is passed into the hepatic vein via the jugular vein. A needle, inserted through the catheter, is passed from the hepatic vein through the liver tissue into a major portal vein branch. This is followed by the placement of a guidewire and withdrawal of the needle. The liver tract is dilated with an angioplasty balloon catheter and the tract is kept open after deployment of an expandable metal stent. (From Krige JEJ, Bornman PC. Endoscopic therapy in the management of esophageal varices: injection sclerotherapy and variceal ligation. In: Fischer JE, Bland KI, et al., eds. *Mastery of Surgery*. 5th ed. Philadelphia, PA: Lippincott Williams & Wilkins; 2007, with permission.)

■ **Splenorenal shunt** – low rate of encephalopathy; need to ligate left adrenal vein, left gonadal vein, inferior mesenteric vein, coronary vein, and pancreatic branches of splenic vein
  • Used only for Child's A cirrhotics who present just with bleeding (rarely used anymore)
  • Contraindicated in patients with refractory ascites, as splenorenal shunts can worsen ascites

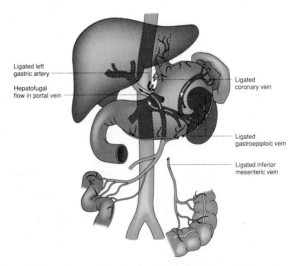

Distal splenorenal Warren shunt. The splenic vein is divided near its junction with the superior mesenteric vein. The distal end of the splenic vein is anastomosed to the renal vein. Varices are selectively decompressed through the stomach and short gastric veins into the splenic vein and then into the vena cava through the renal vein. Portal hypertension is maintained in the portal and superior mesenteric veins to provide enough pressure to drive portal blood through the diseased liver.

- Child's B or C with indication for shunt → **TIPS**
- Child's A that just has bleeding as symptom → **consider splenorenal shunt (more durable); otherwise TIPS**
- **Child's class correlates with mortality after shunt**

- **Portal HTN in children**
  - Usually caused by **extrahepatic thrombosis of the portal vein**
  - Most common cause of massive hematemesis in children

BUDD–CHIARI SYNDROME
- Occlusion of hepatic veins and IVC
- RUQ pain, hepatosplenomegaly, ascites, fulminant hepatic failure, muscle wasting, variceal bleeding
- Dx: angio, CT scan; liver biopsy shows sinusoidal dilatation, congestion, centrilobular congestion
- Tx: portacaval shunt (needs to connect to the IVC above the obstruction)

SPLENIC VEIN THROMBOSIS
- Can lead to isolated gastric varices without elevation of pressure in the rest of the portal system
- These gastric varices can bleed
- Splenic vein thrombosis is most often caused by pancreatitis
- Tx: splenectomy

ABSCESSES
- **Amebic**
  - ↑ LFTs; ↑ in **right lobe** of liver, usually single
  - Primary infection occurs in the colon → amebic colitis
  - Risk factors – travel to Mexico, ETOH; fecal–oral transmission
  - Positive serology for *Entamoeba histolytica* – 90% have infection
  - Symptoms: fever, chills, RUQ pain, ↑ WBCs, jaundice, hepatomegaly
  - Reaches liver via **portal vein**
  - Cultures of abscess often sterile → protozoa exist only in peripheral rim
  - Most do <u>not</u> require aspiration (anchovy paste)
  - Can usually diagnose based on CT characteristics
  - Tx: Flagyl; aspiration if refractory or contaminated; surgery only for free rupture
- *Echinococcus*
  - Forms cyst (hydatid cyst)
  - Positive **Casoni skin test**, positive **indirect hemagglutination**
  - **Sheep** – carriers; **dogs** – human exposure. ↑ in **right lobe** of the liver
  - <u>Do not</u> aspirate → can leak out and cause anaphylactic shock
  - Abdominal CT shows ectocyst (calcified) and endocyst

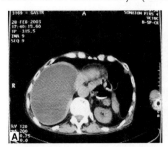 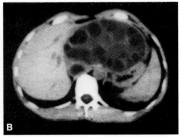

Computerized tomographic images of hydatid cysts. *(A)* A large univesicular cyst. *(B)* Cyst full of daughter cysts (multivesicular, rosette like). *(continued)*

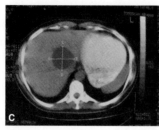
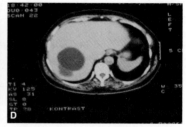

Computerized tomographic images of hydatid cysts. (*Continued*) (*C*) Centrally positioned cyst close to the inferior vena cava. (*D*) Cyst with exogenous vesiculation. (From Milicevic M. Echinococcal cysts: cause, diagnosis, complications, and medical and surgical treatment. In: Fischer JE, Bland KI, et al., eds. *Mastery of Surgery*, 5th ed. Philadelphia, PA: Lippincott Williams & Wilkins; 2007, with permission.)

- Preop ERCP for <u>jaundice</u>, ↑ <u>LFTs</u>, or <u>cholangitis</u> to check for communication with the biliary system
- Tx: preop albendazole, surgical removal (may want to inject cyst with alcohol at time of removal to kill organisms); need to get all of cyst wall

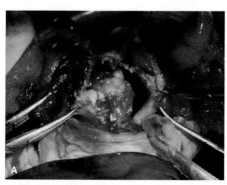
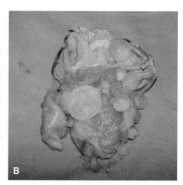

(*A*) The cyst is entered and there is no laminated membrane. Daughter cysts and debris are visible in the bile-stained interior of the cyst. (*B*) Contents of a multivesicular cyst. Fragments of the laminated membrane, daughter cysts, and debris are seen. (From Milicevic M. Echinococcal cysts: cause, diagnosis, complications, and medical and surgical treatment. In: Fischer JE, Bland KI, et al., eds. *Mastery of Surgery*. 5th ed. Philadelphia, PA: Lippincott Williams & Wilkins; 2007, with permission.)

- **Schistosomiasis**
  - Maculopapular rash, ↑ eosinophils
  - Sigmoid colon – fine granulation tissue, petechiae, ulcers
  - Can cause variceal bleeding
  - Tx: praziquantel and control of variceal bleeding
- **Pyogenic abscess**
  - Account for 80% of all abscesses
  - Symptoms: fever, chills, weight loss, RUQ pain, ↑ LFTs, ↑ WBCs, sepsis
  - ↑ in right lobe; 15% mortality with sepsis
  - GNRs – #1 organism (*E. coli*)
  - Commonly secondary to contiguous infection from biliary tract

- Can occur following **bacteremia** from other types of infections (diverticulitis, appendicitis)
- Dx: aspiration
- Tx: CT-guided drainage and antibiotics; surgical drainage for unstable condition and continued signs of sepsis
- May need surgery for biliary obstruction or multiple abscesses

BENIGN LIVER TUMORS
Hepatic adenomas
- Women, steroid use, OCPs, type I collagen storage diseases
- 80% are symptomatic; 10%–20% risk of significant bleeding (rupture)
- Can become malignant
- More common in **right lobe**
- Symptoms: pain, ↑ LFTs, ↓ BP (from rupture), palpable mass
- Dx: no Kupffer cells in adenomas, thus **no uptake on sulfur colloid scan (cold)**
  - MRI demonstrates a hypervascular tumor
  - Has peripheral blood supply
- Tx
  - Asymptomatic – stop OCPs; if regression, no further therapy is needed; if no regression, patient needs resection of the tumor
  - Symptomatic – tumor resection for bleeding and malignancy risk; embolization if multiple and unresectable
Focal nodular hyperplasia
- Has central stellate scar that may look like cancer
- No malignancy risk; very unlikely to rupture
- Dx: abdominal CT; has Kupffer cells, so **will take up sulfur colloid on liver scan**
- MRI/CT scan demonstrates a hypervascular tumor
- Tx: conservative therapy
Hemangiomas
- Most common benign hepatic tumor
- Rupture rare; most asymptomatic; more common in women
- Avoid biopsy → risk of hemorrhage
- Dx: MRI and CT scan show **peripheral to central enhancement**
  - Appears as a **hypervascular** lesion on CT scan/MRI
- Tx: conservative unless symptomatic, then **surgery** +/− **embolization**; XRT and steroids for unresectable disease
- **Rare complications of hemangioma** – consumptive coagulopathy (Kasabach–Merritt syndrome) and CHF
  - These complications are usually seen in children
Solitary cysts
- Congenital; women, right lobe
- Resection needed if bleeding or infected (and cannot be treated percutaneously)
- Complications from these cysts are rare; most can be left alone
- Walls have a characteristic blue hue

MALIGNANT LIVER TUMORS
Metastases:primary ratio is **20:1**
Hepatocellular CA
- **Most common cancer worldwide**
- Risk factors – HBV (#1 cause worldwide), HCV, ETOH, hemochromatosis, alpha-1-antitrypsin deficiency, primary sclerosing cholangitis, aflatoxins, hepatic adenoma, steroids, pesticides
- **Not** **risk factors** – primary biliary cirrhosis, Wilson's disease

- **Clear cell, lymphocyte infiltrative, and fibrolamellar types** (adolescents and young adults) have the best prognosis
- **AFP level** correlates with tumor size
- 30% 5-year survival rate with resection
- Few hepatic tumors are resectable secondary to cirrhosis, portohepatic involvement, or metastases
- Need 1-cm margin
- Tumor recurrence most likely in the liver after resection
- **Hepatic sarcoma**
  - Risk factors – PVC, Thorotrast, arsenic → rapidly fatal
- **Cholangiosarcoma**
  - Risk factors – clonorchiasis infection, ulcerative colitis, hemochromatosis, primary sclerosing cholangitis, choledochal cysts
  - Intrahepatic associated with worse survival than extrahepatic
  - Tumor size and satellite nodules correlate with outcome

- Colon CA metastases – can resect if you leave enough liver for the patient to survive
  - 20% 5-year survival rate
- **Metastatic and primary tumors of the liver** are supplied by the **hepatic arteries**
- **Primary liver tumors** – hypervascular
- **Metastatic liver tumors** – hypovascular

ANATOMY AND PHYSIOLOGY

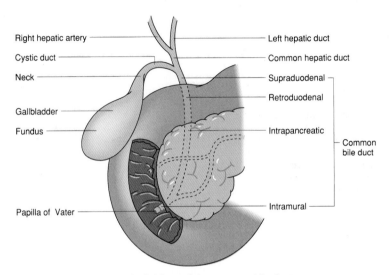

Anatomic divisions of the common bile duct.

- Gallbladder lies between **segments IV and V**
- **Cystic artery** branches off right hepatic artery
- Is found in the triangle of Calot (cystic duct [lateral], common bile duct [medial], liver [superior])
- **Right hepatic (lateral) and retroduodenal branches of the gastroduodenal artery (medial)** supply to the hepatic and common bile duct (9- and 3-o'clock positions when performing ERCP); considered longitudinal blood supply
- **Cystic veins** drain into the right branch of the portal vein and into the liver
- **Lymphatics** are on the right side of the common bile duct
- Parasympathetic fibers from left (anterior) trunk of the vagus
- Sympathetic fibers from T7–10 coursing through the splanchnic and celiac ganglions

- Gallbladder has **<u>no</u> submucosa;** mucosa is columnar epithelium
- Common bile duct and hepatic duct **do not have peristalsis**
- Gallbladder normally fills by **contraction of sphincter of Oddi at the ampulla of Vater**
  - **Morphine** – contracts the sphincter of Oddi
  - **Glucagon** – relaxes the sphincter of Oddi

- **Normal sizes**: CBD < 8 mm (<10 mm after cholecystectomy), gallbladder wall <4 mm, pancreatic duct < 4 mm
- After cholecystectomy, <u>total bile acid pools</u> ↓
- Highest concentration of CCK and secretin cells in the **duodenum**

- **Rokitansky–Aschoff sinuses** – invagination of the epithelium of the wall of the gallbladder; formed from ↑ gallbladder pressure

■ **Ducts of Luschka** – biliary ducts that can leak after a cholecystectomy

■ **Bile excretion regulation**
- ↑ **bile excretion** – CCK, secretin, and vagal input
- ↓ **bile excretion** – VIP, somatostatin, sympathetic stimulation
- **Gallbladder contraction** – CCK causes constant, steady tonic contraction

■ **Essential functions of bile**
- Fat-soluble vitamin absorption
- Bilirubin excretion
- Cholesterol excretion

■ **Gallbladder** – forms concentrated bile by **active resorption of Na and water**

	Na (mEq/L)	Cl (mEq/L)	Bile Salts (mEq/L)	Cholesterol (mEq/dL)
Hepatic bile	140–170	50–120	1–50	50–150
Gallbladder bile	225–350	1–10	250–350	300–700

- Bile salt pool (5–7 g) cycles 4–8 times/day
- Small amount (5%–10%) of bile salts lost in stool
  - Active resorption of conjugated bile acids occurs in the **terminal ileum (50%)**
  - Passive resorption of nonconjugated bile acids can occur in the small intestine (45%) and colon (5%)
- Postprandial emptying maximum at 2 hours (80%)
- Bile secreted by **bile canalicular cells** (20%) and **hepatocytes** (80%)

- Color of bile is mostly due to **conjugated bilirubin**
- **Stercobilin** – breakdown product of conjugated bilirubin in gut; gives stool brown color
- **Urobilin** – breakdown product of conjugated bilirubin in gut; yellow; some gets reabsorbed and released in urine

CHOLESTEROL AND BILE ACID SYNTHESIS
■ HMG CoA → (**HMG CoA reductase**) → cholesterol → (**7-alpha-hydroxylase**) → bile acids
■ **HMG CoA reductase** – rate-limiting step in cholesterol synthesis
■ Stones in obese people – **overactive HMG CoA reductase**
■ Stones in thin people – **underactive 7-alpha-hydroxylase**

GALLSTONES
■ Occur in 10% of the population; most asymptomatic
■ Only 10% of gallstones are radiopaque

■ **Nonpigmented stones**
- ↑ **cholesterol insolubilization** – caused by stasis, calcium nucleation by mucin glycoproteins, and ↑ water reabsorption from gallbladder
- Also caused by ↓ **lecithin and bile acids**
- Found almost exclusively in the gallbladder
- Most common type of stone found in the United States (75%)

- **Pigmented stones** – most common worldwide; 25% of stones in the United States
  - Caused by solubilization of unconjugated bilirubin with precipitation of **calcium bilirubinate** and insoluble salts
  - Dissolution agents do not work on pigmented stones (monooctanoin)

  - **Black stones**
    - Can be caused by **hemolytic disorders or cirrhosis**
    - Can also occur in patients on **chronic TPN** and in patients with **ileal resection**
    - **Important factors for the development of these stones** – ↑ bilirubin load, ↓ hepatic function, and bile stasis
    - Almost always form in gallbladder
    - **Tx:** cholecystectomy

  - **Brown stones** (primary CBD stones, formed in ducts)
    - **Infection** causing deconjugation of bilirubin
    - Increased in Asians
    - **E. coli most common** – produces beta-glucuronidase, which deconjugates bilirubin, causes formation of **calcium bilirubinate**
    - Need to check for ampullary stenosis, duodenal diverticula, abnormal sphincter of Oddi
    - Most commonly form in the bile duct (are primary common bile duct stones)
    - Almost all patients with primary stones need a biliary drainage procedure – sphincteroplasty 90% successful

  - Cholesterol stones and black stones found in the CBD are considered **secondary common bile duct stones**

CHOLECYSTITIS
- Caused by obstruction of the cystic duct by a gallstone
- Results in gallbladder wall distention and wall inflammation
- Symptoms: RUQ pain, referred pain to the right shoulder and scapula, nausea and vomiting, loss of appetite
  - Attacks frequently occur after a fatty meal, and pain is persistent (unlike biliary colic)
- Murphy's sign – patient resists deep inspiration with deep palpation to the RUQ secondary to pain
- Alkaline phosphatase and WBC are frequently elevated

- **Suppurative cholecystitis** associated with frank purulence in the gallbladder → can be associated with sepsis and shock
- Most common organisms in cholecystitis – *E. coli*, *Klebsiella*, *Enterococcus*

- **Stone risk factors** – age >40, female, obesity, pregnancy, rapid weight loss, vagotomy, TPN (pigmented stones), ileal resection (pigmented stones)

- **Ultrasound** – 95% sensitive for picking up stones → hyperechoic focus, posterior shadowing, movement of focus with changes in position
  - Best initial evaluation test for jaundice or RUQ pain
  - **Findings suggestive of acute cholecystitis** – gallstones, gallbladder wall thickening (>4 mm), pericholecystic fluid
  - Dilated CBD (>8 mm) suggests CBD stone and obstruction

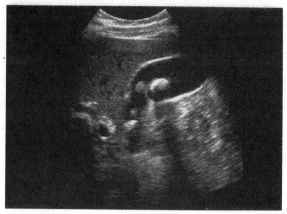

Abdominal ultrasound of gallbladder with multiple echogenic gallstones.

■ **HIDA scan** – technetium taken up by liver and excreted in the biliary tract
  • If gallbladder cannot be seen, it is secondary to cystic duct obstruction by stone → needs cholecystectomy
  • **If <40% of gallbladder volume excreted after CCK over 1 hour** → biliary dyskinesia; although not totally occluded, the excretion is reduced
    • 50% of these patients benefit from cholecystectomy
■ **Indications for preop ERCP (signs that a common bile duct stone is present)** – jaundice, cholangitis, gallstone pancreatitis, ↑ bilirubin (can also be due to primary liver disease), significantly ↑ AST/ALT (can also be due to primary liver disease), stone in CBD on ultrasound
  • **<5%** of patients undergoing cholecystectomy will have a retained CBD stone → 95% of these cleared with ERCP

■ **Tx for cholecystitis** – cholecystectomy; cholecystostomy tube can be placed in patients who are very ill and cannot tolerate surgery
  • When patient is subsequently able to tolerate surgery, cholecystectomy performed

■ **ERCP** – best treatment for late common bile duct stone
  • Sphincterotomy allows for removal of stone
  • Grasper and other tools can then be used to remove the stone
  • Risks: bleeding, pancreatitis, perforation
■ **Biliary colic** – transient cystic duct obstruction caused by passage of a gallstone
  • Resolves within 4–6 hours
■ **Air in the biliary system** most commonly occurs with previous ERCP and sphincterotomy
  • Can also occur with cholangitis or erosion of the biliary system into the duodenum (i.e., gallstone ileus)
■ **Bacterial infection of bile** – dissemination from **portal system** is usual route
  • Can also get retrograde infection from bacteria in duodenum
■ **Highest incidence of positive bile cultures** occurs with **postoperative strictures** (usually *E. coli*, often polymicrobial)

ACALCULOUS CHOLECYSTITIS
■ Thickened wall, RUQ pain, ↑ WBCs
■ Occurs most commonly after severe burns, prolonged TPN, trauma, or major surgery

- Primary pathology is **bile stasis** (narcotics, fasting), leading to distention and ischemia
- Also have ↑ **viscosity secondary to dehydration, ileus, transfusions**
- Ultrasound shows sludge, gallbladder wall thickening, and pericholecystic fluid
- HIDA scan is positive
- Tx: cholecystectomy; percutaneous drainage if patient too unstable

EMPHYSEMATOUS GALLBLADDER DISEASE
- Gas in the gallbladder wall
- Can see on plain film
- ↑ in diabetics; usually secondary to *Clostridium perfringens*
- Symptoms: severe, rapid-onset abdominal pain, nausea, vomiting, and sepsis
- Perforation more common in these patients
- Tx: emergent cholecystectomy; percutaneous drainage if patient is too unstable

GALLSTONE ILEUS
- **Fistula between gallbladder and duodenum** that releases stone, causing small bowel obstruction; elderly
  - Can see **pneumobilia** (air in the biliary system) on plain film
- **Terminal ileum** – most common site of obstruction
- Tx: remove stone with enterotomy proximal to obstruction; perform cholecystectomy and fistula resection if patient can tolerate it

COMMON BILE DUCT INJURIES
- Most commonly occur after laparoscopic cholecystectomy
- Intraoperative cholangiography does not prevent injuries; may limit severity; ↑ early diagnosis of injury
- In 10% of patients, the **right posterior duct** (from segment 6 or 7) **enters the common bile duct separately**
  - Risk of injury with cholecystectomy (confused for cystic duct)
  - If >2 mm, will need to open and perform hepaticojejunostomy

- **Intraoperative CBD injury** – if <50% the circumference of the common bile duct, can probably perform primary repair; in all other cases, will likely need hepaticojejunostomy or choledochojejunostomy

- **Persistent nausea and vomiting or jaundice following laparoscopic cholecystectomy**
  - Ultrasound to look for fluid collection
    - If fluid collection present, may be bile leak → percutaneous drain into the collection
    - If fluid is bilious, get ERCP → sphincterotomy and stent if due to cystic duct remnant leak, small injuries to the hepatic or common bile duct, or a leak from duct of Luschka
    - Larger lesions (i.e., complete duct transection) will require hepaticojejunostomy or choledochojejunostomy
    - If fluid collection not present and the hepatic ducts are dilated, likely have a completely transected common bile duct (see common bile duct or hepatic duct strictures later)

- **Anastomotic leaks** following transplantation or hepaticojejunostomy → usually handled with ERCP and stents

- **Sepsis following laparoscopic cholecystectomy** → fluid resuscitation and stabilize patient
  - May be due to complete transection of the CBD and cholangitis → get ultrasound to look for dilated intrahepatic ducts or fluid collections

- If no fluid collections but bile ducts are dilated → get ERCP and try to stent the strictured area
- If that fails, place a PTC tube

COMMON BILE DUCT OR HEPATIC DUCT STRICTURES

- Most commonly occur after laparoscopic cholecystectomy
- **Ischemia** – most important cause of late postoperative biliary strictures
- Can also be caused by chronic pancreatitis or stricture of a biliary enteric anastomosis
- Dx: ERCP will show stricture; U/S will likely show dilated hepatic ducts
- Symptoms: sepsis, cholangitis, jaundice
- Tx: **ERCP with sphincterotomy** and possible stent placement to decompress; **PTC tube if that fails**

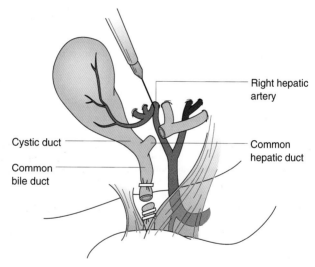

Right hepatic artery

Cystic duct

Common hepatic duct

Common bile duct

Classic laparoscopic bile duct injury. The common bile duct is mistaken for the cystic duct and transected. A variable extent of the extrahepatic biliary tree is resected with the gallbladder. The right hepatic artery, in background, is also often injured.

- For lesions that cause <u>early symptoms (≤7 days)</u> – **hepaticojejunostomy**
- For lesions that cause <u>later symptoms (>7 days)</u> – **hepaticojejunostomy** 6–8 weeks after injury
- Acute injuries are unlikely to be treated sufficiently with ERCP, balloon, and stent
- Late injuries (years later) – can often be treated with ERCP, sphincterotomy, and stent (need to make sure these late injuries do not represent CA – get brushings)

HEMOBILIA

- Fistula between bile duct and hepatic arterial system (most commonly)
- Patients classically present with UGI bleed, jaundice, and RUQ pain
- Most commonly occurs with **trauma** (50% of all cases), infections, primary gallstones, aneurysms, and tumors

- Dx: angiogram
- Tx: resuscitation; angiogram and embolization 1st; operation if that fails

GALLBLADDER ADENOCARCINOMA
- Rare; most common cancer of the biliary tract
- Four times more common than bile duct CA; most have stones
- Liver – most common site of metastasis
- **Porcelain gallbladder** – risk of gallbladder CA (10%–20%) → these patients need cholecystectomy
- 1st spreads to **segments IV and V**; 1st nodes are the cystic duct nodes (right side)
- Symptoms: jaundice 1st, then RUQ pain
- If limited to the mucosa (stage I), cholecystectomy is all that is needed
  - This scenario usually occurs as an incidental finding following laparoscopic cholecystectomy
- If into the muscle (stage II), need wide resection around liver bed at segments IV and V (2–3 cm margins), regional lymphadenectomy, including portal triad; may need Whipple, lobectomy or resection of the CBD
  - 90% of patients present with **stage IV disease**
- High incidence of **tumor implants** in trocar sites when discovered after laparoscopic cholecystectomy
- Laparoscopic approach contraindicated for gallbladder CA
- 5% 5-year survival overall

BILE DUCT CANCER (CHOLANGIOCARCINOMA)
- Occurs in elderly; males
- Risk factors: *C. sinensis* infection, typhoid, ulcerative colitis, choledochal cysts, sclerosing cholangitis, congenital hepatic fibrosis, chronic bile duct infection
- Symptoms: early – painless jaundice most common; can also get cholangitis; late – weight loss, anemia, pruritus
- Persistent ↑ in bilirubin and alkaline phosphatase
- Dx: ERCP 1st; MRI may help define the lesion (these tumors can be hard to find)
- Invades contiguous structures early
- Discovery of a **focal bile duct stenosis** in patients without a history of biliary surgery or pancreatitis is highly suggestive of bile duct CA
- Klatskin tumors – upper ⅓
  - Most common type, worst prognosis, usually unresectable
  - Tx: can try lobectomy and stenting of contralateral bile duct if localized to either the right or left lobe
- Middle ⅓ – hepaticojejunostomy
- Lower ⅓ – Whipple
- Palliative stenting for unresectable disease
- Overall 5-year survival rate – 20%

CHOLEDOCHAL CYSTS (SEE ALSO CHAP. 43)
- Female gender; Asia, Japan; 90% extrahepatic; 15% cancer risk (cholangiocarcinoma)
- Older patients have episodic pain, fever, jaundice, cholangitis
- Most are type I – fusiform or saccular dilatation of extrahepatic ducts (very dilated)
- Infants can have symptoms similar to biliary atresia
- Possibly caused by abnormal reflux of pancreatic enzymes during development secondary to bad angle of insertion
- Occurs during uterine development
- Tx: cyst excision with hepaticojejunostomy and cholecystectomy
- Type IV cysts are partially intrahepatic, and type V (Caroli's disease) are totally intrahepatic → will need partial liver resection

PRIMARY SCLEROSING CHOLANGITIS
- Men in 4th–5th decade
- Can be associated with retroperitoneal fibrosis, Riedel's thyroiditis, pancreatitis, ulcerative colitis, and DM
- Symptoms: fatigue, fluctuating jaundice, pruritus, weight loss, RUQ pain
  - Pruritus caused by bile acids
- Dx: ERCP – multiple strictures and dilatations

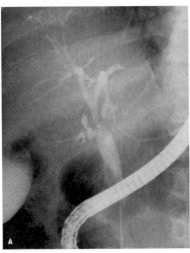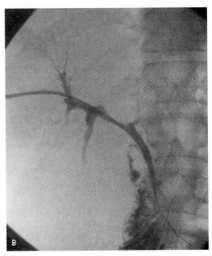

(A) An endoscopic retrograde cholangiopancreatographic image of a patient with primary sclerosing cholangitis that shows the classic features of primary sclerosing cholangitis, including diffuse multifocal strictures involving both the intrahepatic and extrahepatic bile ducts. *(B)* A percutaneous transhepatic cholangiopancreatographic image of a similar patient. (From Pinson CW, Austin MT. Treatment of primary sclerosing cholangitis. In: Fischer JE, Bland KI, et al., eds. *Mastery of Surgery*. 5th ed. Philadelphia, PA: Lippincott Williams & Wilkins; 2007, with permission.)

- Bacterial cholangitis unusual unless biliary tract manipulation has occurred
- Does <u>not</u> get better after colon resection for ulcerative colitis
- Leads to portal HTN and hepatic failure (scarring and patching with progressive fibrosis of intrahepatic and extrahepatic ducts)
- Can have isolated intrahepatic or extrahepatic duct inflammation and fibrosis
- Complications – cirrhosis, cholangiocarcinoma
- Tx: TXP needed long term for most; PTC tube drainage, choledochojejunostomy may be effective for some; balloon dilatation of dominant strictures may provide some symptomatic relief
  - Cholestyramine – can ↓ pruritus symptoms (↓ bile acids)
  - UDCA (urodeoxycholic acid) – can ↓ symptoms (↓ bile acids) and improve liver enzymes

PRIMARY BILIARY CIRRHOSIS
- Women; medium-sized hepatic ducts
- Cholestasis → cirrhosis → portal hypertension
- Symptoms: fatigue, pruritus, jaundice, xanthomas
- **Antimitochondrial antibodies**
- <u>No</u> increased risk for cancer
- Tx: TXP

CHOLANGITIS
- **Charcot's triad** – RUQ pain, fever, jaundice
- **Reynolds' pentad** – Charcot's triad plus mental status changes and shock (suggests sepsis)
- *E. coli* **and** *Klebsiella* – most common organisms
- Cholovenous reflux occurs at 20 mm Hg pressure → systemic bacteremia
- Dx: AST/ALT, bilirubin, alkaline phosphatase, and WBC often ↑
- Ultrasound – CBD will be dilated (>8 mm, >10 mm after cholecystectomy) on ultrasound if due to obstruction of the biliary system
- Stricture and hepatic abscess are late complications of cholangitis
- Renal failure – #1 serious complication; related to **sepsis**
- Gallstones most common etiology
- Other causes – biliary strictures (iatrogenic), neoplasm, chronic pancreatitis, congenital choledochal cysts, duodenal diverticula

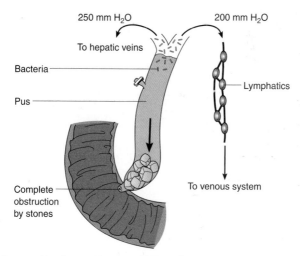

Cholangitis is caused by the combination of biliary obstruction and bactibilia. Bacteria then reflux into the hepatic veins and perihepatic lymphatics, resulting in systemic bacteremia.

- Tx: fluid resuscitation, antibiotics
- Emergent ERCP with sphincterotomy and stone extraction; if ERCP fails, go to PTC tube
- If the patient has cholangitis due to infected PTC tube, change the PTC tube

ORIENTAL CHOLANGIOHEPATITIS
- Asia; recurrent cholangitis from primary CBD stones
- Caused by *C. sinensis*, *A. lumbricoides*, *T. trichiura*, and *E. coli* infections
- Tx: hepaticojejunostomy and antiparasitic medications

SHOCK FOLLOWING LAPAROSCOPIC CHOLECYSTECTOMY
- Early (1st 24 hours) – hemorrhagic shock from clip that fell off cystic artery
- Late (after 1st 24 hours) – septic shock from accidental clip on CBD with subsequent cholangitis

OTHER CONDITIONS
- **Adenomyomatosis** – thickened nodule of mucosa and muscle associated with Rokitansky–Aschoff sinus
  - Not premalignant; does not cause stones, can cause RUQ pain
  - Tx: cholecystectomy
- **Granular cell myoblastoma** – benign neuroectoderm tumor of gallbladder
  - Can occur in biliary tract with signs of cholecystitis
  - Tx: cholecystectomy
- **Cholesterolosis** – speckled cholesterol deposits on the gallbladder wall
- **Gallbladder polyps** – >1 cm, worry about malignancy
  - Polyps in patients > 60 years more likely malignant
  - Tx: cholecystectomy
- **Delta bilirubin** – bound to albumin covalently, half-life of 18 days; may take a while to clear after long-standing jaundice
- **Mirizzi syndrome** – compression of the common hepatic duct by a stone in the infundibulum of the gallbladder or inflammation arising from the gallbladder or cystic duct extending to the contiguous hepatic duct, causing stricture and hepatic duct obstruction
- **Ceftriaxone** – can cause gallbladder sludging and cholestatic jaundice
- **Indications for asymptomatic cholecystectomy** – in patients undergoing liver TXP or gastric bypass procedure

ANATOMY AND PHYSIOLOGY

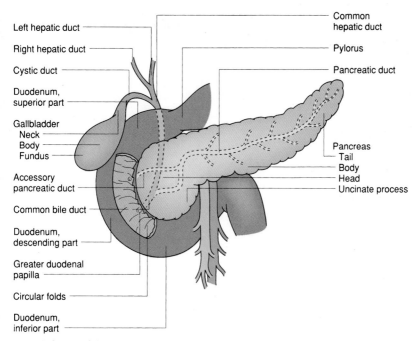

Left hepatic duct

Right hepatic duct

Cystic duct

Duodenum, superior part

Gallbladder
Neck
Body
Fundus

Accessory pancreatic duct

Common bile duct

Duodenum, descending part

Greater duodenal papilla

Circular folds

Duodenum, inferior part

Common hepatic duct

Pylorus

Pancreatic duct

Pancreas
Tail
Body
Head
Uncinate process

Relation of the pancreas to the duodenum and extrahepatic biliary system.

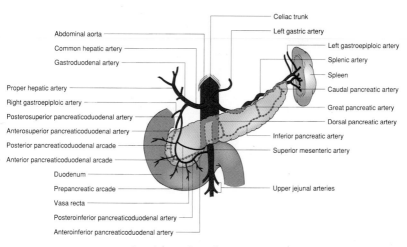

Celiac trunk

Left gastric artery

Abdominal aorta

Common hepatic artery

Gastroduodenal artery

Left gastroepiploic artery

Splenic artery

Spleen

Caudal pancreatic artery

Great pancreatic artery

Dorsal pancreatic artery

Proper hepatic artery

Right gastroepiploic artery

Posterosuperior pancreaticoduodenal artery

Anterosuperior pancreaticoduodenal artery

Posterior pancreaticoduodenal arcade

Anterior pancreaticoduodenal arcade

Duodenum

Prepancreatic arcade

Vasa recta

Posteroinferior pancreaticoduodenal artery

Anteroinferior pancreaticoduodenal artery

Inferior pancreatic artery

Superior mesenteric artery

Upper jejunal arteries

Arterial supply to the pancreas.

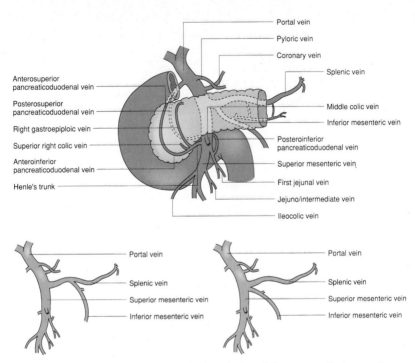

Venous drainage of pancreas. Variations in the relation of the portal, splenic, superior mesenteric, and inferior mesenteric veins are shown at the bottom.

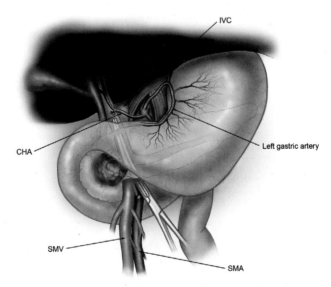

Relationship between the superior mesenteric vein and superior mesenteric artery. (Modified from Evans DB, Lee JE, Tamm EP, et al. Pancreaticoduodenectomy (Whipple operation) and total pancreatectomy for cancer. In: Fischer JE, Bland KI, et al., eds. *Mastery of Surgery*. 5th ed. Philadelphia, PA: Lippincott Williams & Wilkins; 2007, with permission.)

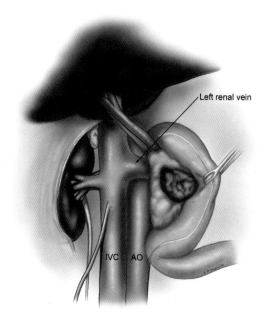

Left renal vein

IVC   AO

Kocher maneuver and relationship between the aorta and inferior vena cava. (Modified from Evans DB, Lee JE, Tamm EP, et al. Pancreaticoduodenectomy (Whipple operation) and total pancreatectomy for cancer. In: Fischer JE, Bland KI, et al., eds. *Mastery of Surgery*. 5th ed. Philadelphia, PA: Lippincott Williams & Wilkins; 2007, with permission.)

- **Head** (including uncinate), **neck, body, and tail**
- **Uncinate process** – rests on aorta, behind SMA
- **SMA and SMV** – lay behind neck of pancreas
- **Portal vein** – forms behind the neck (SMV and splenic vein)
- **Blood supply**
  - **Head** – superior (off GDA) and inferior (off SMA) pancreaticoduodenal arteries (anterior and posterior branches for each)
  - **Body** – great, inferior, and caudal pancreatic artery (all off **splenic artery**)
  - **Tail** – splenic, gastroepiploic, and dorsal pancreatic arteries
- **Venous drainage into the portal system**
- **Lymphatics** – celiac and SMA nodes

- **Ductal cells** – have carbonic anhydrase and secrete HCO_3^- solution
  - ↑ flow leads to ↑ HCO_3^- and ↓ Cl^-
- **Acinar cells** – secrete Cl^- and digestive enzymes

- **Exocrine function of the pancreas** – amylase, lipase, trypsinogen, chymotrypsinogen, carboxypeptidase; HCO_3^-
  - **Amylase** – <u>only pancreatic enzyme secreted in active form</u>; hydrolyzes alpha 1-4 linkages of glucose chains

- **Endocrine function of the pancreas**
  - **Alpha cells** – glucagon
  - **Beta cells (at center of islets)** – insulin
  - **Delta cells** – somatostatin

- **PP or F cells** – pancreatic polypeptide
- **Islet cells** – also produce vasoactive intestinal peptide (VIP), serotonin, neuropeptide Y, gastrin-releasing peptide (GRP)

- ▨ **Islet cells receive majority of blood supply related to size**
- ▨ After islets, blood goes to acinar cells
- ▨ **Enterokinase** – released by the duodenum, activates trypsinogen to trypsin
- ▨ Trypsin activates other pancreatic enzymes including trypsinogen
- ▨ **Hormonal control of pancreatic excretion**
  - **Secretin** – ↑ HCO_3^- mostly
  - **CCK** – ↑ enzymes mostly
  - **Acetylcholine** – ↑ HCO^- and enzymes
  - **Somatostatin and glucagons** – ↓ exocrine function
  - **CCK and secretin** – most released by cells in the duodenum

- ▨ **Ventral pancreatic bud**
  - Connected to duct of Wirsung; migrates posteriorly, to the right, and clockwise to fuse with the dorsal bud
  - Forms uncinate and inferior portion of the head
- ▨ **Dorsal pancreatic bud** – body, tail, and superior aspect of the pancreatic head; has duct of Santorini
- ▨ **Duct of Santorini** – small accessory pancreatic duct that drains directly into duodenum
- ▨ **Duct of Wirsung** – major pancreatic duct that merges with CBD before entering duodenum

ANNULAR PANCREAS
- ▨ 2nd portion of duodenum trapped in pancreatic band; can see double bubble on abdominal x-ray
- ▨ Associated with Down syndrome; forms from the ventral pancreatic bud from failure of clockwise rotation
- ▨ Tx: duodenojejunostomy or duodenoduodenostomy and sphincteroplasty
  - Pancreas <u>not</u> resected

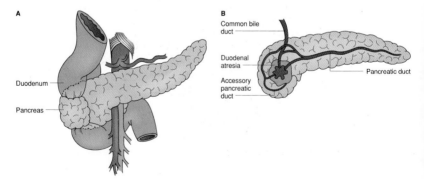

Annular pancreas. *(A)* The associated duodenal atresia is shown. *(B)* The relationships of the annular pancreas to the common bile duct and main and accessory pancreatic ducts are shown in cross section.

PANCREAS DIVISUM
- ▨ Failed fusion of the pancreatic ducts; can result in pancreatitis from duct of Santorini (accessory duct) stenosis

- Most are asymptomatic; some get pancreatitis
- Dx: ERCP – **minor papilla** will show long and large duct of Santorini; **major papilla** will show short duct of Wirsung
- Tx: sphincteroplasty and stent placement if symptomatic
  - May need open sphincteroplasty if that fails
  - If long-standing, sphincteroplasty may not work → then need longitudinal pancreaticojejunostomy

HETEROTOPIC PANCREAS
- Most commonly found in duodenum
- Usually asymptomatic
- Surgical resection if symptomatic

ACUTE PANCREATITIS
- **Stones and ETOH most common causes in the United States**
- **Other causes** – ERCP, trauma, hyperlipidemia, hypercalcemia, viral infection, medications (azathioprine, furosemide, steroids, cimetidine), *Ascaris lumbricoides* and *C. sinensis*

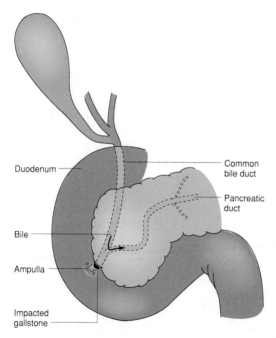

Illustration of the common channel concept. A gallstone lodged at the ampulla of Vater can cause reflux of bile into the pancreatic duct.

- **Symptoms: abdominal pain radiating to the back, nausea, vomiting, anorexia**
  - Jaundice can occur in 40%; can also get left pleural effusion and sentinel loop (dilated small bowel near the pancreas as a result of the inflammation)
- Caused by impaired extrusion of zymogen granules and activation of degradation enzymes → leads to autodigestion
- Mortality rate 10%; hemorrhagic pancreatitis mortality 50%
- Pancreatitis without obvious cause → need to worry about malignancy

■ **Ranson's criteria**   *(liver)*
WALLS 🖤• On admission → age > 55, WBC > 16, glucose > 200, AST > 250, LDH > 350
FO CHUB   • After 48 hours: Hct ↓ 10%, BUN ↑ of 5, Ca < 8, PaO₂ < 60, base deficit > 4, fluid
             sequestration > 6 L
         • 8 Ranson criteria met → mortality rate near 100%
         • ≥ 3 =severe pancreatitis
■ **Labs:** ↑ amylase, lipase, and WBCs
■ **Tx:** NPO, aggressive fluid resuscitation
    • Antibiotics for those with stones, if severe, failure to improve or thought to have
      infection
    • TPN may be necessary during recovery period
    • ERCP may be needed in patients with gallstone pancreatitis and retained stone still
      in the CBD → perform sphincterotomy and stone extraction
    • Patients with gallstone pancreatitis should undergo cholecystectomy when recovered
      from pancreatitis
    • Morphine should probably be avoided in patients with pancreatitis as it can contract
      the sphincter of Oddi and could worsen attack
■ **Abdominal CT** – needed only to check for complications (dead pancreas will not light up)

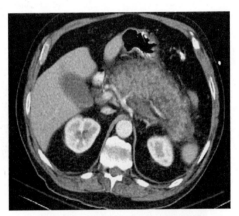

CT scan of acute interstitial pancreatitis.

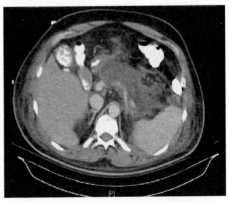

CT scan of acute necrotizing pancreatitis.

- Ultrasound – needed to check for gallstones and possible CBD dilatation
- **Bleeding**
  - **Grey Turner sign** – flank ecchymosis
  - **Cullen's sign** – periumbilical ecchymosis
  - **Fox's sign** – inguinal ecchymosis
- **15% get necrosis** – generally leave sterile necrosis alone
  - 10% of those patients require surgery for infected necrosis (patient not getting better or positive blood cultures) → may need to sample this with CT-guided aspiration
  - CT-guided drainage of pancreatic abscesses is ineffective

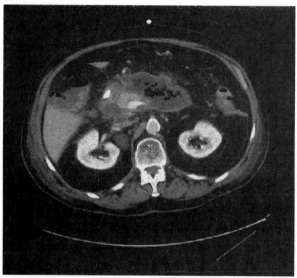

Pancreatic abscess. Overt gas is evident in a zone of infected pancreatic necrosis 8 weeks following initial presentation of gallstone pancreatitis and represents an absolute indication for surgical debridement. (From Vollmer CM Jr. Necrosectomy for acute necrotizing pancreatitis. In: Fischer JE, Bland KI, et al., eds. *Mastery of Surgery*. 5th ed. Philadelphia, PA: Lippincott Williams & Wilkins; 2007, with permission.)

- **Infection** – leading cause of death; usually GNRs
  - Need to remove infected material – see gas in pancreas on abdominal CT
  - May need ultrasound- or CT-guided aspiration to diagnose infection

- Surgery only for infected pancreatitis

- **Obesity** – most important risk factor for necrotizing pancreatitis
- **ARDS** – related to release of phospholipases
- **Coagulopathy** – related to release of proteases
- **Pancreatic/fat necrosis** – related to release of phospholipases
- **Mildly ↑ amylase and lipase can be seen with** cholecystitis, perforated ulcer, sialoadenitis, SBO, and intestinal infarction

PANCREATIC PSEUDOCYSTS
- Most common in patients with chronic pancreatitis
- Symptoms: pain, fever, weight loss, bowel obstruction from compression
- Often occurs in the head of the pancreas; small cysts likely to resolve spontaneously (<5 cm)

- Nonepithelialized sac
- **Expectant management up to 3 months** – allows pseudocyst to mature
- Only need to treat patients with **continued symptoms or pseudocysts that are growing**
- May need to place these patients on TPN if unable to eat
- Usually in head of pancreas
- Can present with persistent **pain, fever, ↑ WBCs, palpable mass, jaundice**

- Patients with symptomatic or growing pseudocyst need <u>MRCP or ERCP</u> to check for duct involvement
  - If <u>duct involved</u>, will need **cystogastrostomy (endoscopic or open)**
  - If <u>duct not involved</u>, may get away with **percutaneous drainage of pseudocyst**
- **Complications of pancreatic pseudocyst** – SBO, infection, portal or splenic vein thrombosis
- **Incidental cysts** should be resected unless associated with pancreatitis or unless the cyst is purely serous

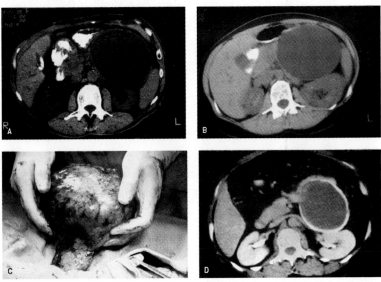

(A) Pseudocyst. *(B)* Serous cystadenoma. These examples are virtually indistinguishable by radiographic criteria, emphasizing the importance of a history consistent with pancre-atitis and aspiration of "cystic" fluid in making a diagnosis. *(C)* The same serous cystade-noma at the time of resection. *(D)* Serous cystadenocarcinoma. Note the presence of a calcified rim, often indicative of malignant disease. (From Warshaw AL, Christison-Lagay ER. Pancreatic cystoenterostomy. In: Fischer JE, Bland KI, et al., eds. *Mastery of Surgery*. 5th ed. Philadelphia, PA: Lippincott Williams & Wilkins; 2007, with permission.)

PANCREATIC FISTULAS
- Most close spontaneously (especially if low output < 200 cc/day)
- Tx: allow drainage, TPN, octreotide
  - If failure to resolve with medical management, can try ERCP, sphincterotomy, and pancreatic stent placement
  - If that fails, for distal lesions perform **distal pancreatectomy**; for proximal lesions **may need Whipple**
- Pancreatitis-associated recurrent pleural effusion or ascites – thoracentesis or paracentesis followed by ERCP and stent placement initially; may need resection if that fails
- Amylase will be elevated in the fluid

CHRONIC PANCREATITIS

- Corresponds to irreversible parenchymal fibrosis
- **ETOH** most common cause; idiopathic 2nd most common
- Pain most common problem; anorexia, weight loss, malabsorption, steatorrhea, recurrent acute pancreatitis
- Exocrine tissue gets calcified and fibrotic; **islet cells usually preserved**
- Advanced disease – **chain of lakes** → alternating segments of dilation and stenosis in pancreatic duct
- Can cause **malabsorption of fat-soluble vitamins**
  - **Stents** – have a temporizing role

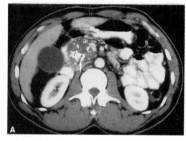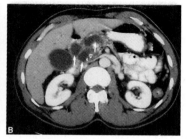

Abdominal computed tomography demonstrates pancreatic calcifications *(arrow)*.

- Dx: abdominal CT will show shrunken pancreas with calcifications
  - Ultrasound – shows pancreatic ducts > 4 mm, cysts, and atrophy
  - ERCP – very sensitive at diagnosing chronic pancreatitis

- Tx: supportive care, including pain control and nutritional support (tube feeds, TPN)
- **Surgical indications** – pain that interferes with quality of life, nutrition abnormalities, addiction to narcotics, failure to rule out malignancy, biliary obstruction, abscess

- **Surgical options**
  - **Puestow procedure** – pancreaticojejunostomy, for ducts > 8 mm (most patients improve) → open along main pancreatic duct and drain into jejunum

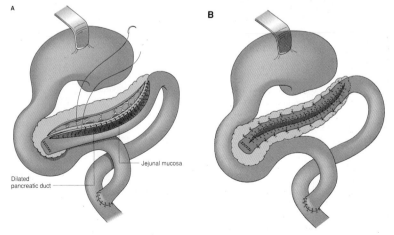

Lateral pancreaticojejunostomy.

- **Distal pancreatic resection** – for normal duct anatomy, failed Puestow procedures, or when only a small portion of the gland is affected
- **Whipple** – may be needed in patients with pancreatic head disease
- Splanchnicectomy or celiac ganglionectomy (ablation) may be used for postop pain control

■ **Common bile duct stricture** – proximal dilation that can occur with chronic pancreatitis
- Tx: hepaticojejunostomy or choledochojejunostomy for pain, jaundice, cholangitis

■ **Splenic vein thrombosis** – chronic pancreatitis most common cause of splenic vein thrombosis
- Can get bleeding from gastric varices that form as collaterals
- Tx: splenectomy for bleeding gastric varices

PANCREATIC INSUFFICIENCY
■ Usually the result of long-standing pancreatitis or occurs after total pancreatectomy (over 90% of the function must be lost)
■ Generally refers to exocrine function
■ Symptoms: malabsorption and steatorrhea
■ Dx: fecal fat testing
■ Tx: high-carbohydrate, high-protein, low-fat diet with pancreatic enzyme replacement
■ **Steatorrhea** – give Pancrease (pancreatic enzymes)

BILIARY STENOSIS (PANCREATIC ETIOLOGIES)
■ Secondary to pseudocysts, fibrosis
■ Complications: biliary cirrhosis, cholangitis
■ Surgery indicated with persistent jaundice, cirrhosis, progressive dilatation of hepatic ducts, or cholangitis; also if cannot exclude pancreatic cancer
■ Tx: hepaticojejunostomy

JAUNDICE WORKUP
■ **Ultrasound 1st**
- **Positive stones, no mass** → ERCP
- **No stones, no mass** → abdominal CT or MRI
- **Positive mass** → abdominal CT or MRI

PANCREATIC ADENOCARCINOMA
■ Male predominance; typically occurs in the 6th–7th decades of life
■ Symptoms: **weight loss (most common symptom), jaundice, pain**
■ **20% 5-year survival rate with resection**
■ Risk factors – **tobacco #1**
■ **CA 19-9** – serum marker for pancreatic CA
■ Lymphatic spread 1st

■ **70% in head**
- 50% invade portal vein, SMV, or retroperitoneum at time of diagnosis (unresectable disease)
- Metastases to peritoneum, omentum, and liver – indicate unresectable disease
- Metastases to celiac or SMA nodal system (nodal systems outside area of resection) – indicate unresectable disease
- Most cures in patients with pancreatic head disease

- **90% ductal adenocarcinoma**
  - Other tumors of the exocrine pancreas (have more favorable prognosis) – papillary cystic adenocarcinoma, serous cystadenomas (vast majority benign), mucinous cystadenomas (considered premalignant)

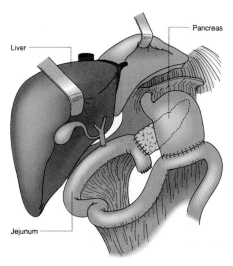

Reconstruction after standard pancreaticoduodenectomy.

- Labs: typically show ↑ conjugated bilirubin and alkaline phosphatase
- **Patients with a resectable mass (no signs of metastatic disease) in the pancreas do <u>not</u> need a biopsy** because you are taking it out regardless. If the patient appears to have metastatic disease, a biopsy is warranted to direct therapy

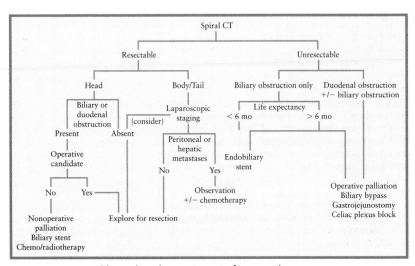

Diagnosis and management of pancreatic cancer.

- ERCP good at differentiating dilated ducts secondary to chronic pancreatitis versus cancer
  - **Signs of CA on ERCP** – duct with irregular narrowing, displacement, destruction
- **Abdominal CT** – may show the lesion and double-duct sign for pancreatic head cancers (dilation of both the pancreatic duct and CBD)
  - May want preop <u>MR angiogram or contrast angiogram</u> if worried about vessel involvement

- Can consider stents, hepaticojejunostomy, or gastrojejunostomy **as palliation** for jaundice or obstruction
- Chemotherapy (**gemcitabine**) **and XRT**

- **Complications from Whipple**
  - **Delayed gastric emptying #1**
    - Tx – metoclopramide
  - Anastomotic breakdown
  - Marginal ulceration
  - Abscess or infection
  - Pancreatitis
  - Fistulas

- **Pancreatic duct leak** – Tx: drain and possible ERCP and stenting of pancreatic duct
- **Celiac plexus block** – for painful unresectable disease
- Prognosis related to vascular and nodal invasion and ability to get a clear margin
- **Bleeding** after Whipple or other pancreatic surgery – go to angio 1st for embolization (the tissue planes are very friable early after surgery and bleeding is hard to control operatively)

NONFUNCTIONAL ENDOCRINE TUMORS
- Represent ⅓ of pancreatic endocrine neoplasms
- **90% of the nonfunctional tumors are malignant**
- Symptoms: pain, weight loss, jaundice
- Tend to have a more indolent and protracted course compared with pancreatic adenocarcinoma
- Dx: abdominal CT or MRI
- Resect these lesions: metastatic disease precludes resection
- 5FU and streptozocin may be effective
- Liver metastases most common
  - 50% 5-year survival rate after resection

FUNCTIONAL ENDOCRINE PANCREATIC TUMORS
- Represents ⅔ of pancreatic endocrine neoplasms
- **Octreotide** – effective for insulinoma, glucagonoma, gastrinoma, VIPoma
- **Most common in pancreatic head** – gastrinoma, somatostatinoma
- All tumors can respond to debulking
- Liver spread – 1st for all

- **Insulinoma**
  - **Most common islet cell tumor of the pancreas**
  - Symptoms: **Whipple's triad** → fasting hypoglycemia (<50), symptoms of hypoglycemia (catecholamine surge → palpitations, ↑ HR, and diaphoresis), relief with glucose
  - **85%–95% benign** and evenly distributed throughout pancreas
  - Dx: Insulin to glucose ratio > 0.4 after fasting, ↑ C peptide and proinsulin → otherwise suspect **Munchausen's syndrome**

- Tx: enucleate if <2 cm; formal resection if >2 cm
  - For metastatic disease → streptozocin, octreotide, 5FU

■ **Gastrinoma (Zollinger–Ellison syndrome [ZES])**
  - **Most common pancreatic islet cell tumor in MEN-1 patients**
  - 50% **malignant** and 50% **multiple**
  - **75% spontaneous and 25% MEN-1**

  - **Majority in gastrinoma triangle** – common bile duct, neck of pancreas, third portion of the duodenum

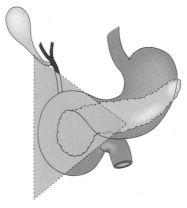

Most gastrinomas are found within the gastrinoma triangle.

- **Symptoms**: **refractory ulcer disease** (abdominal pain) **and diarrhea** (improved with H_2 blockers)

- **Serum gastrin** usually > 200; 1000s is diagnostic

- **Secretin stimulation test** – ZES patients: ↑ gastrin (>200); normal patients: ↓ gastrin
- **Suspect ZES** with refractory ulcer disease, ulcers occurring with diarrhea, bleeding, obstruction, perforation

- Tx: enucleation if <2 cm; formal resection if >2 cm
  - Malignant disease → excise suspicious nodes
  - Cannot find tumor → perform duodenostomy and look inside duodenum for tumor (15% of microgastrinomas there)
  - **Duodenal tumor** – resection with primary closure; may need Whipple if extensive; be sure to check pancreas for primary
  - **Debulking** – can improve symptoms
  - **Somatostatin receptor scintigraphy** – single best study for localizing tumor
  - MRI and CT scan can also be effective
  - Consider vagotomy and pyloromyotomy for patients with unresectable disease and severe symptoms

■ **Somatostatinoma**
  - **Very rare**
  - Symptoms: diabetes, gallstones, steatorrhea, hypochlorhydria
  - Diagnosis: fasting somatostatin level
  - Most **malignant**; most in **head of pancreas**
  - Perform cholecystectomy with resection

■ **Glucagonoma**
- Symptoms: diabetes, stomatitis, dermatitis (necrolytic migratory erythema), weight loss
- Diagnosis: fasting glucagon level
- Most **malignant**; most in **distal pancreas**
- Zinc, amino acids, or fatty acids may treat skin rash

■ **VIPoma (Verner–Morrison syndrome)**
- Symptoms: watery diarrhea, hypokalemia, and achlorhydria (WDHA)
- Hypokalemia from diarrhea
- Dx: exclude other causes of diarrhea; ↑ VIP levels
- Most **malignant**; most in **distal pancreas**, 10% extrapancreatic (retroperitoneal, thorax)
- Can measure VIP levels

Steps in the Management of Patients with Suspected Pancreatic Neuroendocrine Tumor[a]

1. Establish diagnosis biochemically

Insulinoma	Supervised fast with hypoglycemia (<50 mg/dL) and hyperinsulinism (insulin to glucose ratio > 0.3)
Gastrinoma	Fasting high gastrin (>130) with elevated BAO
	Abnormal secretin test
VIPoma	Secretory diarrhea (>3 L/day)
	Elevated serum VIP
Glucagonoma	Rash
	Hypoaminoacidemia
	Type 2 diabetes mellitus
	Elevated fasting serum glucagon (>1,000 pg/mL)

2. Evaluate for familial syndrome

Careful family history with specific attention to evidence for MEN-1 or von Hippel–Lindau syndrome
Check serum levels of calcium and prolactin to screen for MEN-1
If in doubt, may investigate first-degree relatives in whom syndrome is suspected

3. Treat symptoms of hormone excess

Insulinoma	Diet, diazoxide, or octreotide
Gastrinoma	H_2 blockers or proton pump inhibitors
VIPoma	Octreotide and potassium supplements
Glucagonoma	Octreotide, anticoagulation, and IVC filter

4. Perform tumor localization/treatment planning

Insulinoma	Preoperative ultrasound or CT scan
	Consider endoscopic ultrasound
Gastrinoma	Preoperative CT and octreoscan
	Rarely, secretin angiogram
	Consider endoscopic ultrasound
Nonfunctional tumors VIPoma	Preoperative CT scan and octreoscan

5. Prepare for resection

Pneumococcal vaccine (if splenectomy is potentially necessary)
Mechanical bowel preparation (optional)
Insulinoma patients must be on IV glucose during bowel preparation
Zollinger–Ellison syndrome patients must be admitted for IV acid blockade during bowel preparation
Consider somatostatin analog and antibiotics beginning immediately preoperatively

[a]BAO, basal acid output; VIP, vasoactive intestinal polypeptide; MEN-1, multiple endocrine neoplasia type 1; IVC, inferior vena cava; CT, computed tomography; IV, intravenous.
From Doherty GM. Pancreatic neuroendocrine tumors. In: Fischer JE, Bland KI, et al., eds. *Mastery of Surgery*. 5th ed. Philadelphia, PA: Lippincott Williams & Wilkins; 2007, with permission.

ANATOMY AND PHYSIOLOGY

- ▣ Short gastrics and splenic artery are end arteries
- ▣ Splenic vein is posterior and inferior to the splenic artery
- ▣ Spleen serves as antigen-processing center for macrophages; **largest producer of IgM**
- ▣ **85% red pulp** – acts as a filter for aged or damaged RBCs
  - **Pitting** – removal of abnormalities in RBC membrane
    - Howell–Jolly bodies – nuclear remnants
    - Heinz bodies – hemoglobin
  - **Culling** – removal of less deformable RBCs
- ▣ **15% white pulp** – immunologic function; contains lymphocytes and macrophages
  - Major site of **bacterial clearance that lacks preexisting antibodies**
  - Site of removal of **poorly opsonized bacteria, particles, and cellular debris**
  - Antigen processing occurs with interaction between macrophages and helper T cells

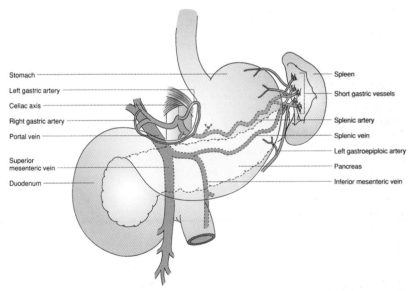

The arterial blood flow to the spleen is derived from the splenic artery, the left gastroepiploic artery, and the short gastric arteries (vasa brevia). The venous drainage into this portal vein is also shown.

- ▣ **Tuftsin** – an opsonin; facilitates phagocytosis → produced in the spleen
- ▣ **Properdin** – activates alternate complement pathway → produced in spleen
- ▣ **Hematopoiesis** – occurs in spleen before birth and in conditions such as myeloid dysplasia
- ▣ **Accessory spleen** – most commonly found at splenic hilum (20%)

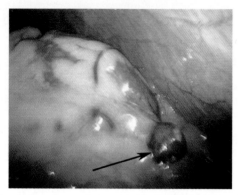

Accessory spleen at lower pole of splenic hilum *(arrow)*.

- **Indication for splenectomy** – ideopathic thrombocytopenic purpura (ITP) far greater than for thrombotic thrombocytopenic purpura (TTP)
- ITP most common nontraumatic condition requiring splenectomy

Normal Functions of the Spleen

HEMATOLOGIC
  Culling or destruction of senescent erythrocytes
  Pitting or removal of cytoplasm inclusive in erythrocytes
  Reservoir for platelets and granulocytes
  Hematopoiesis—as fetus or in conditions with bone marrow destruction

IMMUNOLOGIC
  Filtration and trapping of circulatory antigens
  Lymphocyte stimulation and proliferation
  Antibody production in germinal follicles
  Production of opsonin-tuftsin and properdin
  Opsonins: tuftsin and properdin

IDIOPATHIC THROMBOCYTOPENIC PURPURA

- This can occur from many etiologies – drugs, viruses, etc.
- **Antiplatelet antibodies** (IgG) – bind platelets, cause ↓ platelets
- Petechiae, gingival bleeding, bruising, soft tissue ecchymosis
- **Spleen is normal**
- In children < 10 years, usually resolves spontaneously
- Tx: **steroids** (primary therapy), plasmapheresis, gammaglobulin for steroid-resistant disease
- Splenectomy indicated for those who fail steroids → removes IgG production and source of phagocytosis; 80% respond after splenectomy
- Give platelets 1 hour before surgery

THROMBOTIC THROMBOCYTOPENIC PURPURA

- Associated w/ medical reactions, infections, inflammation, autoimmune disease
- **Loss of platelet inhibition** – leads to thrombosis and infarction, profound thrombocytopenia
- Purpura, fever, mental status changes, renal dysfunction, hematuria, hemolytic anemia
- 80% respond to medical therapy
- Tx: **plasmapheresis** (primary), steroids, ASA
- Death most commonly due to intracerebral hemorrhage or acute renal failure
- Splenectomy rarely indicated

POSTSPLENECTOMY SEPSIS SYNDROME

- ▓ **0.1% risk**; ↑ risk in **children**
- ▓ *S. pneumoniae* (#1), *H. influenzae*, *N. meningitidis* – most common
- ▓ Secondary to specific lack of immunity (immunoglobulin, IgM) to capsulated bacteria
- ▓ Highest in patients with splenectomy for **hemolytic disorders or malignancy**
- ▓ Children also have ↑ risk of mortality after developing postsplenectomy sepsis syndrome
- ▓ Try to wait until at least 5 years old before performing splenectomy → allows antibody formation; child can get fully immunized
- ▓ Most episodes occur within 2 years of splenectomy
- ▓ Children < 10 years should be given prophylactic antibiotics for 6 months (controversial)
- ▓ **Vaccines needed before splenectomy** – *Pneumococcus, Meningococcus, H. influenzae*
  - • Try to give before splenectomy

- ▓ **Postsplenectomy changes** – ↑ RBCs, ↑ WBCs, ↑ platelets; if platelets > 1×10^6, need ASA
- ▓ **Hemangioma** – #1 splenic tumor overall; #1 benign splenic tumor
  - • Splenectomy if symptomatic
- ▓ **Non-Hodgkin's lymphoma** – #1 malignant splenic tumor
- ▓ **Splenic cysts** – surgery if symptomatic or >10 cm

HYPERSPLENISM

- ▓ Results in ↓ platelets, RBCs, and WBCs; splenomegaly occurs as well

Definition of Hypersplenism

Decrease in circulating cell count of erythrocytes and/or platelets and/or leukocytes
and
Normal compensatory hematopoietic responses present in bone marrow
and
Correction of cytopenia by splenectomy
with or without
Splenomegaly

- ▓ **Secondary hypersplenism (most common)**
  - • Associated most commonly with ↑ venous pressure (portal hypertension, CHF), malignant disease (leukemia), chronic inflammatory disease (Felty's syndrome, SLE, sarcoidosis), myeloproliferative disease, infectious disease, amyloidosis, AIDS, hemolytic anemias, polycythemia vera
  - • Splenectomy may be indicated for **symptomatic hypersplenism** associated with CLL, CML, NHL, Hodgkin's, hairy cell leukemia, hemolytic anemias, sarcoidosis
- ▓ **Primary hypersplenism (very rare)** – need to rule out other causes
  - • Splenectomy indicated for primary hypersplenism
- ▓ **Sarcoidosis of spleen** – anemia, ↓ platelets
  - • Tx: splenectomy for symptomatic splenomegaly
- ▓ **Felty's syndrome** – rheumatoid arthritis, hepatomegaly, splenomegaly
  - • Tx: splenectomy for symptomatic splenomegaly
- ▓ **Gaucher's disease** – lipid metabolism disorder leading to splenomegaly
  - • Partial splenectomy may be effective

HEMOLYTIC ANEMIAS – MEMBRANE PROTEIN DEFECTS

- ▓ **Spherocytosis**
  - • **Most common congenital hemolytic anemia requiring splenectomy**
  - • Spectrin deficit (**membrane protein**) deforms RBCs and leads to splenic sequestration
  - • Causes pigmented stones, anemia, reticulocytosis, jaundice, splenomegaly
  - • Try to perform splenectomy after age 5; give immunizations first
  - • Tx: splenectomy and cholecystectomy
  - • Splenectomy curative

- **Elliptocytosis**
  - Symptoms and mechanism similar to spherocytosis; less common
  - Spectrin and protein 4.1 deficit (**membrane protein**)

HEMOLYTIC ANEMIAS – NON–MEMBRANE PROTEIN DEFECTS
- **Pyruvate kinase deficiency**
  - Results in congenital hemolytic anemia
  - Causes altered glucose metabolism; RBC survival enhanced by splenectomy
- **Most common congenital hemolytic anemia <u>not</u> involving a membrane protein that requires splenectomy**
- **G6PD deficiency**
  - Precipitated by infection, certain drugs, fava beans
  - Splenectomy usually not required
- **Warm antibody–type acquired immune hemolytic anemia** – indication for splenectomy
- **Sickle cell anemia** – HgbA replaced with HgbS
  - Spleen usually autoinfarcts and splenectomy <u>not</u> required
- **Beta thalassemia**
  - Most common thalassemia
  - Major – both chains affected; minor – 1 chain, asymptomatic
  - Symptoms: pallor, retarded body growth, head enlargement
  - Persistent HgbF
  - Splenectomy may ↓ hemolysis and symptoms
  - Most die in teens secondary to hemosiderosis

HODGKIN'S DISEASE[1]
- A – asymptomatic
- B – symptomatic (night sweats, fever, weight loss) → unfavorable prognosis
- Stage I – 1 area or 2 contiguous areas on the same side of diaphragm
- Stage II – 2 noncontiguous areas on the same side of diaphragm
- Stage III – involved on each side of diaphragm
- Stage IV – liver, bone, lung, or any other nonlymphoid tissue except spleen

- See **Reed–Sternberg cells**
- **Lymphocyte predominant** – best prognosis
- **Lymphocyte depleted** – worst prognosis
- **Nodular sclerosing** – most common
- Tx: XRT and chemotherapy with vincristine, cyclophosphamide, prednisone, procarbazine

- MCC of Chylous ascites – lymphoma

NON-HODGKIN'S LYMPHOMA
- Worse prognosis than Hodgkin's
- Generally systemic disease by the time the diagnosis is made
- 90% are B-cell lymphomas
- Tx: XRT and chemotherapy with vincristine, cyclophosphamide, prednisone, Adriamycin

Hairy cell leukemia – Tx: splenectomy, INF-γ
Spontaneous splenic rupture – mononucleosis, malaria, sepsis, sarcoid, leukemia, polycythemia vera
Splenosis – splenic implants; usually related to trauma
Hyposplenism – see Howell–Jolly bodies
Pancreatitis – most common cause of splenic artery or splenic vein thrombosis

---

[1] Modified from AJCC. *Cancer Staging Handbook*. 6th ed. New York: Springer-Verlag, 2002:440–441.

Splenic artery aneurysms – females; secondary to fibromuscular dysplasia, atherosclerosis (see Chap. 27)

Results of Splenectomy/Hyposplenic Condition

ERYTHROCYTES
- Howell–Jolly bodies (nuclear fragments)
- Heinz bodies (hemoglobin deposits)
- Pappenheimer bodies (iron deposits)
- Target cells
- Spur cells (acanthocytes)

PLATELETS
- Transient thrombocytosis

LEUKOCYTES
- Transient leukocytosis
- Persistent lymphocytosis
- Persistent monocytosis

Guidelines for Prevention of Postsplenic Sepsis

- Vaccinate with polyvalent pneumococcal vaccine at least 10–14 days prior to splenectomy, if possible
- If splenectomy is urgent, wait until at least 14 days postprocedure to vaccinate
- For high-risk patients (immunosuppressed, children < 10 years of age), meningococcal vaccine and *Haemophilus influenza* vaccine
- Antibiotic prophylaxis for children < 5 years of age
- Early antibiotic treatment for initial signs of infection
- MedicAlert bracelet

Operative Indications for Splenectomy and Whether Total or Partial Splenectomy Is Indicated

Disease	Need for Splenectomy	Partial Splenectomy
Hereditary spherocytosis	Always	Yes
Hereditary elliptocytosis	Sometimes	Yes
Thalassemia	Sometimes	Yes
Sickle cell anemia	Rarely	No
Wiskott–Aldrich syndrome	Sometimes	No
Autoimmune hemolytic anemia	Usually	No
Autoimmune neutropenia	Sometimes	No
Immune thrombocytopenia purpura	Usually	No
Thrombotic thrombocytopenia purpura	Sometimes	No
Hairy cell leukemia	Rarely[a]	No
Chronic lymphocytic leukemia	Sometimes	No
Chronic myelogenous leukemia	Sometimes	No
Non-Hodgkin's lymphoma	Sometimes	No
Angiogenic myeloid metaplasia	Sometimes	Yes
Mastocytosis	Rarely	No
Gaucher's disease	Rarely[a]	Yes
Hodgkin's disease	Rarely[b]	No
Splenic vein thrombosis	Always	No
Splenic abscess	Usually	No
Splenic cyst	Rarely	Yes
Echinococcal cyst	Always	No

[a]Splenectomy rarely indicated in current practice because of effective medical therapy.
[b]Splenectomy rarely indicated because of change in current therapy.

ANATOMY AND PHYSIOLOGY

- **Small intestine** – nutrient and water absorption
- **Large intestine** – water absorption
- **Duodenum**
  - **Bulb (1st)** – 90% of ulcers here
  - **Descending (2nd)** – contains ampulla of Vater (duct of Wirsung) and duct of Santorini
  - **Transverse (3rd)**
  - **Ascending (4th)**
  - Descending and transverse portions are **retroperitoneal**
  - 3rd and 4th portions – transition point at the acute angle between the aorta (posterior) and SMA (anterior)
  - Vascular supply is superior (off gastroduodenal artery) and inferior (off SMA) pancreaticoduodenal arteries
    - Both have anterior and posterior branches
    - Many communications between these arteries

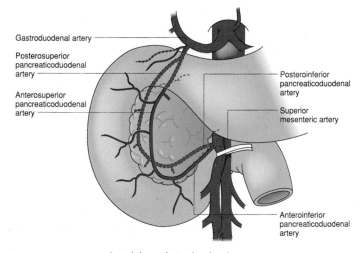

Arterial supply to the duodenum.

- **Jejunum**
  - 100 cm long; long vasa recta, circular muscle folds
  - **Maximum site of all absorption** except B_{12} (terminal ileum), bile acids (ileum – nonconjugated; terminal ileum – conjugated), iron (duodenum), and folate (terminal ileum)
  - 95% NaCl absorbed, 90% water absorbed in jejunum
  - Vascular supply – SMA
- **Ileum** – 150 cm long; short vasa recta, flat
  - Vascular supply – SMA

- **Intestinal brush border** – maltase, sucrase, limit dextrinase, lactase

- **Normal sizes** – small bowel/transverse colon/cecum → **3/6/9 cm**
- SMA eventually branches off **ileocolic artery**

- **Cell types**
  - **Absorptive cells**
  - **Goblet cells** (mucin secretion)
  - **Paneth cells** (secretory granules, enzymes)
  - **Enterochromaffin cells** (APUD, 5-hydroxytryptamine release, carcinoid precursor)
  - **Brunner's glands** (alkaline solution)
  - **Peyer's patches** (lymphoid tissue); increased in the ileum
  - **M cells** – antigen-presenting cells in intestinal wall

- **IgA** – released into gut; also in mother's milk
- **Fe** – both heme and Fe transporters

- **Migrating motor complex (gut motility)**
  - Phase I – rest
  - Phase II – acceleration and gallbladder contraction
  - Phase III – peristalsis
  - Phase IV – deceleration
  - **Motilin** is most important hormone in migrating motor complex

- **Fat and cholesterol**
  - Broken down by cholesterol esterase, phospholipase A_2, lipase, colipase in combination with bile salts
  - Converted to free fatty acids and monacylglycerides → form **micelles**
  - TAGs are re-formed in intestinal cells and released as chylomicrons into the lymphatics via terminal villous lacteals
  - **Chylomicrons** – 90% TAGs, 10% phospholipid, cholesterol, protein; released into lymphatics
  - **Long-chain fatty acids** – released into lymphatics
  - **Short- and medium-chain fatty acids** – released into portal vein
- **Carbohydrate and protein digestion** – see Chap. 10

- **Bile salts**
  - **95% of bile salts are reabsorbed**
    - 50% passive absorption – **45% ileum and 5% colon**
    - 50% active resorption in **terminal ileum** (Na/K ATPase)
    - Conjugated bile is absorbed only in the terminal ileum
  - Bile is conjugated to **taurine and glycine**
  - Can also be deconjugated in the colon by bacteria and absorbed there (small amount)
  - **Primary bile acids** – cholic and chenodeoxycholic
  - **Secondary bile acids** – deoxycholic and lithocholic (from bacterial action on primary bile acids in gut)
  - Gallstones can form after terminal ileum resection from malabsorption of bile acids

SHORT-GUT SYNDROME
- Diagnosis is made on symptoms, not length of bowel
- Symptoms: diarrhea, steatorrhea, weight loss, nutritional deficiency
- Lose fat, B_{12}, electrolytes, water
- **Sudan red stain** – checks for fecal fat
- **Schilling test** – checks for B_{12} absorption (radiolabeled B_{12} in urine)
- Probably need at least 75 cm to survive off TPN; 50 cm with competent ileocecal valve
- Tx: try to restrict fat with diet resumption, H_2 blockers to reduce acid, Lomotil

CAUSES OF STEATORRHEA
- **Gastric hypersecretion of acid** → ↓ pH → ↑ intestinal motility; interferes with fat absorption

- **Interruption of bile salt resorption** interferes with micelle formation (terminal ileum resection)
- Tx: control diarrhea (codeine, Lomotil); ↓ oral intake, especially fats; Pancrease, H_2 blocker

NONHEALING FISTULA

- **"FRIENDS"** – mnemonic for causes of nonhealing fistula: **f**oreign body, **r**adiation, **i**nflammatory bowel disease, **e**pithelialization, **n**eoplasm, **d**istal obstruction, **s**epsis/Infection
- High-output fistulas are more likely with proximal bowel (duodenum or proximal portion of jejunum) and are less likely to close with conservative management
- Colonic fistulas are more likely to close than those in small bowel
- Patients with persistent fever – need to check for abscesses (fistulogram, abdominal CT, upper GI with small bowel follow-through series)
- Most fistulas **iatrogenic** and treated conservatively 1st → TPN, skin protection, NG tube, stoma appliance, octreotide
- 40% close spontaneously
- Surgical options: resect bowel segment containing fistula and perform primary anastomosis

OBSTRUCTION

- **Without previous surgery (most common)**
  - Small bowel – <u>hernia</u>
  - Large bowel – <u>cancer</u>
- **With previous surgery (most common)**
  - Small bowel – <u>adhesions</u>
  - Large bowel – <u>cancer</u>

Symptoms and Signs of Bowel Obstruction

Symptom or Sign	Proximal Small Bowel (Open Loop)	Distal Small Bowel (Open Loop)	Small Bowel (Closed Loop)	Colon and Rectum
Pain	Intermittent, intense, colicky; often relieved by vomiting	Intermittent to constant	Progressive, intermittent constant; rapidly worsens	Continuous
Vomiting	Large volumes; bilious and frequent	Low volume and frequency; progressively feculent with time	May be prominent (reflex)	Intermittent, not prominent; feculent when present
Tenderness	Epigastric or periumbilical; quite mild unless strangulation is present	Diffuse and progressive	Diffuse, progressive	Diffuse
Distention	Absent	Moderate to marked	Often absent	Marked
Obstipation	May not be present	Present	May not be present	Present

Adapted from Schuffler MD, Sinanan MN. Intestinal obstruction and pseudo-obstruction. In: Sleisenger MH, Fordtran JS, eds., *Gastrointestinal Disease*. 5th ed. Philadelphia, PA: WB Saunders; 1993:898.

- Symptoms: nausea and vomiting, crampy abdominal pain, failure to pass gas or stool
- Abdominal x-ray: air–fluid level, distended loops of small bowel, distal decompression

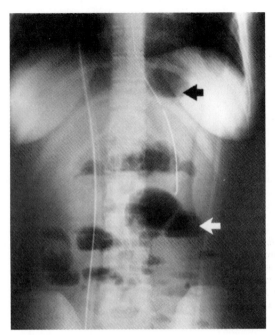

Plain upright abdominal film of a patient with small intestinal obstruction. Note the air–fluid levels in the stomach *(black arrow)*, multiple dilated loops of small intestine *(white arrow)*, and absence of air in the colon or rectum.

- Get bacterial overgrowth; 3rd spacing of fluid into bowel lumen
- Air with bowel obstruction – from **swallowed nitrogen**
- Tx: bowel rest, NG tube, IV fluids → cures 80% of partial SBO, 20%–40% of complete SBO
- Surgical indications: **progressing pain, peritoneal signs, fever, increasing WBCs → signs of strangulation or perforation, failure to resolve**

GALLSTONE ILEUS
- Small bowel obstruction from **gallstone in terminal ileum**
- Classically see **air in the biliary tree** in a patient with small bowel obstruction
- Caused by a **fistula between gallbladder and second portion of duodenum**
- Tx: remove stone from terminal ileum
  - Can leave gallbladder and fistula if patient too sick
  - If not too sick, perform cholecystectomy and close duodenum

MECKEL'S DIVERTICULUM (A TRUE DIVERTICULUM)
- 2 ft from ileocecal valve; 2% of population; usually presents in 1st 2 years of life with bleeding
- Caused by failure of closure of the omphalomesenteric duct
- Accounts for 50% of all **painless lower GI bleeds in children < 2 years**
- **Pancreas tissue** – most common tissue found in Meckel's

- **Gastric mucosa** – most likely to be symptomatic
- **Obstruction** – most common presentation in adults
- **Incidental** → usually not removed unless gastric mucosa suspected (diverticulum feels thick) or has a very narrow neck
- Dx: can get a Meckel's scan (^{99}Tc) if having trouble localizing (mucosa lights up)
- Tx: diverticulectomy for uncomplicated diverticulitis
  - Need segmental resection for complicated diverticulitis or neck > ⅓ the diameter of the normal bowel lumen or if the diverticulitis involves the base

DUODENAL DIVERTICULA
- Need to rule out gallbladder disease (chronic cholecystitis) origin
- Observe unless perforated, bleeding, causing obstruction, or highly symptomatic
- Frequency of diverticula – duodenal > jejunal > ileal
- Tx: segmental resection; may need temporary gastrojejunostomy for duodenal diverticula perforation

CROHN'S DISEASE
- **Intermittent abdominal pain, diarrhea, and weight loss; low-grade fever**
- 15–35 years old at 1st presentation
- ↑ in Ashkenazi Jews
- Can have extraintestinal manifestations (arthritis, arthralgias, pyoderma gangrenosum, erythema nodosum, ocular diseases, growth failure, megaloblastic anemia from folate and vitamin B_{12} malabsorption)
- Can occur anywhere from mouth to anus
- **Terminal ileum** – most commonly involved bowel segment
- **Anal/perianal disease** – 1st presentation in 10%
  - Tx: Flagyl
- **Anal disease most common symptom** – large skin tags
- **Most common sites for initial presentation**
  - Terminal ileum and cecum – 40%
  - Colon only – 35%
  - Small bowel only – 20%
  - Perianal – 5%

- Dx: colonoscopy with biopsies and enteroclysis can help make the diagnosis

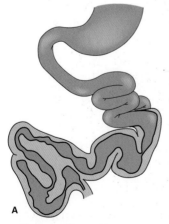 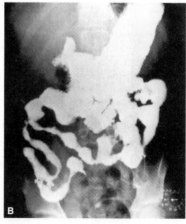

Typical radiographic appearance of extensive jejunoileal Crohn's disease.

- **Pathology** – transmural involvement, segmental disease (skip lesions), cobblestoning, narrow deep ulcers, creeping fat, fistulas; small bowel may be involved, perianal disease common
- **Medical Tx**: **5-ASA, sulfasalazine, steroids, azathioprine, methotrexate, Remicade** (infliximab; TNF-α inhibitor, usually just used for abscess or fistula), **loperamide**
  - **No** agents affect the natural course of disease
- **TPN** – may induce remission and fistula closure with small bowel Crohn's disease
- **90% patients with Crohn's disease eventually need an operation**

- **Surgical indications**
  - **Unlike ulcerative colitis, surgery is not curative**
  - **Obstruction** – usually just partial and can be initially treated conservatively
  - **Abscess** – can usually be treated with percutaneous drainage
  - **Megacolon** – perforation occurs in 15%, usually contained
  - **Hemorrhage** – unusual in Crohn's but can occur
  - **Blind loop obstruction**
  - **Fissures** – <u>no</u> lateral internal sphincterotomy in patients with Crohn's disease
  - **Enterocutaneous fistula** – can usually be treated conservatively
  - **Perineal fistula** – unroof and rule out abscess; let heal on its own
  - **Anorectovaginal fistulas** – may need rectal advancement flap; usually need colostomy
  - Do not need clear margins; just get 2 cm away from gross disease

- **Perirectal disease** may respond to resection of small bowel
- **Patients with diffuse disease of colon and rectum** – proctocolectomy and ileostomy the procedures of choice
- **Incidental finding of inflammatory bowel disease** in patient with presumed appendicitis who has normal appendix – remove **appendix if cecum not involved**

- **Stricturoplasty**
  - Consider if patient has multiple strictures to save small bowel length
  - Probably not good for patient's 1st operation as it leaves disease behind
  - 10% leakage/abscess/fistula rate with stricturoplasty

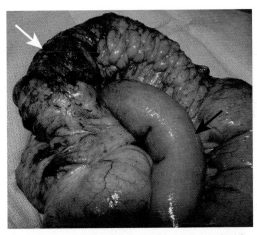

Severe Crohn's disease affecting the terminal ileum *(white arrow)* with normal ileum for comparison *(black arrow)*. (Courtesy of The University of Chicago General Surgery Archives.)

■ 50% recurrence rate requiring surgery for Crohn's disease after resection

■ **Complications from removal of terminal ileum**
  - ↓ **B$_{12}$ uptake** can result in **megaloblastic anemia**
  - ↓ **bile salt uptake** causes osmotic **diarrhea (bile salts) and steatorrhea (fat)** in colon
  - ↓ **oxalate binding** secondary to ↑ **intraluminal fat that binds calcium** → oxalate then gets absorbed in colon → released in urine → **Ca oxalate kidney stones (hyperoxaluria)**
  - **Gallstones** can form after terminal ileum resection from malabsorption of bile acids

CARCINOID
■ **Serotonin** is produced by **Kulchitsky cells** (enterochromaffin cell or argentaffin cell)
  - Part of amine precursor uptake decarboxylase system **(APUD)**
  - **5-HIAA** is a breakdown product of serotonin – can measure this in urine
  - **Tryptophan** is the precursor to serotonin
    - Increased use of tryptophan can lead to **niacin deficiency and pellagra** (diarrhea, dermatitis, dementia)
■ **Bradykinin** – also released by carcinoid tumors

■ **Carcinoid syndrome – caused by bulky liver metastases**
  - Intermittent **flushing and diarrhea – hallmark symptoms**
  - Can also get **asthma-type symptoms and right heart valve lesions**
  - If patient has carcinoid syndrome with small bowel carcinoid primary, it **indicates metastasis to liver** (liver usually clears serotonin)
  - All patients with carcinoid syndrome need abdominal exploration unless unresectable
  - If resection of liver metastases is performed, perform cholecystectomy in case of future embolization
  - **GI symptoms** from **vasoconstriction and fibrosis (desmoplastic reaction)**
  - **Octreotide scan** – good for localizing tumor not seen on CT scan

■ **Appendix carcinoid** – most common site for carcinoid tumor (50% of carcinoids arise here; ileum and rectum next most common)
■ **Small bowel carcinoid** – patients at ↑ risk for **multiple primaries** and **second unrelated malignancies**
  - **Carcinoid in appendix** – <2 cm → appendectomy; ≥2 cm or involving base → right hemicolectomy
  - **Carcinoid anywhere else in GI tract** → treat like cancer (segmental resection with lymphadenectomy)
  - **Chemotherapy – streptozocin and 5FU**; usually just for patients with **unresectable disease and carcinoid syndrome**
  - **Octreotide** – useful for patients with carcinoid syndrome
  - **Bronchospasm** – Tx: **Aprotinin**
  - **Flushing** – Tx: **α-blockers** (phenothiazine)
  - **False 5-HIAA** – fruits
  - **Pentagastrin** – can exacerbate symptoms

INTUSSUSCEPTION IN ADULTS
■ Can occur from small bowel or cecal tumors
■ Most common presentation is bleeding or obstruction
■ Worrisome in adults it often has a malignant lead point (i.e., cecal CA)
■ Tx: resection

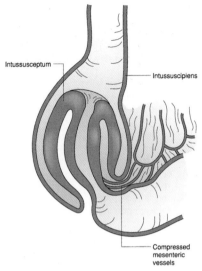

Anatomy of intussusception. The intussusceptum is the segment of bowel that invaginates into the intussuscipiens.

BENIGN SMALL BOWEL TUMORS

- **Rare**
- Benign small bowel tumors are more common than malignant
- **Leiomyomas** – most common benign small bowel tumor; usually extraluminal
- **Adenomas** – most found in ileum; present with bleeding, obstruction
  - Need resection when identified

- **Peutz–Jeghers syndrome (autosomal dominant)** – jejunal and ileal hamartomas; mucocutaneous melanotic skin pigmentation; patients have ↑ extraintestinal malignancies
  - Slight ↑ risk of colon CA in patients who have these polyps
  - Lipomas, neurogenic tumors, and hemangiomas can occur in these patients as well

MALIGNANT SMALL BOWEL TUMORS

Conditions Associated with an Increased Risk of Neoplasia	
Preexisting Condition	**Potential Malignancy**
Adenomatous polyps	Adenocarcinoma
Familial adenomatous polyposis	Adenocarcinoma
Peutz–Jeghers syndrome/ hamartomatous polyps	Adenocarcinoma
Leiomyomas	Possible leiomyosarcoma
Neurofibromatosis	Leiomyosarcoma, carcinoid, adenocarcinoma
Crohn's disease	Adenocarcinoma
Celiac sprue	Lymphoma, adenocarcinoma
Immunosuppression	Lymphoma
HIV infection	Lymphoma, Kaposi sarcoma
Helicobacter pylori infection	Low-grade lymphoma (mucosal-associated lymphoid tissue)
Epstein-Barr virus infection	Lymphoma

- **Adenocarcinoma (rare)** – most common malignant small bowel tumor
  - High proportion is in the **duodenum**
  - Symptoms: obstruction, jaundice
  - Tx: resection and adenectomy; Whipple if in duodenum
- **Duodenal CA** – risk factors: FAP, Gardner's, polyps, adenomas, von Recklinghausen's
- **Leiomyosarcoma**
  - Usually in **jejunum and ileum**; most extraluminal
  - Hard to differentiate compared with leiomyoma (>5 mitoses/HPF, atypia, necrosis)
  - Tx: resection; <u>no</u> adenectomy required
- **Lymphoma**
  - Usually in **ileum**; ↑ incidence in patients with Wegener's disease, SLE, AIDS, Crohn's disease, celiac sprue
  - Posttransplantation – ↑ **risk of bleeding and perforation**
  - Dx: abdominal CT, UGI, node sampling
  - Tx: XRT, chemotherapy, wide en bloc resection may be needed; include nodes
  - 40% 5-year survival rate
  - Usually NHL B cell type
  - **Mediterranean variant** occurs in young males and they get **clubbing**

STOMAS
- **Loop ileostomies** – 1%–2% obstruction rate
- **Parastomal hernias** ↑ with loop colostomies – relocation best treatment
- *Candida* – most common stomal infection
- **Diversion colitis (Hartmann's pouch)** – secondary to ↓ short-chain fatty acids
  - Tx: short-chain fatty acid enemas
- **Ischemia** – most common cause of stenosis of stoma
  - Tx: dilation if mild
- **Crohn's disease** – most common cause of fistula near stoma site
- **Abscesses** – underneath stoma site often caused by irrigation device
- **Gallstones and uric acid kidney stones** – ↑ in patients with ileostomy

APPENDIX
- **Appendicitis** – 1st: anorexia; 2nd: abdominal pain (periumbilical); 3rd: vomiting
- Pain gradually migrates to the RLQ as peritonitis sets in
- Most commonly occurs in patients 20–35 years
- Patients can have normal WBC count
- **CT scan** – <u>diameter > 7 mm or wall thickness > 2 mm</u> (looks like a bull's eye), fat stranding, no contrast in appendiceal lumen; try to give rectal contrast
- **Midpoint of antimesenteric border** – most likely to perforate
- **Hyperplasia** – most common cause in children; can follow a viral illness
- **Fecalith** – most common cause in adults
- Luminal obstruction is followed by distention of the appendix, venous congestion and thrombosis, ischemia, gangrene necrosis, and finally rupture
- **Nonoperative situation** – CT scan shows walled-off perforated appendix
  - Tx: percutaneous drainage and interval appendectomy at later date as long as symptoms are improving
  - Consider follow-up barium enema or colonoscopy to rule out perforated colon CA
- **Children and elderly** have higher propensity to rupture secondary to <u>delayed diagnosis</u>

- Children often have **higher fever and more vomiting and diarrhea**
- **Elderly** – signs and symptoms can be minimal; may need right hemicolectomy if cancer suspected
■ **Appendicitis is infrequent in infants**

■ **Perforation** – patient generally more ill; can have evidence of sepsis

■ **Appendicitis during pregnancy**
- **Most common cause of acute abdominal pain in the 1st trimester**
- **More likely to occur in the 2nd trimester** but is not the most common cause of abdominal pain
- **More likely to perforate in the 3rd trimester** – confused with contractions
- **Need to make the incision where the patient is having pain** – the appendix is displaced superiorly
- May have symptoms of RUQ pain in the 3rd trimester
- 35% fetal mortality with rupture
- Women with suspected appendicitis need beta-HCG drawn +/− abdominal ultrasound to rule out OB/GYN causes of abdominal pain

■ **Mucocele** – can be benign or malignant mucous papillary adenocarcinoma; needs resection
- Need right hemicolectomy if malignant
- Can get pseudomyxoma peritonei with rupture
- MCC of death – SBO from tumor spread

■ **Regional ileitis** – can mimic appendicitis; 10% go on to Crohn's disease

■ **Gastroenteritis** – nausea, vomiting, diarrhea

■ **Presumed appendicitis** but find ruptured ovarian cyst, or thrombosed ovarian vein, or regional enteritis not involving cecum → **still perform appendectomy**

ILEUS
■ Causes include surgery (most common), electrolyte abnormalities (↓ K), peritonitis, ischemia, trauma, drugs
■ Ileus – dilatation is uniform throughout the stomach, small bowel, colon, and rectum without decompression
■ Obstruction – there is bowel decompression distal to the obstruction

TYPHOID ENTERITIS (SALMONELLA)
■ Rare bleeding/perforation; fever, headaches, maculopapular rash, leukopenia, abdominal pain
■ Tx: Bactrim

CHAPTER 36. COLORECTAL

ANATOMY AND PHYSIOLOGY
- Colon secretes **K** and reabsorbs **Na and water** (mostly in right colon and cecum)
- **4 layers** – mucosa (columnar epithelium) → submucosa → muscularis propria → serosa
- Ascending, descending, and sigmoid colon are all **retroperitoneal**
- Peritoneum – covers anterior upper and middle ⅓ of the rectum

- **Muscularis mucosa** – circular/longitudinal interwoven inner layer
- **Muscularis propria** – circular layer of muscle
- **Plicae semilunaris** – transverse bands that form haustra
- **Taenia coli** – 3 bands that run longitudinally along colon. At rectosigmoid junction, the taeniae become broad and completely encircle the bowel as 2 discrete muscle bands

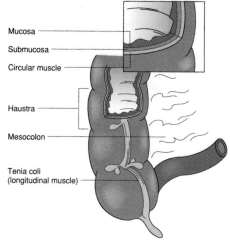

Layers of the colonic wall.

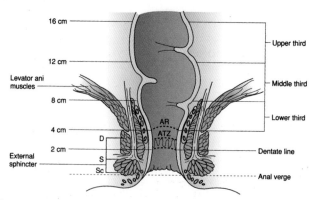

Anorectal anatomy with important landmarks. Approximate measurements are relative to the anal verge. D, deep; S, superficial; Sc, subcutaneous; AR, anorectal ring; ATZ, anal transition zone.

■ **Vascular supply**
  • **Ascending and ⅔ of transverse colon supplied by SMA** (ileocolic, right and middle colic arteries)
  • **⅓ transverse, descending colon, sigmoid colon, and upper portion of the rectum supplied by IMA** (left colic, sigmoid branches, superior rectal artery)
  • **Marginal artery** – runs along colon margin, connecting SMA to IMA (provides collateral flow)
  • **Arc of Riolan** – short direct connection between IMA and SMA
  • 80% of blood flow goes to mucosa and submucosa

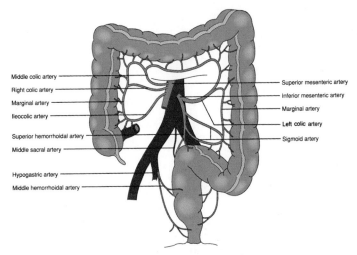

Arterial blood supply of the colon.

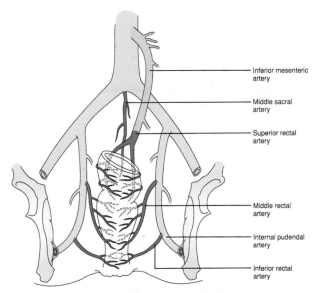

Arterial supply of the rectum and anal canal.

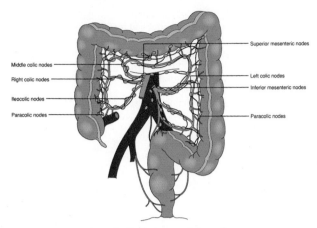

Lymphatic drainage of the colon.

- **Venous drainage** follows arterial except IMV, which goes to the splenic vein
  - Splenic vein joins the SMV to form the portal vein
- **Superior rectal artery** – branch of IMA
- **Middle rectal artery** – branch of internal iliac (the lateral stalks during low anterior resection [LAR] or abdominoperineal resection [APR] contain the middle rectal arteries)
- **Inferior rectal artery** – branch of internal pudendal (which is a branch of internal iliac)

- Superior and middle rectal veins drain into the IMV and eventually the portal vein
- Inferior rectal veins drain into the internal iliac veins and eventually the caval system

- **Superior and middle rectum** – drain to IMA nodal lymphatics
- **Lower rectum** – drains primarily to IMA nodes, also to internal iliac nodes
- Bowel wall contains submucosal and mucosal lymphatics

- **Watershed areas**
  - Splenic flexure (Griffith's point) – SMA and IMA junction
  - Rectum (Sudak's point) – superior rectal and middle rectal junction
  - Colon more sensitive to ischemia than small bowel secondary to ↓ collaterals

- **External sphincter (puborectalis muscle)** – under CNS (voluntary) control
  - Inferior rectal branch of internal pudendal nerve and perineal branch of S4
  - Is the continuation of the levator ani muscle (striated muscle)
- **Internal sphincter** – involuntary control
  - Is the continuation of the circular band of colon muscle (smooth muscle)
  - Is normally contracted

- **Meissner's plexus** – inner nerve plexus
- **Auerbach's plexus** – outer nerve plexus
- **Pelvic nerves** – parasympathetic
- **Lumbar, splanchnic, and hypogastric nerves** – sympathetic

- **From anal verge** – anal canal 0–5 cm, rectum 5–15 cm, rectosigmoid junction 15–18 cm
- **Levator ani** – marks the transition between anal canal and rectum
- **Crypts of Lieberkuhn** – mucus-secreting goblet cells
- **Colonic inertia** – slow transit time; patients may need subtotal colectomy
- **Short-chain fatty acids** – main nutrient of colonocytes
- **Stump pouchitis** (diversion or disuse proctitis) – Tx: short-chain fatty acids

- **Infectious pouchitis** – Tx: metronidazole (Flagyl)
- **Lymphocytic colitis** – watery diarrhea and inflammatory bowel symptoms. Tx: sulfasalazine
- **Denonvilliers fascia (anterior)** – rectovesicular fascia in men; rectovaginal fascia in women
- **Waldeyer's fascia (posterior)** – rectosacral fascia

POLYPS
- **Hyperplastic polyps** – most common polyp; no cancer risk
- **Tubular adenoma** – most common (75%) intestinal neoplastic polyp
  - These are generally pedunculated
- **Villous adenoma** – most likely to produce symptoms
  - These are generally sessile and larger than tubular adenomas
  - 50% of villous adenomas have **cancer**
- >2 cm, sessile, and villous lesions have ↑ cancer risk

Neoplastic Colorectal Polyps

Type	Histologic Features	Incidence (%)	Invasive Malignancy (%)
Adenomatous (tabular adenoma)	Branching tubules embedded in lamina propria	75	5
Villous (villous adenoma)	Finger-like projections of epithelium over lamina propria	10	40
Intermediate (tubulovillous adenoma)	Mixture of adenomatous and villous patterns	15	22

- Polyps have left side predominance
- Most **pedunculated polyps** can be removed endoscopically
- If not able to get all of the polyp (which usually occurs with **sessile polyps**) → need **segmental resection**
- 30% of patients >50 years with guaiac-positive stool have polyps

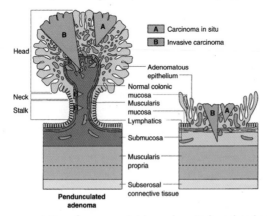

Diagrammatic representation of cancer-containing polyps. Pedunculated adenoma is described on the left and a sessile adenoma on the right. In carcinoma in situ, malignant cells are confined to the mucosa. These lesions are adequately treated by endoscopic polypectomy. Polypectomy is adequate treatment for invasive carcinoma only if the margin is sufficient (2 mm), the carcinoma is not poorly differentiated, and no evidence of venous or lymphatic invasion is found.

- **High-grade dysplasia** – basement membrane is intact (carcinoma in situ)
- **Intramucosal cancer** – into muscularis mucosa (carcinoma in situ → still has not gone through basement membrane)
- **Invasive cancer** – into submucosa (T1)
- Screening

Risk Stratification for Colorectal Cancer Screening

Average Risk for Colorectal Cancer (must fulfill all criteria below)
Age 50 years or older
No personal history of polyps or colorectal cancer
No first-degree relatives with polyps or colorectal cancer
Fewer than two second-degree relatives with colorectal cancer

Moderate Risk for Colorectal Cancer (any criteria below)
First-degree relative with colorectal cancer or polyp at age younger than 60 years
First-degree relative with colorectal cancer or polyp at age 60 years or older
Two or more second-degree relatives with colorectal cancer

Increased Risk for Colorectal Cancer (any criteria below)
Gene carrier or at risk for familial adenomatous polyposis
Gene carrier or at risk for hereditary nonpolyposis colorectal cancer

Surveillance (any criteria below)
Personal history of colorectal polyps
Personal history of colorectal cancer
Personal history of inflammatory bowel disease

Guidelines for Colorectal Cancer Screening[a]

Individuals at Average Risk, Age >50 years

Test[b]	Interval	Comment
Fecal occult blood test	Annually	No rehydration
Flexible sigmoidoscopy	Every 5 years	
Fecal occult blood test and flexible sigmoidoscopy	Fecal occult blood test annually, flexible sigmoidoscopy every 5 years	Fecal occult blood test first; if positive, skip sigmoidoscopy and follow with colonoscopy
Colonoscopy	Every 10 years	
Double contrast barium enema	Every 5 years	

Individuals at Moderate Risk

Risk	Initiate Screening	Comments
First-degree relative with colorectal cancer or polyp at age ≥60 years OR ≥2 or more second-degree relatives with colorectal cancer	Age 40 years	Same screening regimens and intervals as average risk
First-degree relative with colorectal cancer or polyp at age <60 years OR >2 or more first-degree relatives with colorectal cancer	Age 40 years or 10 years younger than youngest family member at the time of diagnosis, whichever comes first	Colonoscopy every 5 years

(continued)

Guidelines for Colorectal Cancer Screening[a] (continued)

Individuals at Increased Risk, Colonoscopy Only

Familial Risk	Initiate Surveillance	Interval if Normal Colonoscopy Result
Familial adenomatous polyposis; consider genetic counseling and testing; colectomy if genetic testing is positive	Age 10–12 years	Annual sigmoidoscopy, stopping at age 40 years if normal
Attenuated adenomatous polyposis coli	Late teens	Annual colonoscopy, no stopping at age 40 years
Hereditary nonpolyposis colon cancer	Age 20–25 years or 10 years younger than earliest family diagnosis	Biennial colonoscopy to age 40 years, then annual

[a]Endorsed by the American Cancer Society, American College of Gastroenterology, American Society of Colon and Rectal Surgeons, American Society for Gastrointestinal Endoscopy, Oncology Nursing Society, and Society of American Gastrointestinal Endoscopic Surgeons.
[b]Diagnostic evaluation with colonoscopy should be performed for any patients with either positive fiindings on screening with fecal occult blood testing or symptoms suggestive of colorectal cancer or polyps.

- **False-positive guaiac** – beef, vitamin C, iron, antacids, and cimetidine
- **No** colonoscopy with recent MI, splenomegaly, pregnancy if fluoroscopy planned

Comparison of Colorectal Cancer Screening Test Characteristics

	Unrehydrated FOBT	Flexible Sigmoidoscopy	Colonoscopy	Double-Contrast Barium Enema
ACCURACY				
Sensitivity	33%–40%	70%	97.5%	70%–85%
Specificity	97%		100%	86%–97%
COST, 2000 $US	$3.50	$400	$695	$296
CONSEQUENCES	Negligible	Perforation = 0%–0.011%	Hemorrhage = 0.15%–4% Perforation = 0.2%–3% Mortality = 0.006%	Negligible
COMPLIANCE	60%–86%	47%–74%	28%–38%	
EFFECTIVENESS (REDUCTION in CRC mortality)	18%–55%	34%–66%	64%–90%	33%–47%

FOBT, fecal occult blood test, unrehydrated; CRC, colorectal cancer.

- **Polypectomy shows T1 lesion** – polypectomy is adequate if margins are clear (2 mm), is well differentiated, and has no vascular/lymphatic invasion; otherwise, need formal colon resection
- **Extensive low rectal villous adenomas with atypia** – transanal excision (can try mucosectomy) as much of the polyp as possible
  - **No** APR unless cancer is present

- **Pathology shows T1 lesion after transanal excision of rectal polyp** → transanal excision is adequate if margins are clear (2 mm), is well differentiated, or has no vascular/lymphatic invasion
- **Pathology shows T2 lesion after transanal excision of rectal polyp** → patient needs APR or LAR

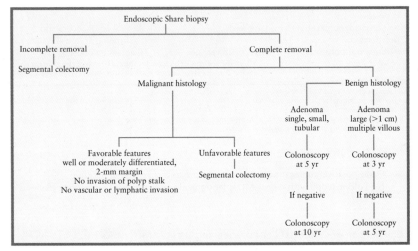

Management of colonic adenoma.

Guidelines for Colorectal Cancer Endoscopic Surveillance[a]		
Personal History Risk	**Initiate Surveillance**	**Interval**
Following resection of single <1 cm adenoma	5 years postpolypectomy	If first colonoscopy is normal, resume average-risk recommendations
Following resection of ≥1 cm or high-risk adenoma	3 years postpolypectomy	Repeat colonoscopy in 3 years; if normal, return to average-risk recommendations
Following curative resection for colorectal cancer	Within 1 year postoperatively	Repeat in 3 years, then every 5 years
Inflammatory bowel disease	Within 8 years of diagnosis	Survey for dysplasia Every 1–2 years

[a]Endorsed by the American Cancer Society, American College of Gastroenterology, American Society of Colon and Rectal Surgeons, American Society for Gastrointestinal Endoscopy, Oncology Nursing Society, and Society of American Gastrointestinal Endoscopic Surgeons.

COLORECTAL CANCER
- **2nd leading cause of CA death**
- Symptoms: **anemia, constipation, and bleeding**
- Fat → O_2 radicals are thought to have a role

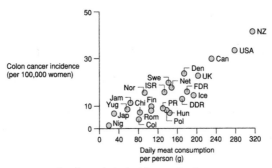

Correlation between meat intake and the incidence of colon cancer among women in 23 countries.

■ Colon CA has had an association with *Clostridium septicum* infection
■ **Colon CA** – main gene mutations are **APC, DCC, p53, and k-ras**

■ **Sigmoid colon** – most common site of primary

Prognostic Factors for Primary Colorectal Cancer	
Factor	Association
Age	Patients <40 years old often present with more advanced stage of disease
Symptoms	Symptomatic patients tend to have more advanced stage of disease
Obstruction and perforation	Poorer prognosis when present
Location of primary	Rectosigmoid and rectal cancers have lower cure rates compared with cancers elsewhere in the colon
Tumor configuration	Exophytic tumors are associated with less advanced stage of cancer compared with ulcerative tumor
Blood vessel invasion	Poorer prognosis when present
Lymphatic vessel invasion	Poorer prognosis when present
Perineural invasion	Poorer prognosis when present
Lymphocytic infiltration	Improved prognosis when present
Carcinoembryonic antigen study	Poorer prognosis when elevated before primary tumor resection
Aneuploidy	Poorer prognosis when present

■ **Disease spread**
  • **Spreads to nodes first**
  • **Nodal status** – most important prognostic factor
  • **Liver** – #1 site of metastases; lung – #2 site of metastases
    ∘ Portal vein → **liver metastases**; iliac vein → **lung metastases**
    ∘ **Liver metastases** – if resectable and leaves adequate liver function, patients have 25% 5-year survival rate
    ∘ **Lung metastases** – 20% 5-year survival rate in selected patients
    ∘ **Isolated liver and lung metastases should be resected**

  • 5% get drop metastases to **ovaries**
  • **Rectal CA** – can metastasize to **spine directly via Batson's plexus (venous)**
  • **Colon CA** typically does not go to bone
  • Colorectal CA growing into adjacent organs can be resected en bloc with a portion of the adjacent organ (i.e., partial bladder resection)

- **Lymphocytic penetration** – patients have an improved prognosis
- **Mucoepidermoid** – worst prognosis

- **Rectal ultrasound** – good at assessing depth of invasion (sphincter involvement), recurrence, and presence of enlarged nodes
- Need **colonoscopy** to rule out **synchronous** lesions

- **Goals of resection**
  - En bloc resection, adequate margins, and regional adenectomy
  - **Most right-sided colon CAs** can be treated with primary anastomosis without ostomy
  - **Rectal pain with rectal CA** – patient needs APR
  - Need 2-cm margins

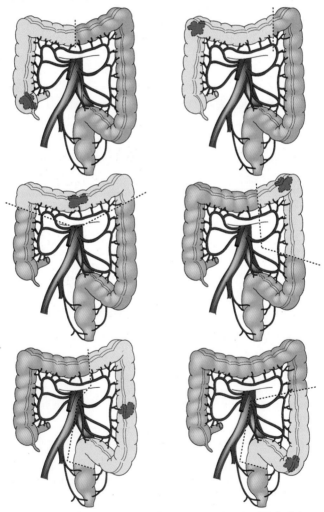

Segmental resections for cancers of the colon and upper third of the rectum.

■ **Intraoperative ultrasound** – best method of picking up intrahepatic metastases
  • Conventional ultrasound: 10 mm
  • Abdominal CT: 5–10 mm
  • Abdominal MRI: 5–10 mm (better resolution than CT)
  • Intraoperative ultrasound: 3–5 mm

■ **Abdominoperineal resection (APR)**
  • Permanent colostomy; anal canal is excised along with the rectum
  • Can have impotence and bladder dysfunction
  • Indicated for malignant lesions only (not benign tumors) that are not amenable to LAR
  • Need at least a 2-cm margin (2 cm from levator ani muscles) for LAR
  • High rate of impotence in men after rectal resection, especially with APR, due to disruption of nerve supply
  • Risk of local recurrence higher with rectal CA than with colon CA in general
  • Unresectable large liver metastases at time of APR → may not need APR
    • If obstructed or nearly obstructed → place colostomy and mucous fistula
    • Avoid morbidity of APR in patient with terminal CA
    • If bleeding was a significant symptom, probably best to proceed with APR
    • If rectal pain was a significant symptom, probably best to proceed with APR
  • Unresectable large liver metastases during preop workup for colon or rectal CA → no resection unless obstructed or nearly obstructed, or unless bleeding is a significant symptom

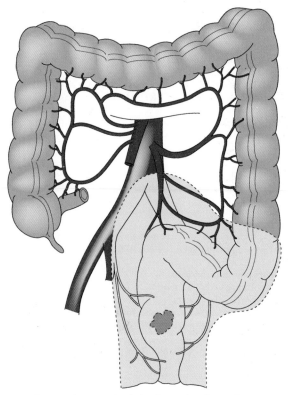

Extent of surgery in abdominoperineal resection.

■ **Preoperative chemotherapy/XRT** – produces complete response in some patients with rectal CA; preserves sphincter function in some

---

TNM STAGING SYSTEM FOR COLORECTAL CANCER
- **T1**: into submucosa. **T2**: into muscularis propria. **T3**: into serosa or through muscularis propria if no serosa is present. **T4**: through serosa into free peritoneal cavity or into adjacent organs/structures if no serosa is present
- **N0**: nodes negative. **N1**: 1–3 nodes positive, **N2**: ≥4 nodes positive, **N3**: central nodes positive
- **M1**: distant metastases

Neoplastic	
Stage	TNM Status
I	T1–2, N0, M0
II	T3–4, N0, M0
III	Any N1 disease
IV	Any M1 disease

Modified from AJCC. *Cancer Staging Handbook.* 6th ed. New York, NY: Springer-Verlag; 2002:131–132.

■ **Low rectal T1** (limited to submucosa) – can be excised transanally if <4 cm, has negative margins (need 1 cm), is well differentiated, and there is no neurologic or vascular invasion; otherwise patient needs APR or LAR
■ **Low rectal T2 or higher** – Tx: APR or LAR

■ **Chemotherapy**
- **Stage III and IV colon CA** (nodes positive or distant metastases) → **postop chemo**, no XRT
- **Stage II and III rectal CA** → **preop or postop chemo and XRT**
- **Stage IV rectal CA** → **chemo and XRT +/−surgery** (possibly just colostomy)

- **Stages II (rectal) and III (colon or rectal)** – 5FU, leucovorin, and oxaliplatin
- **Stage IV (colon or rectal)** – 5FU and leucovorin

■ **XRT**
- ↓ local recurrence and ↑ survival when combined with chemotherapy
- **Postop XRT for rectal CA** – needed for T3 tumors or positive nodes (stage II or higher)
- **XRT damage** – rectum most common site of injury → vasculitis, thrombosis, ulcers, strictures
- Preop XRT and chemotherapy may help shrink tumor, allowing downstaging of the tumor and possibly allowing LAR versus APR

■ **20% of patients have a recurrence**
- 50% have recurrence within 6 months
- 100% have recurrence by 3 years
- 5% have another primary – **main reason for surveillance colonoscopy**

■ **Follow-up**
- History and physical exam, CEA, and stool guaiac – every 6 months for 3 years, then annually
- Yearly LFTs, abdominal CT, colonoscopy, CXR
- These vary and there is no consensus
- Colonoscopy mainly to check for new colon CAs (metachronous)

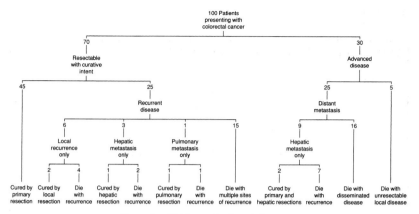

The natural history of colorectal cancer.

FAMILIAL ADENOMATOUS POLYPOSIS (FAP)

- Autosomal dominant; all have cancer by age 40
- **APC gene** – chromosome 5
- 20% of FAP syndromes are spontaneous
- Polyps <u>not</u> present at birth; are present in puberty
- Do <u>not</u> need colonoscopy for surveillance in patients with suspected FAP → just need flexible sigmoidoscopy to check for polyps
- Need **total colectomy prophylactically at age 20**
- Also get duodenal polyps → need to check duodenum for cancer with esophagogastroduodenoscopy every 2 years
- **Surgery – proctocolectomy, rectal mucosectomy, and ileoanal pouch** (J-pouch)
  - Need lifetime surveillance of residual rectal mucosa
  - Following colectomy, most common cause of death in FAP patients is **periampullary tumors of duodenum**
  - **Total proctocolectomy with end ileostomy** is also an option

- **Gardner's syndrome** – patients get colon CA (associated with APC gene) and desmoid tumors/osteomas
- **Turcot's syndrome** – patients get colon CA (associated with APC gene) and brain tumors

LYNCH SYNDROMES (HEREDITARY NONPOLYPOSIS COLON CANCER)

- 5% of population, autosomal dominant
- Associated **with DNA mismatch repair gene**
- Predilection for right-sided and multiple cancers
- **Lynch I** – just colon CA risk
- **Lynch II** – patients also have ↑ risk of ovarian, endometrial, bladder, and stomach cancer
- **Amsterdam criteria** – "3, 2, 1" → at least **3** first-degree relatives, over **2** generations, **1** with cancer before age 50
- Need surveillance colonoscopy starting at age 25 or 10 years before primary relative got cancer
- 50% get metachronous lesions within 10 years; often have multiple primaries
- Women need **endometrial biopsy** every 3 years and annual pelvic exams; earlier mammograms
- Consider **total abdominal hysterectomy and bilateral salpingoophorectomy** after childbearing years
- Consider subtotal colectomy with first cancer operation

JUVENILE POLYPOSIS
- Hamartomatous polyps – cancer is dependent on adenomatous change in these polyps
- Symptoms: anemia, ↓ energy, failure to thrive, and anergy
- Colonic surveillance every 2 years; total colectomy probably best option if CA develops
- Juvenile polyps do not have malignant potential, but **patients with juvenile polyposis do have ↑ CA risk**

PEUTZ-JEGHERS SYNDROME
- Gastrointestinal (GI) hamartoma polyposis and dark pigmentation around mucous membranes
- Now believed to ↑ risk of GI CAs
- These patients need polypectomy if possible (may be too many polyps to resect) – 2% colon/duodenal CA risk
- ↑ risk of other cancers – gonadal, breast, and biliary

CRONKITE-CANADA SYNDROME
- Hamartomatous polyps; get atrophy of nails and hair, hypopigmentation
- Thought to have <u>no</u> malignant potential

SIGMOID VOLVULUS
- More common with high-fiber diets (Iran, Iraq)
- Occurs in debilitated, psychiatric patients; neurologic dysfunction, laxative abuse
- Symptoms: pain, distention, and obstipation
- Causes closed loop obstruction
- Abdominal x-ray – bent inner tube sign; Gastrografin enema may show bird's beak sign (tapered colon)
- Do not attempt decompression with gangrenous bowel or peritoneal signs → go to OR for sigmoidectomy
- Tx: decompress with colonoscopy (80% reduce, 50% will recur), give bowel prep, and perform sigmoid colectomy during same admission

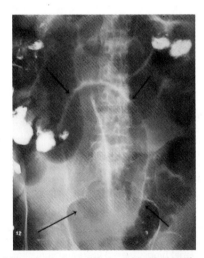

Plain supine abdominal film of a patient with sigmoid volvulus. The centrally located sigmoid loop is outlined by trapped air. The proximal small intestine is dilated as well, suggesting that the volvulus has been present for sufficient time to cause accumulation of air and fluid proximally. (Courtesy of John Braver, M.D., Department of Radiology, Brigham and Women's Hospital, Harvard Medical School, Boston, MA.)

CECAL VOLVULUS
- Less common than sigmoid volvulus; occurs in 20-30s
- Can appear as an SBO, with dilated cecum in the RLQ
- Can try to decompress with colonoscopy but unlikely to succeed (only 20%)
- Tx: OR → right hemicolectomy probably best treatment; can try cecopexy if colon is viable and patient is frail

ULCERATIVE COLITIS
- Symptoms: **bloody diarrhea, abdominal pain, fever, and weight loss**
- **Involves the mucosa and submucosa**
- Strictures and fistulae unusual with ulcerative colitis

Pathologic Features of Crohn's Disease and Ulcerative Colitis

Pathology	Crohn's Disease	Ulcerative Colitis
Transmural inflammation	Yes	Uncommon
Granulomas	50%-75%	No
Fissures	Common	Rare
Submucosal thickening, fibrosis	Common	No
Submucosal inflammation	Common	Uncommon

Distinguishing Characteristics of Crohn's Colitis and Ulcerative Colitis

Characteristic	Crohn's Colitis	Ulcerative Colitis
Location	Small bowel involvement	Colon only (rare backwash ileitis) 10%
Anatomic distribution	Asymmetric distribution (skip lesions)	Contiguous involvement beginning distally
Rectal involvement	Rectal sparing common 50%	Involved 90%
Gross bleeding	Absent in 25%-30%	Universal
Perianal disease	≤75%	Rare, may be severe
Fistulization	Yes	No
Granulomas	50%-75%	No

Endoscopic Features of Crohn's Disease and Ulcerative Colitis

Endoscopic Feature	Crohn's Disease	Ulcerative Colitis
Mucosal involvement	Discontinuous	Contiguous
Discrete ulcers (aphthous ulcers)	Common	Rare
Surrounding mucosa	Relatively normal	Abnormal
Longitudinal ulcer	Common	Rare
Cobblestoning	In severe cases	No
Rectal involvement	Sparing common	Involved in 90%
Mucosal friability	Uncommon	Common
Vascular pattern	Normal	Distorted

- **Spares anus** – unlike Crohn's disease
  - Starts distally in **rectum**, is contiguous (<u>no</u> skip areas like Crohn's disease)
  - Bleeding is universal and has mucosal friability with <u>pseudopolyps and collar button ulcers</u>
  - Always need to rule out infectious etiology
  - Backwash ileitis can occur with proximal disease
- **Barium enema** – with chronic disease see loss of haustra, narrow caliber, short colon, and loss of redundancy

- **Medical Tx**: sulfasalazine, 5-ASA, steroids, methotrexate, azathioprine (Imuran), infliximab (Remicade), and loperamide
- 5-ASA and sulfasalazine have been shown to maintain remission in ulcerative colitis

- **Toxic megacolon**
  - **Clinical Dx**: fever, ↑ HR, bloating, abdominal radiographs → dilated colon
  - **Initial Tx**: NGT, fluids, steroids, bowel rest, TPN, and antibiotics will treat 50% adequately; other 50% require surgery
    - Follow clinical response and abdominal radiographs

Indications for Surgery

Absolute	Relative
Pneumoperitoneum	Inability to promptly control sepsis
Diffuse peritonitis	Increasing megacolon
Localized peritonitis with increasing abdominal pain and/or colonic distension >10 cm	Failure to improve within 24–48 h
	Increasing toxicity or other signs of clinical deterioration
Uncontrolled sepsis	Continued transfusion requirements
Major hemorrhage	

From Rothenberger DA, Bullard KM. Surgery for toxic megacolon. In: Fischer JE, Bland KI, et al., eds. *Mastery of Surgery*. 5th ed. Philadelphia, PA: Lippincott Williams & Wilkins; 2007, with permission.

- **Perforation with ulcerative colitis** – transverse colon more common
- **Perforation with Crohn's** – distal ileum most common

- **Surgical indications**: hemorrhage, toxic megacolon, acute fulminant ulcerative colitis (occurs in 15%), obstruction, any dysplasia, cancer, intractability, systemic complications, failure to thrive, and long-standing disease (>10 years) as prophylaxis against colon CA

- Emergent/urgent resections – total proctocolectomy and bring up ileostomy
  - Perform definitive hookup later

- Elective resections
  - **Ileoanal anastomosis** – rectal mucosectomy, J-pouch, and ileoanal (low rectal) anastomosis; not used with Crohn's disease
    - Protects bladder and sexual function
    - Needs lifetime surveillance of residual rectal area
    - Many ileoanal anastomoses need resection secondary to cancer, dysplastic changes, or refractory proctitis
    - Needs temporary diverting ileostomy (6–8 weeks) while pouch heals
    - **Leak** – most common major morbidity after surgery → can lead to sepsis
    - **Infectious pouchitis** – Tx: Flagyl

  - **APR with ileostomy** – can also be performed

- **Cancer risk is 1%–2% per year starting 10 years after initial diagnosis**
  - Cancer more evenly distributed throughout colon
  - Needs yearly colonoscopy starting 8–10 years after diagnosis

- **Extraintestinal manifestations**
  - Most common extraintestinal manifestation requiring total colectomy – **failure to thrive in children**
  - Do **not** get better with colectomy → primary sclerosing cholangitis, ankylosing spondylitis

- **Get better with colectomy** → most ocular problems, arthritis, and anemia
- **50% get better** → pyoderma gangrenosum
- **HLA B27** – sacroiliitis and ankylosing spondylitis
- Can get **thromboembolic disease**
- **Pyoderma gangrenosum** – Tx: steroids

CARCINOID OF THE COLON AND RECTUM
- Represents 15% of all carcinoids; infrequent cause of carcinoid syndrome
- Metastases related to size of tumor
- ⅔ of colon carcinoids have either local or systemic spread
- Low rectal carcinoids – <2 cm → wide local excision with negative margins; >2 cm or invasion of muscularis propria → APR
  - Colon or high rectal carcinoids – formal resection with adenectomy

COLONIC OBSTRUCTION
- **Colon perforation with obstruction** – most likely to occur in cecum
  - Law of LaPlace: tension = pressure × diameter
- **Closed-loop obstructions** – can be worrisome; can have rapid progression and perforation with minimal distention
  - Competent ileocecal valve can lead to closed-loop obstruction
- **Colonic obstruction** – #1 cancer; #2 diverticulitis
- **Pneumatosis intestinalis** – air on the bowel wall, associated with ischemia and dissection of air through areas of bowel wall injury; most often an indication for surgery
- **Air in the portal system** – usually indicates significant infection or necrosis of the large or small bowel; often an ominous sign

OGILVIE'S SYNDROME
- Pseudoobstruction of colon
- Associated with opiate use, bedridden or older patient's recent surgery, infections, and trauma
- Get a massively dilated colon
- Check electrolytes; discontinue drugs that slow the gut, such as morphine
- Tx: **colonoscopy with decompression and neostigmine**; cecostomy if that fails

AMOEBIC COLITIS
- 10% become carriers for **Entamoeba histolytica**; from contaminated food and water with feces that contain cysts
- **Primary infection** – occurs in colon; **secondary infection** – occurs in liver
- Risk factors – travel to Mexico, ETOH; fecal–oral transmission
- Symptoms: similar to ulcerative colitis (dysentery); chronic more common form (3–4 bowel movements/day, cramping, and fever)
- Dx: endoscopy → ulceration, trophozoites; 90% have antiamebic antibodies
- Tx: Flagyl, diiodohydroxyquin

ACTINOMYCES
- Can present as a mass, abscess, fistula, or induration; suppurative and granulomatous
- Cecum most common location
- Tx: tetracycline or penicillin, drainage

LYMPHOGRANULOMA VENEREUM
- Chlamydia; homosexuals
- Causes proctitis, tenesmus, and bleeding; may produce fistulas
- Tx: doxycycline, hydrocortisone

DIVERTICULA
- Herniation of mucosa through the colon wall at sites where arteries enter the muscular wall
- Thickening of circular muscle adjacent to diverticulum with luminal narrowing
- Caused by **straining (↑ intraluminal pressure)**
- More diverticula occur on **left side** (80%) in the sigmoid colon
  - **Bleeding** is more likely with right-sided diverticula (50% of bleeds occur on right)
  - **Diverticulitis** is more likely to present on left side
- Present in 35% of the population

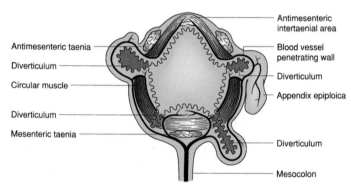

Cross section of the colon illustrating the relation of diverticula to the blood vessels penetrating the circular muscle layer, the taeniae, and the appendices epiploicae.

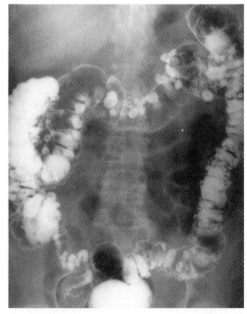

Barium enema showing multiple diverticula of the colon.

LOWER GI BLEEDING

- Stool guaiac can stay positive up to 3 weeks after bleed
- **Hematemesis** – pharynx to ligament of Treitz
- **Melena** – passage of tarry stools; need as little as 50 cc

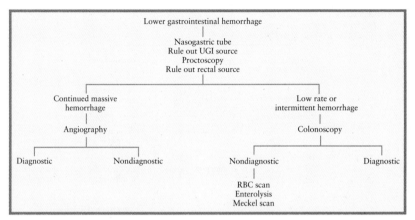

Diagnostic steps in the evaluation of acute lower gastrointestinal hemorrhage. UGI, upper gastrointestinal; RBC, red blood cell.

- **Azotemia after GI bleed** – caused by production of urea from bacterial action on intraluminal blood (↑ BUN, total bilirubin)
- **Arteriography** – bleeding must be ≥0.5 cc/min
- **Tagged RBC scan** – bleeding must be ≥0.1 cc/min

DIVERTICULITIS

- Result of perforations in the mucosa in the diverticulum with adjacent fecal contamination
- Denotes infection and inflammation of the colonic wall as well as surrounding tissue
- LLQ pain, tenderness, fever, ↑ WBCs
- Dx: CT scan is needed only if worried about complications of disease
- **Need follow-up barium enema to rule out cancer**
- 25% of patients will have a complication, **most likely abscess formation,** which can usually be percutaneously drained
  - **Signs of complication** – obstruction symptoms, fluctuant mass, peritoneal signs, temperature >39, and WBCs >20
- **Uncomplicated diverticulitis** – Tx: Flagyl and sulfamethoxazole and trimethoprim (Bactrim), bowel rest for 3–4 days

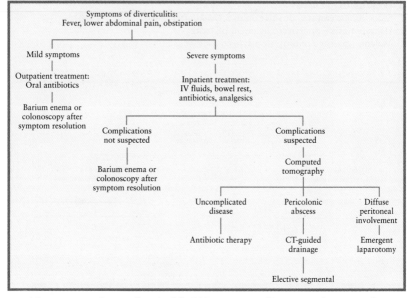

Management of acute diverticulitis. IV, intravenous; CT, computed tomography.

- **Surgery for recurrent disease** (2nd attacks associated with 50% recurrence rate), **significant emergent complications** (obstruction, perforation, or abscess formation not amenable to percutaneous drainage), and **inability to exclude cancer**
  - Some say that patients with any complicated diverticulitis (i.e., abscess formation) or if young should undergo sigmoidectomy with 1st time diverticulitis
  - Need to resect all of the sigmoid colon up to the superior rectum
- **Right-sided diverticulitis** – 80% discovered at the time of incision for appendectomy
  - Tx: right hemicolectomy

- **Colovesicular fistula** – fecaluria, pneumonuria
  - Occurs in men; women are more likely to get **colovaginal fistula**
  - **Cystoscopy** is more likely to identify
  - Tx: close bladder opening, resect involved segment of colon, and perform reanastomosis, diverting ileostomy

DIVERTICULOSIS BLEEDING
- Most common cause of lower GI bleed
- Usually causes significant bleeding
- 75% stops spontaneously; recurs in 25%
- Caused by disrupted vasa rectum; creates **arterial bleeding**
- Dx: **colonoscopy 1st** or **angio 1st** if massive bleed → these can be therapeutic and will localize the bleeding should surgery be required
  - **Go to operating room** if hypotensive and not responding to resuscitation → subtotal colectomy if bleeding source has not been localized
  - **Tagged RBC scan** for intermittent bleeds that are hard to localize
  - **NG tube to rule out upper GI source**

- ■ Tx: with colonoscopy can coagulate bleeder
  - With arteriography can use vasopressin or highly selective coil embolization
  - Vasopressin can allow time for resuscitation
  - May need segmental colectomy or even subtotal colectomy when bleeding is not localized and not controlled
- ■ Patients with recurrent diverticular bleeds should have resection of the area if it can be localized or they may need subtotal colectomy if the area cannot be localized

ANGIODYSPLASIA BLEEDING
- ■ ↑ on right side of colon
- ■ Bleeds are usually less severe than diverticular bleeds but are more likely to recur (80%)
- ■ Causes **venous bleeding**
- ■ Soft signs of angiodysplasia on angiogram – tufts, slow emptying
- ■ 20%–30% of patients with angiodysplasia have **aortic stenosis**

ISCHEMIC COLITIS
- ■ Symptoms: abdominal pain, bright red bleeding
- ■ Can be caused by a low-flow state, ligation of the IMA at surgery (i.e., AAA repair), embolus or thrombosis of the IMA, sepsis, and MI
- ■ **Splenic flexure and descending colon** most vulnerable to low-flow state
- ■ **Griffith's point** – SMA and IMA junction
- ■ **Sudeck's point** – superior rectal and middle rectal artery junction
- ■ Dx: made by endoscopy → cyanotic edematous mucosa covered with exudates
  - Lower ⅔ of the rectum is spared → supplied by the middle (off the internal iliac) and inferior (off the internal pudendal) rectal artery
  - If gangrenous colitis is suspected (peritonitis), <u>no</u> colonoscopy and go to OR → sigmoid or left hemicolectomy usual

PSEUDOMEMBRANOUS COLITIS (*C. DIFFICILE* COLITIS)
- ■ Symptoms: watery, green, mucoid diarrhea; pain and cramping
- ■ Can occur up to 3 weeks after antibiotics; increased in postop, elderly, and ICU patients
- ■ Carrier state not eradicated; 15% recurrence
- ■ Key finding – **PMN inflammation of mucosa and submucosa**
  - Pseudomembranes, plaques, and ringlike lesions
- ■ Most common in the distal colon
- ■ Dx: fecal leukocytes, stool cultures for *C. difficile*, *C. difficile* toxin
  - Only ⅓ of patients with *C. difficile* colitis are positive for fecal leukocytes with each test
  - If tests are negative at first, need to repeat if your suspicion is high or just treat empirically
- ■ Tx: oral – vancomycin or Flagyl. IV – Flagyl
  - Lactobacillus can also help; stop other antibiotics or change them

NEUTROPENIC TYPHLITIS (ENTEROCOLITIS)
- ■ Follows chemotherapy when WBCs are low
- ■ Can mimic surgical disease
- ■ Can often see pneumatosis on plane film
- ■ TX: antibiotics; patients will improve when WBCs ↑

OTHER COLON DISEASES
- ■ Other causes of colitis – *Salmonella*, *Shigella*, *Campylobacter*, CMV, *Yersinia* (can mimic appendicitis in children), other viral infections, *Giardia*
- ■ **TB enteritis** – presents like Crohn's disease (stenoses)
  - Tx: INH, rifampin; surgery with obstruction

- *Yersinia* – can mimic appendicitis; comes from contaminated food (feces/urine)
  - Tx: tetracycline or Bactrim
- **Megacolon** – propensity for volvulus; enlargement is proximal to nonperistalsing bowel
  - **Hirschsprung's disease** – rectosigmoid most common. Dx: rectal biopsy
  - *Trypanosoma cruzi* – most common acquired cause, secondary to destruction of nerves

Arterial supply to the anus – inferior rectal artery
Venous drainage – above the dentate is internal hemorrhoid plexus and below the
  dentate is external hemorrhoid plexus

HEMORRHOIDS

- Left lateral, right anterior, and right posterior hemorrhoidal plexuses
- **External hemorrhoids** cause pain when they thrombose
  - Distal to the dentate line, covered by sensate squamous epithelium; can cause pain, swelling, and itching
- **Internal hemorrhoids** cause bleeding or prolapse
  - **Primary** – slides below dentate with strain
  - **Secondary** – prolapse that reduces spontaneously
  - **Tertiary** – prolapse that has to be manually reduced
  - **Quaternary** – not able to reduce
- Tx: fiber and stool softeners; sitz baths
- Thrombosed external hemorrhoid → lance open to relieve pain
- Surgical indications: recurrent disease (bleeding), thrombosis multiple times, large external component
- Can band primary, secondary, and tertiary internal hemorrhoids
- Surgery needed for some tertiary and quaternary internal hemorrhoids – 3 quadrant resection
- Need to resect down to the internal sphincter
- Postop needs sitz baths, stool softener, and high-fiber diet
- Do not band external hemorrhoids (painful)

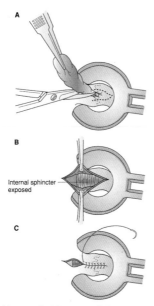

Technique of interanal closed hemorrhoidectomy. *(A)* Exposure of hemorrhoid with elliptic excision starting at perianal skin and extending to anorectal ring. *(B)* Submucosal hemorrhoidal plexus dissected from the internal sphincter, anoderm, and mucosa. *(C)* Wound closed with a running suture.

RECTAL PROLAPSE
- Starts 6–7 cm from anal verge
- Secondary to pudendal neuropathy and laxity of the anal sphincters
- ↑ with female gender, straining, chronic diarrhea, previous pregnancy, and redundant sigmoid colons

Anatomic Defects or Abnormalities in Patients with Chronic Rectal Prolapse
- Abnormally deep rectovaginal or rectovesical pouch
- Lax and atonic musculature of the pelvic floor
- Lack of normal fixation of the rectum and an elongated mesorectum
- Redundant sigmoid colon
- Lax and atonic anal sphincter

- Prolapse involves all layers of the rectum

- Tx: high-fiber diet
  - Rectosigmoid resection (Altmier) transanally if patient is older and frail
  - LAR; in the absence of a large redundant colon or constipation symptoms may perform just rectopexy

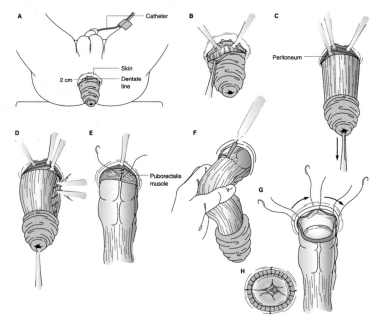

Perineal rectosigmoidectomy. The patient is placed in the lithotomy position with both legs in gynecologic stirrups. *(A and B)* A circular incision is made on the prolapsed rectum 2 cm proximal to the dentate line. *(C)* The peritoneal attachment is dissected from the anterior rectal wall, thus opening into the peritoneal cavity. *(D)* The mesorectum or mesosigmoid is clamped and divided laterally and posteriorly. *(E)* The previously opened peritoneum is sutured to the anterior wall of the rectum or sigmoid colon as high as possible. This is followed by approximation of the puborectalis (optional). *(F)* The anterior wall of the protruding rectum is cut 1 cm distal to the anal verge. *(G)* Stay sutures of 3-0 synthetic absorbable material are placed in four quadrants. *(H)* Anastomosis with running stitches.

CONDYLOMATA ACUMINATA
- Cauliflower mass; papillomavirus (HPV)
- Tx: laser surgery

ANAL FISSURE
- Caused by a split in the anoderm
- **90% in posterior midline**
- Causes pain and bleeding after defecation; chronic ones will see a **sentinel pile**
- Medical Tx: **Sitz baths, bulk, lidocaine jelly, and stool softeners** (90% heal)
- Surgical Tx: **lateral subcutaneous internal sphincterotomy**
- Fecal incontinence is the most serious complication of surgery
- Do <u>not</u> perform surgery if secondary to Crohn's disease or ulcerative colitis
- **Lateral or recurrent fissures** – worry about inflammatory bowel disease

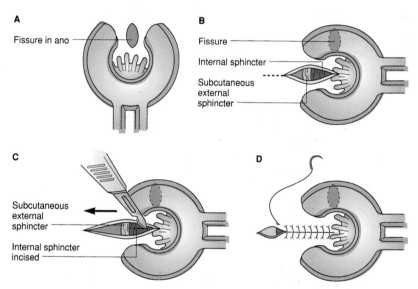

A
Fissure in ano

B
Fissure
Internal sphincter
Subcutaneous external sphincter

C
Subcutaneous external sphincter
Internal sphincter incised

D

Lateral internal sphincterotomy (open method). *(A)* The fissure in the midline is left alone. *(B)* With a speculum used to expose the left lateral quadrant, an incision is made through the subcutaneous tissue to expose both the subcutaneous external sphincter and the internal sphincter. *(C)* The internal sphincter is incised to its full thickness; care is taken not to cut the external sphincter. *(D)* The wound is closed.

ANORECTAL ABSCESS
- Can cause severe pain
- **Perianal, intersphincteric, and ischiorectal abscesses** can be drained through the skin (all are below the levator muscles)
  - **Intersphincteric and ischiorectal abscesses** can form horseshoe abscess
- **Supralevator abscesses** need to be drained transrectally
- Antibiotics are needed for cellulitis, patient with DM, immunosuppressed, or artificial valve

PILONIDAL CYSTS
- Sinus or abscess formation over the sacrococcygeal junction; ↑ in men
- Tx: drainage and packing; follow-up surgical resection of cyst

FISTULA-IN-ANO
- Unroof fistula and eliminate the primary opening with rectal advancement flap
- Do **not** need to excise the tract
- Often occurs after anorectal abscess formation
- **Goodsall's rule** – anterior fistulas connect with rectum in a straight line
  - Posterior fistulas go toward a midline internal opening in the rectum

RECTOVAGINAL FISTULAS

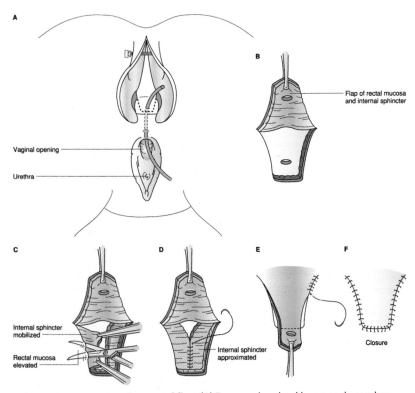

Endorectal advancement of anorectal flap. *(A)* Exposure is gained by an anal speculum, and the fistula is identified. Outline of endorectal flap, extending proximally to 7 cm from the anal verge. *(B)* The full-thickness flap is created to include the internal sphincter muscle. *(C)* Lateral mobilization is made on each side in the submucosal plane. *(D)* Anorectal wall on each side is approximated. *(E and F)* The endorectal flap is pulled down to cover the wound and sutured. The fistula is excised. The aperture in the vagina is not sutured but is left open for drainage.

- **Simple** – secondary to infection or obstetrical trauma, low to midvagina, and <2.5 cm
  - Tx: transanally unroof and place rectal mucosa advancement flap
  - Many obstetrical fistulas heal spontaneously

- **Complex** – secondary to inflammatory bowel disease, XRT, neoplasm, or high in vagina or >2.5 cm
  - Tx: abdominal or combined approach usual; resection and reanastomosis with placement of colostomy; need good tissue for anastomosis

ANAL INCONTINENCE

- **Neurogenic (gaping hole)** – no good treatment
- **Abdominoperineal descent** – damage to levator ani muscle and anus falls below levators, also stretches the pudendal nerves
  - Tx: high-fiber diet, limit to 1 bowel movement a day; sphincteroplasty if related to trauma (childbirth)

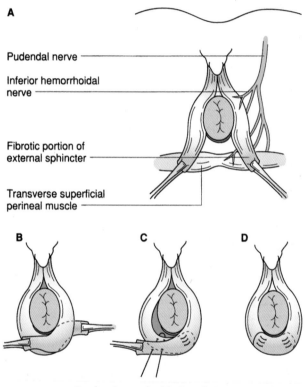

A

Pudendal nerve

Inferior hemorrhoidal nerve

Fibrotic portion of external sphincter

Transverse superficial perineal muscle

B   **C**   **D**

Overlapping anal sphincteroplasty.

AIDS ANORECTAL PROBLEMS

- **Kaposi's sarcoma** – see nodule with ulceration; most common cancer in patients with AIDS
- **CMV** – see shallow ulcers; similar presentation as appendicitis. Tx: ganciclovir
- **HSV** – #1 rectal ulcer
- **B cell lymphoma** – can look like abscess or ulcer
- Need biopsies of ulcers to rule out cancer

ANAL CANCER

- Association with **HPV and XRT**
- Anal canal – above dentate line
- Anal verge – below dentate line

- **Anal canal lesions (above dentate line)**
  - **Squamous cell CA (type of epidermal CA)**
    - **Symptoms**: pruritus, bleeding, and palpable mass
    - Tx: **chemotherapy 1st line** (Nigro protocol, chemo – 5FU and mitomycin, and XRT), **not** surgery
    - If the patient has inguinal adenopathy, need to get FNA – if positive, need to extend the radiation field to the inguinal nodes
    - Cures 80%
    - APR for persistent or recurrent cancer

Modified Nigro Regimen for Squamous Cell Carcinoma of the Anal Canal		
Treatment	Dose	Schedule
External radiation	50 Gy to the primary carcinoma and 35–45 Gy to pelvic inguinal nodes	Start day 1 (2 Gy/day, 5 days a week for 5 weeks)
Systemic chemotherapy	Fluorouracil, 1,000 mg/m^2/24 hr as a continuous infusion for 4 days	Start day 1; repeat 4-day infusion starting day 28
Mitomycin C	10–15 mg/m^2 as intravenous bolus	Day 1 only

  - **Basaloid (cloacogenic) CA, mucoepidermoid CA**
    - Tx: same as squamous cell CA
  - **Adenocarcinoma**
    - Tx: APR usual; WLE if <3 cm, <⅓ circumference, limited to submucosa (T1), well differentiated, and no vascular/lymphatic invasion; needs about 1-cm margin
    - Postoperative chemo/XRT same as rectal CA
  - **Melanoma**
    - 3rd most common site for melanoma (skin and eyes #1 and #2)
    - ⅓ has spread to mesenteric lymph nodes
    - Hematogenous spread to the liver and the lung is early and accounts for most deaths
    - Symptomatic disease is often associated with significant metastatic disease
    - Most common symptom – rectal bleeding
    - Most tumors are lightly pigmented or not pigmented at all
    - Tx: APR usual; margin dictated by depth of lesion standard for melanoma

- **Anal margin lesions (below dentate line)** – have better prognosis than anal canal lesions
  - **Squamous cell CA**
    - Ulcerating, slow growing; men with better prognosis
    - Metastases – go to inguinal nodes
    - Tx: WLE for lesions <3 cm and can get 0.5-cm margin
    - May need APR for larger lesions or if sphincter is involved
    - Need inguinal node dissection if clinically positive
  - **Basal cell CA** – central ulcer, raised edges, rare metastases
    - Tx: WLE usually sufficient, only need 3-mm margins; rare need for APR unless sphincter involved
  - **Bowen's disease (malignant)**
    - Intraepidermal squamous cell CA
    - Many of these patients have or will develop 1 or more primary internal malignancies or will develop a primary cancer of the skin with internal metastases

- Tx: local therapy, possible WLE with clear margins; check for other internal malignancies
- **Paget's disease (rare)**
  - Intraepidermal apocrine gland CA
  - Slow growing; has positive PAS stain
  - Many of these patients have intractable itching
  - Many of these patients have or will develop a rectal or colon CA
  - Tx: WLE with clear margins; groin dissection for positive nodes; check for other internal malignancies

NODAL METASTASES
- Superior and middle rectum – IMA nodes
- Lower rectum – primarily IMA nodes, also to internal iliac nodes
- Upper ⅔ of anal canal – internal iliac and pelvic nodes
- Lower ⅓ of anal canal – inguinal nodes

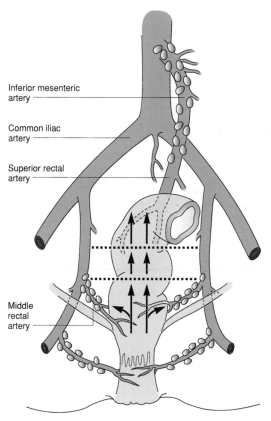

Inferior mesenteric artery

Common iliac artery

Superior rectal artery

Middle rectal artery

Lymphatic drainage of the rectum.

INGUINAL HERNIAS

- **External abdominal oblique** – forms external abdominal oblique fascia and shelving edge
- **Internal abdominal oblique** – forms cremasteric muscles
- **Transversalis muscle** – forms inguinal canal floor
- **Inguinal ligament** (Poupart's ligament) – from external abdominal oblique, runs from anterior superior iliac spine to the pubis
  - **Lacunar ligament** – where the inguinal ligament splays out to insert in the pubis
- **Ileopubic tract** – from transversalis, runs from anterior, superior, iliac spine to the pubis
  - Is below the inguinal ligament
- **Cooper's ligament** – pectineal ligament
- **Conjoined tendon** – composed of the aponeurosis of the internal abdominal oblique and transversus abdominis muscles
- **Vas deferens** – runs medial to cord structures

- **Hesselbach's triangle** – rectus muscle, inferior inguinal ligament, and inferior epigastrics
  - Direct hernias are inferior/medial to the epigastric vessels
  - Indirect hernias are superior/lateral to the epigastric vessels

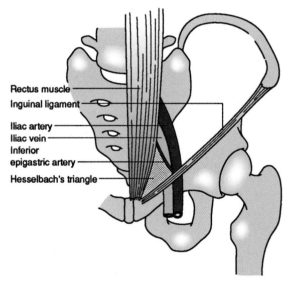

Rectus muscle
Inguinal ligament
Iliac artery
Iliac vein
Inferior epigastric artery
Hesselbach's triangle

The inguinal (Hesselbach's) triangle.

- **Risk factors for inguinal hernia in adults**: age, obesity, heavy lifting, COPD (coughing), chronic constipation, straining (BPH), ascites, pregnancy, and peritoneal dialysis

- **Indirect hernias** – most common; from persistently patent processus vaginalis
- **Direct hernias** – lower risk of incarceration; rare in females, higher recurrence than indirect
- **Pantaloon hernia** – direct and indirect components

- **Incarcerated hernia** – can lead to bowel strangulation; should be repaired emergently

- **Sliding hernias**
  - **Females** – ovaries or fallopian tubes most common
  - **Males** – cecum or sigmoid most common
  - Bladder can also be involved

- **Females with ovary in canal**
  - Ligate the round ligament
  - Return ovary to peritoneum
  - Perform biopsy if looks abnormal

- **Hernias in infants and children**
  - Just perform high ligation (nearly always indirect)
  - Open sac prior to ligation

- **Lichtenstein repair** = mesh; recurrence ↓ with use of **mesh** (↓ tension)

- **Bassini repair** – approximation of the conjoined tendon and transversalis fascia (superior) to the free edge of the inguinal ligament (inferior)
- **McVay (Cooper's ligament) repair** – approximation of the conjoined tendon and transversalis fascia (superior) to Cooper's ligament (pectineal ligament, inferior)
  - Needs a relaxing incision in the external abdominal oblique fascia

- **Laparoscopic hernia repair** – indicated for bilateral or recurrent inguinal hernia

- **Urinary retention** – most common early complication following hernia repair
- **Wound infection** – 2%
- **Recurrence rate** – 2%
- **Testicular atrophy** – usually secondary to dissection of the distal component of the hernia sac causing vessel disruption
  - Thrombosis of **spermatic cord veins**
  - Usually occurs with indirect hernias
- **Pain after hernia** – usually compression of ilioinguinal nerve
  - Tx: local infiltration can be diagnostic and therapeutic
- **Ilioinguinal nerve injury** – loss of cremasteric reflex; numbness on ipsilateral penis, scrotum, and thigh
  - Nerve is usually injured at the external ring; nerve runs on top of cord
- **Genitofemoral nerve injury** – usually injured with laparoscopic hernia repair
  - Genital branch – cremaster (motor) and scrotum (sensory)
  - Femoral branch – upper lateral thigh (sensory)
- **Cord lipomas** – should be removed
- **Trapezoid of doom**
  - Laparoscopic hernia repairs – femoral branch of genitofemoral nerve, lateral cutaneous nerve, and femoral artery
  - Need to dissect lateral to vessels; stay along inguinal ligament

FEMORAL HERNIA

- Most common in males
- Femoral canal boundaries – Cooper's ligament, inguinal ligament, and femoral vein (Poupart's ligament is medial)
- **Femoral hernia** is medial to the femoral vein and lateral to the lymphatics (in empty space)
- High risk of incarceration → **may need to divide the inguinal ligament to reduce the bowel**

■ Hernia passes under the inguinal ligament
■ Characteristic bulge on the anterior–medial thigh below the ligament
■ Hernia is usually repaired through an inguinal approach with McVay or Bassini repair

OTHER HERNIAS
■ **Umbilical hernia**
  • ↑ incidence in African-Americans
  • Delay repair until age 5 years
  • Risk of incarceration in adults, not children
■ **Spigelian hernia**
  • Lateral border of rectus muscle, **through linea semilunaris**
  • Almost always inferior to the semicircularis
  • Occurs between the muscle fibers of the internal abdominal oblique muscle and line of insertion of the external abdominal oblique aponeurosis into the rectus sheath
■ **Richter's hernia** – noncircumferential incarceration of the nonmesenteric bowel wall
■ **Littre's hernia** – incarcerated Meckel's
■ **Petit's hernia** – inferior lumbar hernia
  • External abdominal oblique
  • Latissimus dorsi (or lumbodorsal aponeurosis)
  • Iliac crest
■ **Grynfeltt's hernia** – superior lumbar hernia
  • Internal abdominal oblique
  • Lumbodorsal aponeurosis
  • 12th rib (or posterior lumbocostal ligament)
■ **Sciatic hernia (posterior pelvis)**
  • Herniation through the greater sciatic foramen; high rate of strangulation
■ **Obturator hernia (anterior pelvis)**
  • **Howship–Romberg sign** – inner thigh pain with internal rotation
  • Elderly women, previous pregnancy, and bowel gas below superior pubic ramus
  • Tx: operative reduction, may need mesh; check other side for similar defect
  • Diagnosis is usually made at the time of surgery for small bowel obstruction
■ **Incisional hernia** – most likely to recur; inadequate closure is the most common cause
■ **Peristomal hernia**
  • True hernias – need to remove and place in rectus muscle (missed the rectus)
  • Prolapse – keep stoma at same site, fix mesentery (is in rectus but prolapsing through)
  • Pseudohernia – secondary to being in the oblique muscle; need to move to rectus

RECTUS SHEATH
■ Anterior – complete
■ Posterior – absent below semicircularis (below umbilicus)
■ The posterior aponeurosis of the internal abdominal oblique and transversalis aponeurosis move anterior
■ **Rectus sheath hematomas**
  • Most common after trauma; epigastric vessel injury
  • Painful abdominal wall mass
  • Mass more prominent and painful with flexion of the rectus muscle (Fothergill's sign)
  • Tx: nonoperative usual, surgery if expanding

DESMOID TUMORS
■ Women, benign but locally invasive; ↑ recurrences
■ Gardner's syndrome

- Painless mass
- Tx: wide local excision; if involving small bowel, excision may not be indicated → often not completely resectable and can cause worsening fibrosis
- NSAIDs and antiestrogens may help

RETROPERITONEAL FIBROSIS
- Can occur with hypersensitivity to methysergide
- IVP most sensitive test
- Symptoms usually related to **trapped ureters and lymphatic obstruction**
- Tx: steroids, nephrostomy if infection is present, and surgery if renal function becomes compromised (free up ureters and wrap in omentum)

MESENTERIC TUMORS
- Of the primary tumors, most are cystic
  - **Malignant tumors** – closer to the **root** of the mesentery
  - **Benign tumors** – more **peripheral**
- Malignant – **liposarcoma**, leiomyosarcoma
- Most solid tumors of the mesentery are benign
- Dx: abdominal CT
- Tx: resection

RETROPERITONEAL TUMORS
- 15% in children, others in 5th–6th decade
- Malignant > benign
- Most common malignant retroperitoneal tumor – #1 **lymphoma**, #2 liposarcoma
- Symptoms: vague abdominal and back pain
- **Retroperitoneal sarcomas**
  - <25% resectable; local recurrence in 40%; 10% 5-year survival rate
  - Have pseudocapsule but cannot shell out → leave residual tumor
  - Metastases go to the lung

OMENTAL TUMORS
- Most common omental solid tumor is metastatic disease
- Omentectomy for metastatic cancer has a role for some cancers (e.g., ovarian CA)
- Omental cysts are usually asymptomatic, can undergo torsion
- Primary solid omental tumors are rare; 1/3 malignant
- No biopsy → can bleed
- Tx: resection

PERITONEAL MEMBRANE
- Saline absorbed at 35 cc/hr
- Blood absorbed through fenestrated lymphatic channels
- Most drugs are not removed with peritoneal dialysis; NH_3, Ca, Fe, and lead are removed
- Movement into the peritoneal cavity with hypertonic intraperitoneal saline load → 300–500 cc/hr; can cause hypotension

CO_2 PNEUMOPERITONEUM
- Cardiopulmonary dysfunction can occur with intra-abdominal pressure > 20
- ↑ pulmonary artery pressure, HR, systemic vascular resistance, central venous pressure, mean airway pressure, peak inspiratory pressure, and CO_2

- ↓ pH, venous return (IVC compression), renal flow secondary to renal vein compression, and cardiac output
- Hypovolemia lowers pressure necessary to cause compromise
- PEEP has additive effect → pressure causes ↓ renal blood flow and can ↑ renin production
- CO_2 can cause some ↓ in myocardial contractility
- **CO_2 embolus** – head down, turn patient to the left (sudden rise in $ETCO_2$ hypotension)

Physiologic Effects of Pneumoperitoneum	
Parameter	**Effect**
Mean arterial pressure	↑
Systemic vascular resistance	↑
Pulmonary vascular resistance	↑
Heart rate	↑
Central venous pressure	↑
Venous return	↓
Cardiac output	↓
Cardiac index	↓

SURGICAL TECHNOLOGY
- **Harmonic scalpel**
  - Cost-effective for medium vessels (short gastrics)
  - Disrupts protein H-bonds, causes coagulation
- **Ultrasound**
  - B-mode used most commonly (B = brightness; assesses relative density of structures)
  - **Shadowing** – dark area posterior to object indicates mass
  - **Enhancement** – brighter area posterior to object indicates fluid-filled cyst
  - **Duplex**
    - **Lower frequencies** – deep structures
    - **Higher frequencies** – superficial structures
- **Argon beam** – energy transferred across argon gas
  - Depth of necrosis related to power setting (2 mm); pretty superficial coagulation
  - Noncontact – good for hemostasis of the liver and spleen; smokeless
- **Laser** – return of electrons to ground state releases energy as heat → coagulates and vaporizes
  - Used for condylomata acuminata (wear mask)
- **Nd:YAG laser** – good for deep tissue penetration; good for bronchial lesions
  - 1–2 mm cuts, 3–10 mm vaporizes, and 1–2 cm coagulates
  - **Gore-Tex** (PTFE) – cannot get fibroblast ingrowth
  - **Dacron** (polypropylene) – allows fibroblast ingrowth
  - **Incidence of vascular or bowel injury with Veress needle or trocar – 0.1%**

CHAPTER 39. UROLOGY

ANATOMY AND PHYSIOLOGY
- **Gerota's fascia** – around kidney
- **Anterior to posterior** – renal vein, renal artery, and renal pelvis
  - **Right renal artery** crosses posterior to the IVC
- **Ureters cross over iliac vessels**
- **Left renal vein** – can be ligated from IVC secondary to increased collaterals (left adrenal vein, left gonadal vein, and left ascending lumbar vein)
- **Epididymis** – connects to vas deferens
- **Hypotension** – most common cause of acute renal insufficiency following surgery

KIDNEY STONES
- **Symptoms**: severe colicky pain, restlessness
- **Urinalysis** – blood or stones
- **Abdominal CT** – can demonstrate stones and associated hydronephrosis
- **Calcium oxalate (phosphate) stones** – most common (75%); radiopaque
- Mg ammonium phosphate (struvite) stones – 15%; radiopaque
- Uric acid stones – 7%; radiolucent
- Cysteine stones – 2%; radiolucent to radiopaque

- **Calcium oxalate stones** – ↑ in patients with terminal ileum resection due to ↑ oxalate absorption in colon
- **Struvite stones** – occur with infections (*Proteus mirabilis*) that are <u>urease</u> producing
  - Can cause <u>staghorn calculi</u> (fill the renal pelvis)
- **Uric acid stones** – ↑ in patients with ileostomies, gout, and myeloproliferative disorders
- **Cysteine stones** – associated with congenital disorders in the reabsorption of cysteine

- **Surgery for kidney stones**
  - Intractable pain or infection
  - Progressive obstruction
  - Progressive renal damage
  - Solitary kidney
  - 90% of kidney stones opaque; >6 mm not likely to pass
  - Tx: ESWL, ureteroscopy with stone extraction or placement of stent past the stone obstruction, percutaneous nephrostomy tube, open nephrolithotomy, or urethrotomy

TESTICULAR CANCER
- **#1 cancer killer** in men 25–35
- **Symptom**: painless hard mass
- **Testicular mass** – patient needs an **orchiectomy** through an **inguinal incision** (<u>not</u> a transscrotal incision → does not want to disrupt lymphatics)
  - The testicle and attached mass constitute the biopsy specimen
- Most testicular masses are **malignant**
- **Ultrasound** can help with diagnosis
- Chest x-ray – to check for pulmonary metastases
- Chest and abdominal CT – to check for retroperitoneal and mediastinal burden
- **LDH** correlates with tumor bulk
- **Needs a B-HCG and AFP level**
- 90% of tumors are germ cells – seminoma or nonseminoma

- **Undescended testicles (cryptorchidism)** – ↑ risk of testicular CA
  - Most likely to get seminoma

- **Seminoma**
  - #1 testicular tumor
  - 10% of seminomatous tumors have beta-HCG elevation
  - Should not have AFP elevation (if elevated, need to treat like nonseminomatous)
  - Spreads to retroperitoneum
  - **Seminoma is extremely sensitive to XRT**
  - Tx: all stages get **orchiectomy and retroperitoneal XRT** – some patients have occult retroperitoneal metastases
    - If the paraaortic nodes in the abdomen are enlarged, need to extend XRT to the mediastinum
    - **Positive nodes, metastatic disease, or bulky retroperitoneal disease** → chemo (cisplatin, bleomycin, VP-16)
    - If the patient still has disease after XRT and chemo, needs to go with surgery

- **Nonseminomatous testicular CA**
  - **Types** – embryonal, teratoma, choriocarcinoma, and yolk sac
  - **Alpha fetoprotein and beta-HCG** – 90% have these markers
  - Spreads hematogenously to **lungs**
  - Also spreads to **retroperitoneum**
  - Classically, tumors with ↑ teratoma components are more likely to metastasize to the retroperitoneum
  - Surgical Tx
    - **Stage I – orchiectomy**, prophylactic **retroperitoneal node dissection**
    - **Stage II or greater – orchiectomy, XRT, and chemo (cisplatin, bleomycin, VP-16); surgical resection of residual metastases**

PROSTATE CANCER
- **Posterior lobe** – most common site
- **Bone** – most common site of metastases
  - **Osteoblastic; x-ray demonstrates hyperdense areas**
- Many patients become impotent after resection; can get incontinence
- Can also get urethral strictures
- Dx: transrectal Bx, CXR, Abd/pelvic CT, PSA, alkaline phosphatase; possible bone scan
- **Intracapsular tumors and no metastases (T1 and T2)** → XRT, radical prostatectomy with pelvic lymph node dissection (if life span > 10 years), or nothing depending on age and health
- **Extracapsular invasion or metastatic disease**
  - **Hormonal Tx**: leuprolide (LH-RH blocker), flutamide (testosterone blocker), bilateral orchiectomy, ketoconazole, and XRT for bone pain
  - **Chemotherapy**: reserved for metastatic disease not responding to hormonal therapy
- **Stage IA disease found with TURP** – Tx: nothing
- **With prostatectomy, PSA should go to 0 after 3 weeks** → if not, get bone scan to check for metastases
- **Normal PSA <4 in a patient who has a prostate gland**
  - **PSA** can be ↑ with prostatitis, BPH, and chronic catheterization
- ↑ **alkaline phosphatase** in a patient with prostate CA → metastases or extracapsular disease

RENAL CELL CARCINOMA (HYPERNEPHROMA)
- #1 primary tumor of kidney (15% calcified)
- Risk factor: smoking
- **Abdominal pain, mass, and hematuria**
- ⅓ have metastatic disease at the time of diagnosis → can perform **wedge resection of isolated lung and colon metastases**
- **Lung** – most common location for RCC metastases

- **Erythrocytosis** can occur secondary to $\uparrow$ erythropoietin (HTN)
- Tx: radical nephrectomy with regional nodes; XRT, chemotherapy
  - Radical nephrectomy takes kidney, adrenal, fat, Gerota's fascia, and regional nodes
  - Predilection for growth in the IVC; can still resect even if going up IVC → can pull the tumor thrombus out of the IVC
  - Partial nephrectomies should be considered only for patients who would require dialysis after nephrectomy
  - Embolization can be used to palliate large tumors or as preop for large tumors to facilitate removal

- Most common tumor in kidney – **metastasis from the breast**
- **Paraneoplastic syndromes associated with RCC** – erythropoietin, PTHrp, ACTH, and insulin
- **Transitional cell CA of renal pelvis** – Tx: radical nephroureterectomy
- **Oncocytomas** – benign
- **Angiomyolipomas** – hamartomas; can occur with tuberous sclerosis; large tumors (>4 cm) may be symptomatic and require excision or embolization
- **Von Hippel–Lindau syndrome** – multifocal and recurrent RCC, renal cysts, CNS tumors, and pheochromocytomas

BLADDER CANCER
- Usually transitional cell CA
- **Painless hematuria**
- Males; prognosis based on stage and grade
- Risk factors: smoking, aniline dyes, and cyclophosphamide
- Dx: cystoscopy, IVP
- Tx: **intravesical BCG or transurethral resection if muscle is not involved (T1)**
  - **If muscle wall is invaded (T2 or greater)** → cystectomy with ileal conduit, chemotherapy (MVAC: methotrexate, vinblastine, Adriamycin [doxorubicin], and cisplatin), and XRT
  - Metastatic disease – chemotherapy
- **Ileal conduit standard** – avoid stasis as this predisposes to infection, stones (calcium resorption), and ureteral reflux
- **Reservoirs or neobladders may also be options**
- **Squamous cell CA of bladder** – schistosomiasis infection

TESTICULAR TORSION
- Peaks in 15-year-olds
- Involved testis almost never viable
- Usually has intravaginal torsion of the spermatic cord if viable
- Torsion is usually toward the midline
- Tx: **bilateral orchiopexy**
  - If not, resection and orchiopexy of contralateral testis

URETERAL TRAUMA
- If going to repair end-to-end
  - Spatulate ends
  - Use **absorbable suture** to avoid stone formation
  - **Stent the ureter** to avoid stenosis
  - **Place drains** to identify and potentially help treat leaks
- Avoid stripping the soft tissue on the ureter, as it will compromise blood supply

URETHRAL AND BLADDER TRAUMA – SEE CHAP. 15

BENIGN PROSTATIC HYPERTROPHY (BPH)
- Arises in **transitional zone**
- **Symptoms**: nocturia, frequency, dysuria, weak stream, and urinary retention
- **Initial therapy**
  - **Alpha blockers** – terazosin, doxazosin (relax smooth muscle)
  - **5-alpha-reductase inhibitors** – finasteride → inhibits the conversion of testosterone to dihydrotestosterone (inhibits prostate hypertrophy)
- **Surgery (TURP)**: for recurrent UTIs, gross hematuria, stones, renal insufficiency, and failure of medical therapy
  - **Post-TURP syndrome** – hyponatremia secondary to irrigation with water; can precipitate **seizures** from cerebral edema
  - Tx: careful correction of Na with diuresis
- Most patients with TURP have retrograde ejaculation

NEUROGENIC BLADDER
- Most commonly secondary to spinal compression
- Patient urinates all the time
- Injury above T-12
- Tx: surgery to improve bladder resistance

NEUROGENIC OBSTRUCTIVE UROPATHY
- Incomplete emptying
- Injury below T-12; can occur with APR
- Tx: intermittent catheterization

INCONTINENCE
- **Stress incontinence (cough, sneeze)**
  - Because of hypermobile urethra or loss of sphincter mechanism
  - Tx: Kegel exercises, alpha-adrenergic agents, and surgery for urethral suspension or pubovaginal sling
- **Urge incontinence**
  - Sense of urgency or frequency
  - Because of involuntary detrusor contraction without neurologic disorder
  - Tx: anticholinergics, behavior modification, cystoplasty, and urinary diversion (last resort)
- **Neuropathic incontinence**
  - Urgency or frequency
  - ↓ bladder capacity; associated with neurologic conditions → spinal cord dysfunction, stroke, and multiple sclerosis.
    - Tx: underlying neurologic disorder, behavior modification; surgical options – cystoplasty or urinary diversion
- **Overflow incontinence**
  - Incomplete emptying and enlarged bladder
  - Obstruction (BPH) leads to the distention and leakage
  - Tx: TURP
- **Congenital incontinence**
  - Continuous leakage and nocturnal enuresis; sphincter mechanism is bypassed
  - Tx: surgical correction (bladder exstrophy, ureteral diversion)

OTHER UROLOGIC DISEASES
- **Ureteropelvic obstruction** – Tx: pyeloplasty
- **Vesicoureteral reflux** – Tx: reimplantation with long bladder portion
- **Ureteral duplication** – most common urinary tract abnormality. Tx: reimplantation
- **Ureterocele** – Tx: resect and reimplant

- **Hypospadias** – ventral. Tx: repair at 6 months with penile skin
- **Epispadias** – dorsal. Tx: surgery
- **Horseshoe kidney** – usually joined at lower poles
  - Complications: UTI, urolithiasis, and hydronephrosis
  - Tx: may need pyeloplasty
- **Polycystic kidney disease** – resection only if symptomatic
- **Failure of closure of urachus** – connection between umbilicus and bladder; occurs in patients with bladder outlet obstructive disease (wet umbilicus)
  - Tx: resection of sinus/cyst and closure of the bladder; relieve obstruction
- **Epididymitis** – sterile epididymitis can occur from ↑ abdominal straining
- **Varicocele** – worrisome for <u>renal cell CA</u> (left gonadal vein inserts into left renal vein; obstruction by renal tumor causes varicocele); could also be caused by another retroperitoneal malignancy
- **Hydrocele in adult** – if acute, suspect tumor elsewhere; translucent
- **Pneumaturia** – most common cause is diverticulitis and subsequent formation of colovesical fistula
- **WBC casts** – pyelonephritis, glomerulonephritis
- **RBC casts** – glomerulonephritis
- **Interstitial nephritis** – fever, rash, arthralgias, and eosinophils
- **Vasectomy** – 50% pregnancy rate after repair of vasectomy
- **Priapism** – Tx: aspiration of the corpus cavernosum with dilute epinephrine or phenylephrine
  - May need to create a communication through the glans with scalpel
  - Risk factors: sickle-cell anemia, hypercoagulable states, trauma, and intracorporeal injections for impotence
- **SCC of penis** – penectomy with 2-cm margin
- **Indigo carmine or methylene blue** – used to check for urine leak
- **Phimosis found at time of laparotomy** – Tx: dorsal slit
- **Erythropoietin** – ↓ production in patients with renal failure
- **Spermatocele** – fluid-filled cystic structure separate from and superior to the testis along the epididymis; Tx: surgical removal

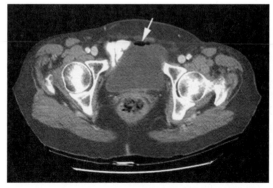

CT scan: Air in bladder from sigmoid-vesicle fistula complicating diverticulitis. (From Fry RD, Mahmoud NN. Segmental resection for diverticulitis. In: Fischer JE, Bland KI, et al., eds. *Mastery of Surgery*, 5th ed. Philadelphia, PA: Lippincott Williams & Wilkins; 2007, with permission.)

LIGAMENTS
- **Round ligament** – allows anteversion of the uterus
- **Broad ligament** – contains uterine vessels
- **Infundibular ligament** – contains ovarian artery, nerve, and vein
- **Cardinal ligament** – holds cervix and vagina

ULTRASOUND
- Very good at diagnosing disorders of the female genital tract

PREGNANCY
- Can see most pregnancies on ultrasound at 6 weeks
- Fetal pole usually is seen with beta-HCG of 6,000
- Gestational sac is seen with beta-HCG of 1,500

ABORTIONS
- **Missed** – 1st trimester bleeding, closed os, positive sac on ultrasound, and no heart-beat
- **Threatened** – 1st trimester bleeding, positive heartbeat
- **Incomplete** – tissue protrudes through os
- **Ectopic** – acute abdominal pain; positive beta-HCG, negative ultrasound for sac (life-threatening); missed period, vaginal bleeding, and hypotension
  - **Risk factors for ectopic pregnancy**: previous tubal manipulation, PID, and previous ectopic pregnancy
  - Significant shock and hemorrhage can occur from an ectopic pregnancy

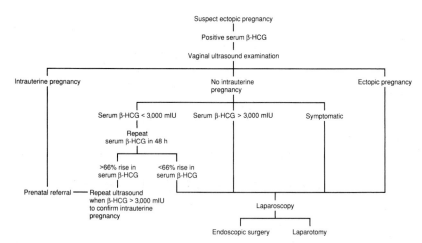

Management of suspected ectopic pregnancy. The level of serum beta-HCG, human chorionic gonadotropin; at which intrauterine pregnancy is detected by vaginal ultrasound examination can vary according to institution.

ENDOMETRIOSIS
- Symptoms: dysmenorrhea, infertility, and dyspareunia
- Can involve the rectum and cause bleeding during menses → endoscopy shows **blue mass**
- Ovaries – most common site
- Tx: OCPs

PELVIC INFLAMMATORY DISEASE
- Has ↑ risk of infertility and ectopic pregnancy
- Symptoms: pain, nausea, vomiting, fever, and vaginal discharge
  - Most commonly occurs in the first ½ of the menstrual cycle
- Risk factors: multiple sexual partners
- Dx: cervical motion tenderness, cervical cultures, and Gram's stain
- Tx: ceftriaxone, doxycycline
- **Gonococcus** – diplococci
- **Chlamydia** – granuloma lymphadenopathy
- **Complications**: persistent pain, infertility, and ectopic pregnancy

HSV – condylomata, vesicles
Syphilis – positive dark-field microscopy, chancre

MITTELSCHMERZ
- Rupture of graafian follicle
- Causes pain that can be confused with appendicitis
- Occurs 14 days after the 1st day of menses

VAGINAL CANCER
- #1 primary – squamous cell CA
- DES – can cause clear cell CA of vagina
- Botryoides – rhabdosarcoma that occurs in young girls
- XRT – used for most cancers of vagina

VULVAR CANCER
- Elderly, nulliparous, obese
- Usually unilateral
- Tx: <2 cm (stage I) – WLE and ipsilateral inguinal node dissection; >2 cm (stage II or greater) – vulvectomy with bilateral inguinal dissection, **postop XRT if close margins** (<1 cm)
  - Paget's VIN III or higher – **premalignant**

OVARIAN CANCER
- **Leading cause of gynecologic death**

Presenting Symptoms of Ovarian Cancer
Abdominal bloating and distention
Abdominal or pelvic pain
Pelvic pressure
Change in stool habits
Change in urinary habits
Abnormal vaginal bleeding

- ↓ **risk** with OCPs and bilateral tubal ligation
- ↑ **risk** with nulliparity, late menopause, and early menarche

Risk Factors for and Prevention of Ovarian Cancer

INCREASES RISK
Early menarche
Late menopause
Long-term (>12 cycles) and high-dose ovulation induction
Lack of oral contraceptive use
Low parity
Advanced age (>30 y) at the time of first term delivery
Lack of or late (>30 y of age) breast feeding
Personal or family history of breast, colon, or endometrial cancer
Perineal talc use

DECREASES RISK
Opposite of above, plus tubal ligation

- **Types** – teratoma, granulosa-theca (estrogen secreting, precocious puberty); Sertoli-Leydig (androgens, masculinization); struma ovarii (thyroid tissues); choriocarcinoma (beta-HCG); mucinous; serous; and papillary
- **Clear cell type** – worst prognosis

Staging of Ovarian Cancer

Stage	Location
I	One or both ovaries only
II	Limited to pelvis
III	Spread throughout abdomen
IV	Distant metastases

Modified from AJCC. *Cancer Staging Handbook*. 6th ed. New York, NY: Springer-Verlag; 2002:309–310.

- **Bilateral ovary involvement still stage I**
- **MC initial site of regional spread** – other ovary
- **Debulking tumor** – can be effective; including omentectomy (helps chemo and XRT)
- Tx: **total abdominal hysterectomy and bilateral oophorectomy for all stages**
  - Pelvic and para-aortic LN dissection
  - Omentectomy
  - 4 quadrant washes
  - Chemotherapy: cisplatin and paclitaxel (Taxol)
- **Krukenberg tumor** – stomach CA that has metastasized to ovary
  - Pathology classically shows **signet ring cells**
- **Meige's syndrome** – pelvic ovarian fibroma that causes ascites and hydrothorax
  - Excision of tumor cures syndrome

ENDOMETRIAL CANCER
- **Most common malignant tumor in female genital tract**
- **Risk factors** – nulliparity, late 1st pregnancy, obesity, tamoxifen, and unopposed estrogen
- Vaginal bleeding in postmenopausal patient is endometrial CA until proved otherwise
- Uterine polyps have very low chance of malignancy (0.1%)
- **Serous and papillary** subtypes – worst prognosis

Staging and Treatment

Stage	Location	Treatment
I	Endometrium	Total abdominal hysterectomy and BSO or XRT
II	Cervix	Total abdominal hysterectomy and BSO or XRT
III	Vagina, peritoneum, and ovary	Total abdominal hysterectomy and BSO and XRT
IV	Bladder and rectum	Total abdominal hysterectomy and BSO and XRT

BSO, bilateral salpingo-oophorectomy; XRT. Modified from AJCC. *Cancer Staging Handbook*. 6th ed. New York, NY: Springer-Verlag; 2002:301–302.

CERVICAL CANCER
- Goes to **obturator nodes 1st**
- Associated with **HPV 16 and 18**
- Squamous cell CA – most common

Staging of Cervical Cancer

Stage	Location
I	Cervix
II	Upper ⅔ of vagina
III	Pelvis, side wall, and lower ⅓ of vagina; hydronephrosis
IV	Bladder and rectum

Modified from AJCC. *Cancer Staging Handbook*. 6th ed. New York, NY: Springer-Verlag; 2002:294–296.

- Tx: microscopic disease without basement membrane invasion – cone biopsy (conization)
  - **Stages I and IIa** – total abdominal hysterectomy (TAH)
  - **Stages IIb to IV** – XRT

OVARIAN CYSTS
- **Postmenopausal patient**
  - **If septated, has ↑ vascular flow on Doppler, has solid components, or has papillary projections** → oophorectomy with intraoperative frozen sections; TAH if ovarian CA
  - If none of the above are present, follow with ultrasound for 1 year → if persists or gets larger → oophorectomy with intraoperative frozen sections; TAH if ovarian CA
- **Premenopausal patient**
  - **If septated, has ↑ vascular flow on Doppler, has solid components, or has papillary projections** → oophorectomy with intraoperative frozen sections
    - Algorithm becomes very complicated after this, weighing how aggressive the cancer is (based on histology and stage at the time of operation) compared with whether the patient desires future pregnancy
  - If none of the above are present → can follow with ultrasound; surgery if suspicious findings appear

INCIDENTAL OVARIAN MASS AT THE TIME OF LAPAROTOMY FOR ANOTHER PROCEDURE
- **Postmenopausal patient**
  - Oophorectomy, frozen section, TAH, and BSO if ovarian CA at the time of initial surgery
- **Premenopausal patient**
  - Much more complicated; likely will need partial oophorectomy and frozen section
  - If cancer → removal of the tube and ovary (need to have gynecologist look at this)
  - Then determine whether patient wants children → if not, go with TAH (usually at 2nd procedure)

ABNORMAL UTERINE BLEEDING
- <40 years old – **anovulation**. Tx: medroxyprogesterone; if leiomyomas → GnRH
- >40 years old – **cancer or menopause** → need biopsy

OTHER GYNECOLOGIC CONSIDERATIONS
- **Contraindications to estrogen therapy** – endometrial CA, active thromboembolic disease, undiagnosed vaginal bleeding, and breast CA
- **Uterine endometrial polyp** – can present as progressively heavier menses
- **Uterine fibroids (leiomyomas)** – under hormonal influence; recurrent abortions, infertility, and bleeding
- **Most common vaginal tumor** – invasion from surrounding or distant structure
- **Appendicitis with pregnancy** – ↑ risk of premature labor and fetal mortality

Variation in Signs and Symptoms of Appendicitis during Pregnancy

Signs and Symptoms	First Trimester (%)	Second Trimester (%)	Third Trimester (%)
Right lower quadrant pain	100	50	14
Right upper quadrant pain	0	17	57
Guarding (muscle spasm)	80	50	43
Nausea and vomiting	53	60	23
Tenderness on rectal examination	60	17	0
Perforation rate	20	49	70

- **Hydatidiform mole** – malignancy risk with partial mole; complete mole is of paternal origin
  - Tx: chemo (methotrexate)
- **Toxic shock syndrome** – fever, erythema, diffuse desquamation, nausea, and vomiting; associated with highly absorbent tampons
- **Ovarian torsion** – Tx: remove torsion and check for viability
- **Adnexal torsion with vascular necrosis** – Tx: adnexectomy
- **Ruptured tuboovarian abscess** – Tx: drainage
- **Ovarian vein thrombosis** – Dx: CT scan. Tx: heparin
- **Postpartum pelvic thrombophlebitis** – Tx: heparin and antibiotics

Also see Chap. 15

CIRCLE OF WILLIS
▨ **Vertebral arteries** – come together to form a single **basilar artery**, which branches into 2 **posterior cerebral arteries**
▨ **Posterior communicating arteries** – connect **middle cerebral arteries** to **posterior cerebral arteries**
▨ **Anterior cerebral arteries** – branches off **middle cerebral arteries** and are connected to each other through the 1 **anterior communicating artery**

NERVE INJURY
▨ **Neurapraxia** – no axonal injury (temporary loss of function, foot falls asleep)
▨ **Axonotmesis** – disruption of **axon** with preservation of axon sheath, will improve
▨ **Neurotmesis** – disruption of **axon and axon sheath (whole nerve is disrupted)**, may need surgery for recovery
▨ Regeneration of nerves occurs at a rate of **1 mm/day**
▨ **Nodes of Ranvier** – bare sections; allow salutatory conduction

ANTIDIURETIC HORMONE (ADH)
▨ Release controlled by **supraoptic nucleus of hypothalamus**, which descends into the posterior pituitary gland
▨ Released in response to high plasma osmolarity; ↑ water absorption in collecting ducts
▨ **Diabetes insipidus (↓ ADH)** – ↑ urine output, ↓ urine specific gravity, ↑ serum Na, and ↑ serum osmolarity
  • Can occur with ETOH, head injury
  • Tx: DDAVP, free water
▨ **SIADH (↑ ADH)** – ↓ urine output, concentrated urine, ↓ serum Na, and ↓ serum osmolarity
  • Can occur with head injury
  • Tx: fluid restriction, then diuresis; can give hypertonic saline if initial treatment fails

HEMORRHAGE
▨ **Arteriovenous malformations** – 50% present with hemorrhage
  • Usually in patients <30; sudden headache and loss of consciousness; are congenital
  • Tx: resection if possible for both symptomatic and asymptomatic AVMs
  • Can coil embolize these prior to resection

▨ **Cerebral aneurysms** – usually occur in patients >40
  • Can present with bleeding, mass effect, seizures, or infarcts
  • Occur at branch points in artery, most in carotid or anterior circulation; most congenital
  • Often place coils before clipping and resecting the aneurysm if elective resection

▨ **Subdural hematoma** – caused by **torn bridging veins**
  • Has crescent shape on head CT and conforms to brain
  • Higher mortality than epidural hematoma

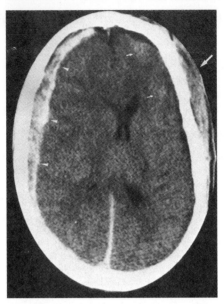

Acute subdural hematoma imaged by noncontrast computed tomography.

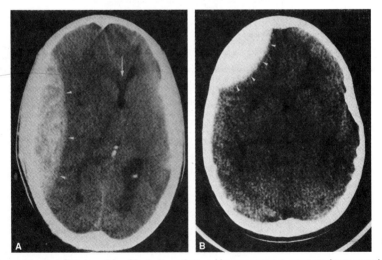

Two examples of acute epidural hematoma imaged by noncontrast computed tomography.

▨ **Epidural hematoma** – caused by injury to **middle meningeal artery**
  • Has lens shape on head CT and pushes brain away
  • Patients classically lose consciousness, have a lucid interval, and then lose consciousness again

▨ **Subarachnoid hemorrhage (nontraumatic)**
  • Caused by cerebral aneurysms (50% middle cerebral artery) and AVMs

- Symptoms: stiff neck (nuchal rigidity), severe headache, photophobia, and neurologic defects
- Goal is to isolate the aneurysm from systemic circulation (clipping vascular supply), maximize cerebral perfusion to overcome vasospasm, and prevent rebleeding
- Tx: hypervolemia, calcium channel blockers
- Go to **OR only if neurologically intact**
- **Can get subarachnoid hemorrhages with trauma as well**

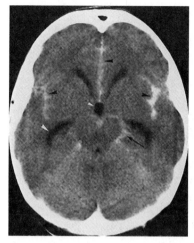

This patient presented with severe headache, nausea, and lethargy of acute onset. A noncontrast computed tomography scan reveals diffuse subarachnoid hemorrhage with blood in the interhemispheric and bilateral sylvian fissures (*black arrowheads*) and in the subarachnoid spaces around the brain stem (*arrow*). Early hydrocephalus is evidenced by the rounding of the third ventricle (*small white arrowhead*) and visualization of the temporal horns (*large white arrowhead*).

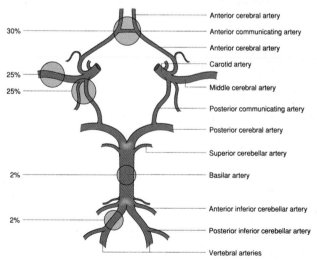

Locations of aneurysms of the circle of Willis and their relative occurrence.

■ **Intracerebral hematomas** – temporal lobe most often affected
  • Those that are large and cause focal deficits should be drained

CEREBRAL PERFUSION PRESSURE

■ Cerebral perfusion pressure (CPP) = mean arterial pressure *minus* intracranial pressure
■ Keep >60–70
■ Head trauma and ↓ CPP
  • Elevate head of bed
  • Sedate and paralyze
  • Moderate hyperventilation (P_{CO_2} 30–35)
  • Mannitol to ↓ brain edema
  • May need craniectomy if these measures fail
■ **Maximum brain swelling occurs 48–72 hours after trauma**
■ **Symptoms of** ↑ ICP – stupor, headache, nausea and vomiting, and stiff neck
■ **Signs of** ↑ ICP – hypertension, HR lability, and slow respirations
  • **Intermittent bradycardia** is a sign of severely elevated ICP and impending herniation
  • **Cushing's triad** – hypertension, bradycardia, and slow respiratory rate
■ **Dilated pupil after trauma** – ipsilateral temporal herniation onto 3rd cranial nerve

SPINAL CORD INJURY

■ **Cord injury with deficit** → give **high-dose steroids (↓ swelling)**
■ **Complete cord transection** – areflexia, flaccidity, anesthesia, and autonomic paralysis below the level of the lesion
■ **Spinal shock – hypotension, normal or slow heart rate, and warm extremities (vasodilated)**
  • Occurs with spinal cord injuries above T5 (loss of sympathetic tone)
  • Tx: fluids initially, may need phenylephrine drip (alpha agonist)
■ **Anterior spinal artery syndrome** – most commonly occurs with acutely ruptured cervical disc
  • **Bilateral loss of motor, pain, and temperature sensation** below the level of lesion
  • **Preservation of position–vibratory sensation and light touch**
  • About 10% recover to ambulation

■ **Brown-Sequard syndrome** – incomplete cord transection (hemisection of cord); most commonly due to penetrating injury
  • **Loss of ipsilateral motor, contralateral pain, and temperature** below level of lesion
  • About 90% recover to ambulation

■ **Central cord syndrome** – most commonly occurs with hyperflexion of the cervical spine
  • **Bilateral loss motor, pain, and temperature sensation in upper extremities**; lower extremities spared

■ **Cauda equina syndrome** – pain and weakness in lower extremities due to compression of lumbar nerve roots

■ Spinothalamic tract – carries pain and temp sensory neurons
■ Corticospinal tract – carries motor neurons
■ Rubrospinal tract – carries motor neurons
■ Dorsal nerve roots – are generally afferent; carry sensory fibers
■ Ventral nerve roots – are generally efferent; carry motor neuron fibers

BRAIN TUMORS
▨ **Symptoms**: **headache**, seizures, progressive neurologic deficit, and persistent vomiting
▨ Adults – ⅔ supratentorial
▨ Children – ⅔ infratentorial

▨ **Gliomas** – most common primary brain tumor
  • **Glioma multiforme** – most common subtype, uniformly fatal
▨ **Lung** – #1 metastasis to brain

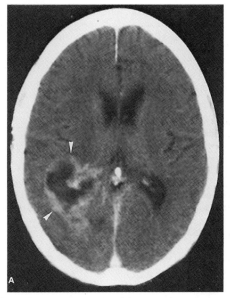

Glioblastoma multiforme (astrocytoma grade IV) discovered on contrast-enhanced computed tomography. Typical appearance is that of a low-attenuation lesion with peripheral enhancement (*arrowheads*).

▨ Most common brain tumor in children – medulloblastoma
▨ Most common metastatic brain tumor in children – neuroblastoma

▨ **Acoustic neuroma** – arises from the 8th cranial nerve
  • Symptoms – hearing loss, unsteadiness, vertigo, nausea, and vomiting
  • Tx: surgery

SPINE TUMORS
▨ Overall most are benign, #1 tumor overall **neurofibroma**
▨ **Intradural tumors** are more likely benign and **extradural tumors** are more likely malignant
▨ **Paraganglionoma** – check for metanephrine in urine; MIBG for extramedullary chromatin tissue

PEDIATRIC NEUROSURGERY
▨ **Intraventricular hemorrhage** (subependymal hemorrhage)
  • Seen in premature infants secondary to rupture of the fragile vessels in germinal matrix
  • Patients go on to get intraventricular hemorrhage

- Risk factors: ECMO, cyanotic congenital heart disease
- Symptoms: bulging fontanelle, neurologic deficits, ↓ BP, and ↓ Hct
- Tx: ventricular catheter for drainage and prevention of hydrocephalus
■ **Myelomeningocele**
  - Neural cord defect – herniation of spinal cord and nerve roots through defect in vertebra
  - If sac ruptured – surgery needed to prevent infection of spinal cord
  - Most commonly occurs in the lumbar region

Wernicke's area – speech comprehension, temporal lobe
Broca's area – speech motor, posterior part of anterior lobe
Pituitary adenoma, undergoing XRT, patient now in shock
   Dx: pituitary apoplexy
   Tx: steroids
Cervical nerves roots 3–5 innervate diaphragm
Microglial cells – act as brain macrophages

Cranial Nerves

Nerve	Name	Function	Muscle
I	Olfactory	Smell	
II	Optic	Sight	
III	Oculomotor		Motor to eye
IV	Trochlear		Superior oblique (eye)
V	Trigeminal: ophthalmic, maxillary, and mandibular branches	Sensory to face	Muscles of mastication
VI	Abducens		Lateral rectus (eye)
VII	Facial	Taste to anterior ⅔ of tongue	Motor to face
VIII	Vestibulocochlear	Hearing	
IX	Glossopharyngeal	Taste to posterior ⅓ of tongue	Swallowing muscles
X	Vagus	Many functions	
XI	Accessory		Trapezius Sternocleidomastoid
XII	Hypoglossal		Tongue

Also see Chap. 15

BACKGROUND
- **Osteoblasts** – synthesize nonmineralized bone cortex
- **Osteoclasts** – reabsorb bone
  - Stages of bone healing – inflammation, soft callus formation, mineralization of the callus, and removal of the callus
- Cartilage receives nutrients from synovial fluid

- **Salter-Harris fractures III, IV, and V** – cross the epiphyseal plate and can affect the growth plate of the bone; need open reduction and internal fixation (ORIF)
- **Salter-Harris types I and I – closed reduction**

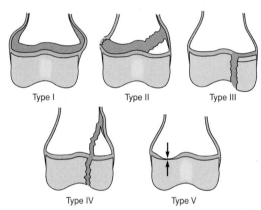

Type I   Type II   Type III

Type IV   Type V

Salter-Harris classification of epiphyseal injuries. Type I injury is an epiphysiolysis of the involved growth plate without associated fracture. Type II has an additional metaphyseal fracture fragment; Type I and II injuries have a good prognosis and are usually treated with closed reduction and casting. Type III injury results in a fracture through the growth plate and epiphysis. Type IV fracture crosses the epiphysis, growth plate (physis), and metaphysis. Type III and IV injuries require careful open reduction and internal fixation if displaced. Type V injury involves a crush of the growth plate without a fracture and is usually detected late by asymmetric or premature closure of the growth plate.

- **Fractures associated with AVN** – scaphoid, femoral neck, and talus
- **Fractures associated with nonunion** – clavicle, 5th metatarsal fracture (Jones' fracture)
- **Fractures associated with compartment syndrome** – supracondylar humerus and tibia
- **Biggest risk factor for nonunion** – smoking

LOWER EXTREMITY NERVES
- **Obturator nerve** – hip adduction
- **Superior gluteal nerve** – hip abduction
- **Inferior gluteal nerve** – hip extension
- **Femoral nerve** – knee extension

LUMBAR DISC HERNIATION
- Presents with back pain, sciatica
- Herniated **nucleus pulposus**

■ Nerve root compression affects 1 nerve root below disc
  • **L3 nerve** compression (L2–3 disc) – weak hip flexion
  • **L4 nerve** compression (L3–4 disc) – weak knee extension (quadriceps), weak patellar reflex
  • **L5 nerve** compression (L4–5 disc) – weak dorsiflexion (foot drop)
    ∘ ↓ sensation in big toe web space
  • **S1 nerve** compression (L5–S1 disc) – weak plantar flexion, weak Achilles reflex
    ∘ ↓ sensation in lateral foot
■ Dx: patients with neurologic findings need MRI
■ Tx: NSAIDs, heat, and rest; surgery for substantial/progressive neurologic deficit, refractory cases, severe sciatica, and disc fragments that have herniated into the cord

TERMINAL BRANCHES OF BRACHIAL PLEXUS
■ **Ulnar nerve**
  • **Motor** – <u>intrinsic musculature of hand</u> (palmar interossei, palmaris brevis, adductor pollicis, and hypothenar eminence); finger abduction (spread fingers); wrist flexion
  • **Sensory** – all of 5th and ½ 4th fingers, back of hand
  • Injury results in **claw hand**
■ **Median nerve**
  • **Motor** – thumb apposition (anterior interosseous muscle, OK sign); thumb abduction; and finger flexors
  • **Sensory** – most of palm and 1st 3½ fingers on palmar side
  • Nerve is involved in **carpal tunnel syndrome**
■ **Radial nerve**
  • **Motor** – wrist extension, finger extension, thumb extension, and triceps; <u>no</u> hand muscles
  • **Sensory** – 1st 3½ fingers on dorsal side
■ **Musculocutaneous nerve** – motor to biceps, brachialis, and coracobrachialis
■ **Axillary nerve** – motor to deltoid (abduction)

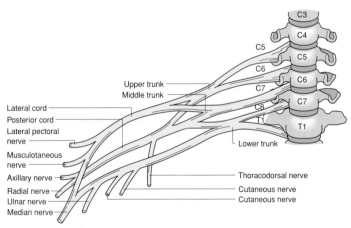

Anatomy of the brachial plexus.

CERVICAL RADICULOPATHY
■ **C1, C2, C3, and C4 nerve compression** (C1-2, C2-3, C3-4 discs) – neck and scalp pain
■ **C5 nerve compression** (C4–5 disc) – weak deltoid and biceps
  • Weak biceps reflex

- **C6 nerve compression** (C5–6 disc) – weak deltoid and biceps, weak wrist extensors
  - Weak biceps reflex and brachioradialis reflex
- **C7 nerve compression** (most common, C6–7 disc) – weak triceps
  - Weak triceps reflex
- **C8 nerve compression** (C7–T1 disc) – weak triceps, weak intrinsic muscles of hand and wrist flexion
  - Weak triceps reflex
- **Radial nerve** – C5–C8
- **Median nerve** – C6–T1
- **Ulnar nerve** – C8–T1
- **Musculocutaneous nerve** – C5–C7
- **Axillary nerve** – C5–C6

- **Radial nerve roots** – on the superior portion of the brachial plexus
- **Ulnar nerve roots** – on the inferior portion of the brachial plexus

UPPER EXTREMITY
- **Clavicle fracture** – usually just treated with sling (risk of vascular impingement)
- **Shoulder dislocation**
  - **Anterior** (85%–95%) risk of **axillary nerve injury**. Tx: closed reduction
  - **Posterior** (seizures, electrocution) risk of **axillary artery injury**. Tx: closed reduction
- **Acromioclavicular separation** – Tx: sling (risk of brachial plexus and subclavian vessel injury)
- **Scapula fracture** – sling unless glenoid fossa involved, then need internal fixation
- **Midshaft humeral fracture** – often treated just with sling
- **Supracondylar humeral fracture** – adults → internal fixation; children → closed reduction, internal fixation if severe
- **Monteggia fracture** – proximal ulnar fracture and radial head dislocation
  - Tx: ORIF
- **Colles fracture** – fall on outstretched hand, distal radius. Tx: closed reduction
- **Nursemaid's elbow** – subluxation of the radius at the elbow caused by a pulling on an extended, pronated arm. Tx: closed reduction
- **Combined radial and ulnar fracture**
  - **Adults** – ORIF
  - **Children – closed reduction**

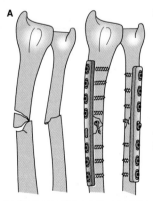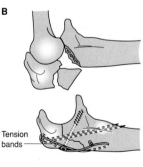

(*A*) Both bone fractures of the radius and the ulna in adults are best treated by anatomic open reduction and internal fixation. (*B*) Displaced fractures of the olecranon require open reduction and internal fixation. Tension-band technique and interfragmentary fixation are illustrated. (*continued*)

C

Brachioradialis
Superficial radial nerve
Cut edge of supinator
Flexor digitorum
superficialis

Radial artery

Flexor carpi radialis
Cut edge of radial periosteum

Posterior interosseous
nerve in arcade of Frohse

Brachialis
Bicepital
aponeurosis

Radial
recurrent artery
Biceps tendon

(*Continued*) (*C*) Open reduction and internal fixation of a proximal radius fracture. This fracture may be associated with a dislocation of the radial head (Monteggia fracture). An anterior approach is illustrated, although a posterior approach is more commonly used. The posterior interosseous branch of the radial nerve is at risk because it lies in the supinator muscle. It must be carefully identified and protected.

■ **Scaphoid fracture** – snuffbox tenderness; can have negative x-ray
  • Tx: all patients require cast to elbow, may need fixation; risk of **avascular necrosis**
■ **Volkmann's contracture**– supracondylar humerus fracture → occluded **anterior interosseous artery** → closed reduction of humerus → artery opens up → reperfusion injury, edema, and **forearm compartment syndrome (flexor compartment)**
  • Patients have pain in forearm with passive extension, weakness, tense forearm, and hypesthesia
  • **Median nerve** affected by swelling
  • Tx: **fasciotomy**
■ **Dupuytren's contracture** – associated with diabetes, ETOH
  • Progressive proliferation of the **palmar fascia of hand** results in contractures that usually affect the **4th and 5th digits** (cannot extend fingers)
  • Tx: NSAIDs, steroid injections; excision of involved fascia for significant contraction
■ **Carpal tunnel syndrome** – median nerve compression by transverse carpal ligament
  • Tx: splint, NSAIDs, and steroid injections; transverse carpal ligament release if that fails
■ **Trigger finger** – tenosynovitis of the flexor tendon that catches at the MCP joint when trying to extend finger
  • Tx: splint, tendon sheath steroid injections (not the tendon itself); if that fails can release the pulley system at the MCP joint
■ **Suppurative tenosynovitis**
  • Infections that spread along the flexor tendon sheaths
  • **4 classic signs**: tendon sheath tenderness, pain with passive motion, swelling along sheath, and semiflexed posture of the involved digit
  • Tx: elevation, splinting, and antibiotics
    • If improvement not prompt → midaxial longitudinal incision and drainage
■ **Rotator cuff tears** – supraspinatus, infraspinatus, teres minor, and subscapularis
  • Acutely → sling and conservative treatment
  • Surgical repair if the patient needs to retain a high level of activity or if ADL affected

▣ **Forearm fasciotomies** – need to open volar and dorsal compartments
▣ **Paronychia** – infection under nail bed; painful. Tx: antibiotics; remove nail if purulent
▣ **Felon** – infection in the terminal joint space of the finger
  • **Tx**: incision over the tip of the finger and along the medial and lateral aspects to prevent necrosis of tip of finger

LOWER EXTREMITY
▣ **Hip dislocation**
  • **Posterior** (85%–95%) – patients have internal rotation and adduction of leg; risk of **sciatic nerve injury**. Tx: closed reduction
  • **Anterior** – patients have external rotation and abduction of leg; risk of injury to **femoral artery.** Tx: closed reduction

▣ **Hip fracture (isolated anterior ring with minimal ischial displacement)** – Tx: weight-bearing as tolerated
▣ **Femoral shaft fracture** – ORIF with intramedullary rod
▣ **Femoral neck fracture** – ORIF → risk of avascular necrosis if open reduction delayed
▣ **Lateral knee trauma** – can result in injury to **anterior cruciate ligament, posterior cruciate ligament, and medial meniscus**
▣ **Anterior cruciate ligament injury** – positive anterior drawer test
  • **Present with knee effusion and pain with pivoting action;** MRI confirms diagnosis
  • Tx: surgery with knee instability (reconstruction with patellar tendon or hamstring tendon); otherwise physical therapy with leg-strengthening exercise
▣ **Posterior cruciate ligament injury** – positive posterior drawer test
  • Much less common than ACL injury; present with knee pain and joint effusion
  • Tx: conservative therapy initially; surgery for failure of medical management
▣ **Medial collateral ligament injury** – lateral blow to knee
▣ **Lateral collateral ligament injury** – medial blow to knee
  • Tx: **small tear** – brace; **large tear** – surgery
  • These injuries are associated with injuries to the corresponding **meniscus** (medial and lateral meniscus, respectively)
  • **Meniscus tears** – joint line tenderness; can treat with arthroscopic repair or debridement
▣ **Posterior knee dislocation** – all patients need angiogram to rule out popliteal artery injury
▣ **Patellar fracture** – long leg cast unless comminuted, then need internal fixation
▣ **Tibial plateau fracture and tibia–fibula fracture** – ORIF fixation unless open, then need external fixator until tissue heals
▣ **Plantaris muscle rupture** – pain and mass below popliteal fossa (contracted plantaris) and ankle ecchymosis
▣ **Ankle fracture** – most treated with cast and immobilization; bimalleolar or trimalleolar fractures need ORIF
▣ **Metatarsal fracture** – cast immobilization or brace for 6 weeks
▣ **Calcaneus fracture** – cast and immobilization if nondisplaced; ORIF for displacement
▣ **Talus fracture** – closed reduction for most; ORIF for severe displacement
▣ **Nerve most commonly injured with lower extremity fasciotomy** – superficial peroneal nerve (foot eversion); can also injure the common peroneal
▣ **Footdrop after lithotomy position or after crossing legs for long periods or fibula head fracture** – common peroneal nerve

LEG COMPARTMENTS
▣ **Anterior** – anterior tibial artery, deep peroneal nerve
  • **Muscles** – anterior tibialis, extensor hallucis longus, extensor digitorum longus, and communis

- **Lateral** – superficial peroneal nerve
  - **Muscles** – peroneal muscles
- **Deep posterior** – posterior tibial artery, peroneal artery, and tibial nerve
  - **Muscles** – flexor hallucis longus, flexor digitorum longus, and posterior tibialis
- **Superficial posterior** – sural nerve
  - **Muscles** – gastrocnemius, soleus, and plantaris

COMPARTMENT SYNDROME
- Most likely to occur in the **anterior compartment of leg (get footdrop) after vascular compromise**
- Can also occur from crush injuries

- **Distal pulses can be present with compartment syndrome** → last thing to go
- **Pain with passive motion**
- Pressure >20–30 mm Hg abnormal → consider fasciotomies; leave open 5–10 days
- Dx: based on clinical suspicion

PEDIATRIC ORTHOPAEDICS
- **Osteomyelitis** – can occur in metaphysis of long bones in children; most commonly staph
  - Symptoms: pain, ↓ use of extremity
  - Dx: MRI, bone biopsy
  - Tx: antibiotics, incision, and drainage
- **Idiopathic adolescent scoliosis** – prepubertal females, right thoracic curve most common, usually asymptomatic
  - Curves >20 to 45 degrees need bracing to slow progression, which can occur with growth spurt
  - Curves >45 degrees or those likely to progress → spinal fusion
- **Osgood–Schlatter disease** – tibial tubercle apophysitis; caused by traction injury from the quadriceps in adolescents aged 13–15; most commonly have pain in front of the knee
  - X-ray: irregular shape or fragmenting of the tibial tubercle
  - Tx: mild symptoms → activity limitation; severe symptoms → cast 6 weeks followed by activity limitation
- **Legg–Calvé–Perthes disease** – AVN of the femoral head; children 2 years and older
  - Can result from a hypercoagulable state; bilateral in 10%
  - Symptoms: painful gait limp
  - X-ray: flattening of the femoral head
  - Tx: maintain range of motion with limited exercise; **femoral head will remodel without sequelae**
  - Surgery if femoral head is not covered by the acetabulum
- **Slipped capital femoral epiphysis**
  - Males aged 10–13; ↑ risk of AVN of the femoral head; painful gait
  - X-ray: widening and irregularity of the epiphyseal plate
  - Tx: surgical pinning
- **Congenital dislocation of the hip**
  - More common in females
  - Tx: Pavlik harness, which keeps the legs abducted and the femoral head reduced in the acetabulum
- **Clubfoot** – Tx: serial casting

BONE TUMORS
- Most common is metastatic disease (#1 breast, #2 prostate)
  - Tx: internal fixation with impending fracture (>50% cortical involvement); followed by XRT

- Multiple myeloma – most common primary malignant tumor of bone
  - Tx: chemotherapy for systemic disease; internal fixation for impending fractures
- **Pathologic fractures** – treat with internal fixation
  - XRT can be used for pain relief in patients with painful bony metastases
- **Osteogenic sarcoma** – most common primary bone sarcoma, usually around the knee
  - 80% in patients <20 years
  - X-ray: <u>Codman's triangle → periosteal reaction</u>
  - Tx: limb-sparing resection; XRT and doxorubicin-based chemotherapy can be used preoperatively to increase chance of limb-sparing resection; also often given post-operatively
- **Benign bone tumors treated with curettage +/− bone graft** – osteoid osteoma, endochondroma (may be able to observe), osteochondroma (resection only if cosmetic defect or causing symptoms), chondroblastoma, nonossifying fibroma (may be observed), and fibrodysplasia
- **Giant cell tumor of bone** – total resection +/− XRT (benign but 30% risk of recurrence; also has malignant degeneration risk)

OTHER ORTHOPAEDICS CONDITIONS

- **Spondylolisthesis** – formed by subluxation or slip of one vertebral body over another
  - Most commonly occurs in lumbar region
  - Most common cause of lumbar pain in adolescents (gymnasts)
  - Tx: depends on degree of subluxation and symptoms – ranges from conservative treatment to surgical fusion
- **Cervical stenosis** – surgical decompression if significant myelopathy present
- **Lumbar stenosis** – surgical decompression for cases refractory to medical treatment
- **Torus fracture** – buckling of the metaphyseal cortex seen in children (i.e., distal radius)
- **Open fractures** – need incision and drainage, antibiotics, fracture stabilization, and soft tissue coverage

Foregut – lungs, esophagus, stomach, pancreas, liver, gallbladder, bile duct, and duodenum proximal to ampulla
Midgut – duodenum distal to ampulla, small bowel, and large bowel to distal ⅓ of transverse colon
Hindgut – distal ⅓ of transverse colon to anal canal
Midgut rotates 270 degrees counterclockwise normally

Low birth weight <2,500 g; premature <37 weeks

Immunity at birth – **IgA** from mother's milk; **IgM** synthesized in child

#1 cause of childhood death – **trauma**
Trauma bolus – 20 cc/kg × 2, then give blood 10 cc/kg
Tachycardia – best indicator of shock (neonate >150; <1 year >120; rest >100)
Urine output 2–4 cc/kg/hr
Children (<6 months) have **25% GFR capacity of adults** – poor concentrating ability

↑ alkaline phosphatase in children compared with adults → **bone growth**
Umbilical vessels – 2 arteries and 1 vein

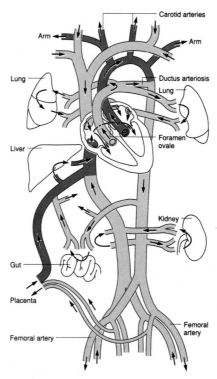

Persistent fetal circulation.

MAINTENANCE INTRAVENOUS FLUIDS

- 4 cc/kg/hr for 1st 10 kg
- 2 cc/kg/hr for 2nd 10 kg
- 1 cc/kg/hr for everything after that

CALORIC NEED

Age (yr)	Calories (kcal/day)
0–1	90–120
1–12	70–90
12–18	30–60

CONGENITAL CYSTIC DISEASE OF THE LUNG

- **Pulmonary sequestration**
  - Lung tissue has systemic arterial supply (aorta) and either systemic venous or pulmonary vein drainage
  - Can be **intralobar** (more likely pulmonary venous drainage) **or extralobar** (more likely systemic venous drainage)
  - Neither communicates with tracheobronchial tree
  - Most commonly presents with infection; can also have respiratory compromise or an abnormal CXR
  - Tx: lobectomy
- **Congenital lobar overinflation (emphysema)**
  - Cartilage fails to develop in bronchus, leading to air trapping with expiration
  - Vascular supply and other lobes are normal (except compressed by hyperinflated lobe)
  - Can develop hemodynamic instability (same mechanism as tension PTX) or respiratory compromise
  - LUL or RML most commonly affected
  - Tx: lobectomy
- **Congenital cystic adenoid malformation**
  - Communicates with airway
  - Alveolar structure is not well developed although lung tissue is present
  - Symptoms: respiratory compromise or recurrent infection
  - Tx: lobectomy
- **Bronchiogenic cyst**
  - Extrapulmonary cysts formed from bronchial tissue and cartilage wall
  - Usually present with a mediastinal mass filled with milky liquid
  - Can compress adjacent structures or become infected
  - Occasionally are intrapulmonary
  - Tx: resect cyst

MEDIASTINAL MASSES IN CHILDREN

- **Neurogenic tumors (neurofibroma, neuroganglionoma, neuroblastoma)** – most common mediastinal tumor in children; usually located posteriorly
- **Respiratory symptoms, dysphagia** – common to all mediastinal masses regardless of location
- **Anterior** – T cell lymphoma, teratoma and other germ cell tumors (most common type of anterior mediastinal mass in children), thymoma, thyroid CA
- **Middle** – T cell lymphoma, teratoma, and cyst (cardiogenic or bronchiogenic)
- **Posterior** – T cell lymphoma, neuroblastoma, and neurogenic tumor

Choledochal Cysts			
Type	%	Description	Treatment
I	85%	Fusiform dilation of entire common bile duct, mildly dilated common hepatic duct, normal intrahepatic ducts	Resection, hepaticojejunostomy
II	3%	A true diverticulum that hangs off the common bile duct	Resection off common bile duct; may be able to preserve common bile duct and avoid hepaticojejunostomy
III	1%	Dilation of distal intramural common bile duct; involves sphincter of Oddi	Resection, choledochojejunostomy
IV	10%	Multiple cysts, both intrahepatic and extrahepatic	Resection; may need liver lobectomy
V	1%	Caroli's disease: intrahepatic cysts; get hepatic fibrosis; may be associated with congenital hepatic fibrosis and medullary sponge kidney	Resection; may need lobectomy

CHOLEDOCHAL CYST
- Need to resect – risk of cholangiocarcinoma, pancreatitis, cholangitis, and obstructive jaundice. Thought to be caused by **reflux of pancreatic enzymes** into the biliary system

LYMPHADENOPATHY
- Usually acute suppurative adenitis associated with URI or pharyngitis
- **If fluctuant** → FNA, culture and sensitivity, and antibiotics; may need incision and drainage if it fails to resolve
  - **Chronic causes** – cat scratch fever, atypical mycoplasma
- **Asymptomatic** – antibiotics for 10 days → excisional biopsy if no improvement
  - This is lymphoma until proved otherwise
- **Cystic hygroma** (lymphangioma) – found in lateral cervical and submandibular regions in neck; gets infected
  - Tx: resection

DIAPHRAGMATIC HERNIAS
- Overall survival 50%
- Increased on **left side (80%)**; abdominal approach; can have severe **pulmonary HTN**
- 80% have associated anomalies (cardiac and neural tube defects mostly; malrotation)
- Diagnosis can be made with prenatal ultrasound
- Symptoms: respiratory distress
- CXR – bowel in chest
- Tx: high-frequency ventilation; may need ECMO, prostacyclin (pulmonary vasodilator)
  - Stabilize these patients before operating on them
  - Need to reduce bowel and repair defect +/− mesh
  - Look for visceral anomalies (run the bowel)
- **Bochdalek's hernia** – most common, located posteriorly
- **Morgagni's hernia** – rare, located anteriorly
- **Eventration** – failure of diaphragm to fuse

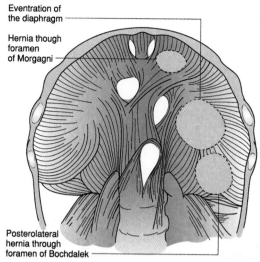

Anatomy of the diaphragm showing the location of congenital diaphragmatic defects.

<u>**PECTUS EXCAVATUM**</u> (sinks in) – sternal osteotomy, need strut; performed if causing respiratory symptoms or emotional stress

<u>**PECTUS CARINATUM**</u> (pigeon chest) – strut not necessary; repair for emotional stress

BRANCHIAL CLEFT CYST
- Leads to cysts, sinuses, and fistulas
- **1st branchial cleft cyst** – angle of mandible; may connect with external auditory canal
  - Often associated with facial nerve
- **2nd branchial cleft cyst (most common)** – on anterior border of SCM muscle
  - Goes through carotid bifurcation into tonsillar pillar
- **3rd branchial cleft cyst** – lateral neck
- Tx for all cysts: resection

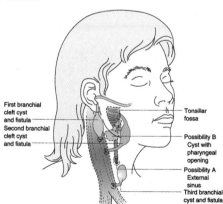

Types of first, second, and third branchial cleft remnants. Sinuses and fistulas are seen most often in infants and young children, whereas cysts usually appear at a later age.

THYROGLOSSAL DUCT CYST
- From the descent of the thyroid gland from the **foramen cecum**
- May be only thyroid tissue patient has
- Presents as a midline cervical mass
- Goes through the hyoid
- Tx: excision of **cyst, tract, and hyoid bone**

HEMANGIOMA
- Appears at birth or shortly after
- Rapid growth during first 6–12 months of life, then begins to involute
- Tx: **observation** – most resolve by age 7–8
- If lesion has **uncontrollable growth, impairs function** (eyelid or ear canal), or is **persistent after age 8** → can treat with **steroids** → laser or resection if steroids are not successful

NEUROBLASTOMA
- **#1 solid abdominal malignancy in children**
- Usually presents as asymptomatic mass
- Can have secretory diarrhea, raccoon eyes (orbital metastases), **HTN,** and opsomyoclonus syndrome (unsteady gait)
- Most often on **adrenals**; can occur anywhere along the sympathetic chain
- Most common in **1st 2 years of life**
  - Children <1 year have best prognosis
- Most have ↑ **catecholamines, VMA, HVA, and metanephrines**
- Derived from **neural crest cells**
- Encases vasculature rather than invades
- **Rare metastases** – go to lung and bone

- **Abdominal x-ray**: may show stippled calcifications in the tumor
- NSE, LDH, HVA, diploid tumors, and **N-myc** – have worse prognosis

Risk Status Determinants in Neuroblastoma		
Parameters	Low Risk	High Risk
Age	<1 y (especially <6 mo)	>1 y at diagnosis
Stage	1, 2A, 2B, 4S	3, 4
Shimada classification	Favorable	Unfavorable
N-myc amplification	<3 Copies	>3 Copies
Expression of TRK	TRK Expressed	No TRK expression
Flow cytometry	Hyperdiploid, triploid	Diploid
Cytogenetics	No 1p abnormality	1p Deletion
Ferritin at diagnosis	<142 ng/mL	≥142 ng/mL
Lactate dehydrogenase	≤1,500 U/mL	>1,500 U/mL
Neuron-specific enolase	≤100 ng/mL	>100 ng/mL

- **NSE ↑ in all patients with metastases**
- Tx: resection (30%–40% cured)
- Initially unresectable tumors may be resectable after chemotherapy

Staging of Neuroblastoma	
Stage	**Description**
I	Localized, complete
II	Incomplete excision but does not cross midline
III	Crosses midline +/− regional nodes
IV	Distant metastases (nodes or solid organ)
IV-S	Localized tumor with distant metastases

WILMS TUMOR (NEPHROBLASTOMA)

- Usually presents as asymptomatic mass; can have hematuria or HTN; 10% bilateral
- Mean age at diagnosis – **3 years**
- **Prognosis based on tumor grade** (anaplastic and sarcomatous variations have worse prognosis)
- **Frequent metastases** to **bone and lung**
- Can resect pulmonary metastases if resectable
- May be associated with Beckwith–Wiedemann syndrome (hemihypertrophy, cryptorchidism, Drash syndrome, aniridia)
- Abdominal CT – replacement of renal parenchyma and <u>not</u> displacement (as seen with neuroblastoma)

- Tx: nephrectomy (80%–90% cured)
  - If venous extension occurs in the renal vein, the tumor can be extracted from the vein
  - Need to examine the contralateral kidney and look for peritoneal implants
  - Avoid rupture of tumor with resection, which will ↑ stage
  - All patients except stage I tumor weighing <500 g get **actinomycin and vincristine**
  - Patients with stage II tumor or greater or tumors >500 g get **actinomycin and vincristine plus doxorubicin**
  - Patients with stage III tumor or greater get **actinomycin, vincristine, and doxorubicin plus abdominal XRT**

Staging of Wilms Tumor	
Stage	**Description**
I	Limited to kidney, completely excised
II	Beyond kidney but completely excised
III	Residual nonhematogenous tumor
IV	Hematogenous metastases
V	Bilateral renal involvement

HEPATOBLASTOMA

- Most common malignant liver tumor in children; ↑ AFP in 90%
- Fractures, precocious puberty (from beta-HCG release)
- Better prognosis than hepatocellular CA
- Associated with Beckwith–Wiedemann syndrome
- Can be pedunculated; vascular invasion common; may develop areas of extramedullary hematopoiesis

- Tx: resection optimal; otherwise doxorubicin- and cisplatin-based chemotherapy → may downstage tumors and make them resectable
- Survival is primarily related to resectability
- **Prefetal histology** has best prognosis

#1 children's malignancy overall – **leukemia (ALL)**
#1 solid tumor class – **CNS tumors**
#1 general surgery tumor – **neuroblastoma**
    #1 in child <2 years → **neuroblastoma**
    #1 in child >2 years → **Wilms tumor**
#1 cause of duodenal obstruction in newborns (<1 week) – **duodenal atresia**
#1 cause of duodenal obstruction after newborn period (>1 week) and overall –
malrotation
#1 cause of colon obstruction – **Hirschsprung's disease**; some say constipation
#1 liver tumor in children – **hepatoblastoma**; ⅔ of liver tumors in children are
malignant
#1 lung tumor in children – **carcinoid**
Painful lower GI bleeding – **#1 benign anorectal lesions** (fissures, etc.)
Painless lower GI bleeding – **#1 Meckel's diverticulum**
Upper GI bleeding – 0–1 year → **gastritis, esophagitis**;
    1 year to adult → **esophageal varices, esophagitis**

MECKEL'S DIVERTICULUM
- Found on **antimesenteric border** of small bowel
- Embryology – **persistent vitelline duct**
- Rule of 2s – 2 feet from ileocecal valve, 2% population, 2% symptomatic, 2 tissue types (<u>pancreatic</u> – most common; <u>gastric</u> – most likely to be symptomatic), and 2 presentations (diverticulitis and bleeding)
- **#1 cause of painless lower GI bleeding in children**
- Can get Meckel's diverticulum scan with pertechnetate if suspicious of Meckel's diverticulum and having trouble locating
- Tx: resection with symptoms, suspicion of gastric mucosa, or narrow neck
  - Diverticulitis involving the base or if the base is >⅓ the size of the bowel, need to perform segmental resection

PYLORIC STENOSIS
- 3–12 weeks, firstborn males
- Projectile vomiting
- Can feel olive mass in stomach
- Get <u>hypochloremic, hypokalemic metabolic alkalosis</u>
- Ultrasound – pylorus ≥4 mm thick, ≥14 mm long
- For severe dehydration, resuscitate with normal saline boluses until making urine, then switch to D5 normal saline with 10 mEq K maintenance
  - Avoid fluid resuscitation with K containing fluids in children with severe dehydration as hyperkalemia can quickly develop
  - Avoid nonsalt-containing solutions in infants as hyponatremia can quickly develop
  - Infants should always have a maintenance fluid with glucose because of their limited reserves for gluconeogenesis and vulnerability for hypoglycemia
- Tx: pyloromyotomy (RUQ incision; proximal extent should be the circular muscles of stomach)

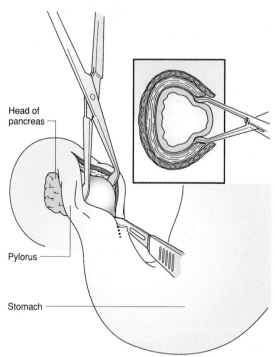

Head of
pancreas

Pylorus

Stomach

Ramstedt pyloromyotomy for infantile hypertrophic pyloric stenosis. The cross-sectional view shows herniation of the submucosa into the myotomy site, indicative of an adequate myotomy.

INTUSSUSCEPTION
- Usually 3 months to 3 years
- Currant jelly stools (from vascular congestion, <u>not</u> an indication for resection), sausage mass, abdominal distention, RUQ pain, and vomiting

- Invagination of one loop of intestine into another
- Lead points in children – enlarged Peyer's patches (#1), lymphoma, and Meckel's diverticulum
- 15% recurrence after reduction
- Tx: reduce with air-contrast enema → 80% successful; <u>no</u> surgery required if reduced
  - Max pressure with air-contrast enema – **120 mm Hg**
  - Max column height with barium enema – **1 meter (3 feet)**
  - High perforation risk beyond these values → need to proceed to OR if you have reached these values
  - Need to go to OR with peritonitis or free air, or if unable to reduce
    - When reducing in OR, do <u>not</u> place traction on proximal limb of bowel; apply pressure to the distal limb
    - Usually do not require resection unless associated with lead point (Meckel's, etc.)

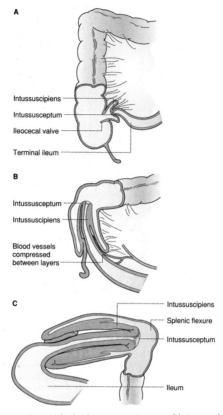

A

Intussuscipiens
Intussusceptum
Ileocecal valve
Terminal ileum

B

Intussusceptum
Intussuscipiens

Blood vessels
compressed
between layers

C

Intussuscipiens
Splenic flexure
Intussusceptum

Ileum

Ileocolic intussusception with the intussusceptum and intussuscipiens indicated.

- **Adults presenting with intussusception** – patient most likely has **malignant lead point** (i.e., colon CA in cecum) → OR

INTESTINAL ATRESIAS
- Develop as a result of **intrauterine vascular accidents**
- Symptoms: bilious emesis, distention; most do not pass meconium
- More common in jejunum; can be <u>multiple</u>
- Get barium enema to R/O Hirschsprung's before surgery
- Tx: resection

DUODENAL ATRESIA
- #1 cause of duodenal obstruction in newborns (<1 week)
- Usually distal to ampulla of Vater and causes **bilious vomiting,** feeding intolerance
- Associated with polyhydramnios in mother
- Associated with cardiac, renal, and other GI anomalies
- 20% of these patients have **Down's syndrome (check chromosomal studies)**
- Abdominal x-ray – shows **double-bubble sign**

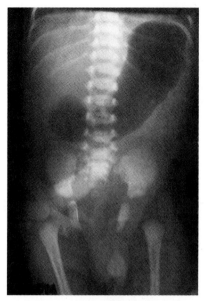

A typical plain film of a newborn with duodenal obstruction demonstrating the "double bubble" sign. (From Oldham KT, Aiken JJ. Congenital pyloric stenosis and duodenal obstruction. In: Fischer JE, Bland KI, et al., eds. *Mastery of Surgery*, 5th ed. Philadelphia, PA: Lippincott Williams & Wilkins; 2007, with permission.)

■ Tx: resuscitation; duodenoduodenostomy or duodenojejunostomy

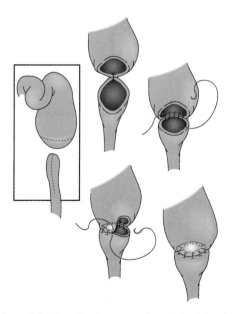

Diamond-shaped duodenoduodenostomy for repair of duodenal atresia.

TRACHEOESOPHAGEAL (TE) FISTULAS
- **Type C** – most common type (80%–90%)
  - **Proximal esophageal atresia (blind pouch) and distal TE fistula**
  - Symptoms: newborn spits up feeds, has excessive drooling, and respiratory symptoms with feeding; cannot place NG tube in stomach
- **Type A** – second most common type (5%–10%)
  - Esophageal atresia and no fistula
  - Symptoms: similar to type C
  - Abdominal x-ray – patients have gasless abdomen
- **Type E** – most likely to present in adulthood (H configuration of esophagus and trachea), not associated with atresia

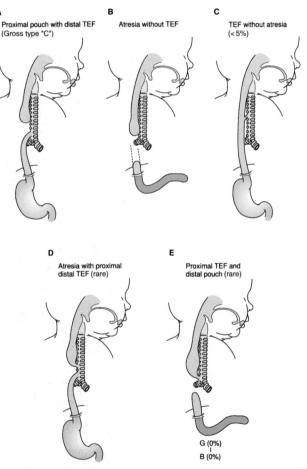

A Proximal pouch with distal TEF (Gross type "C")

B Atresia without TEF

C TEF without atresia (<5%)

D Atresia with proximal distal TEF (rare)

E Proximal TEF and distal pouch (rare)

G (0%)
|
B (0%)

The anatomy of the variants of esophageal atresia (EA) and tracheoesophageal fistula (TEF). (*A*) Proximal pouch with distal TEF (most common type occurring in 85% of patients; gross type "C"). (*B*) Esophageal atresia without TEF (5%). (*C*) TEF without esophageal atresia (<5%). (*D*) Esophageal atresia with proximal and distal TEF (rare). (*E*) Proximal TEF and distal pouch (rare).

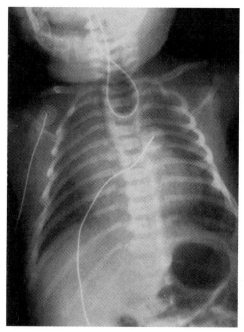

Radiograph demonstrating coiled orogastric tub in the proximal atretic pouch and air below the diaphragm. (From Engum SA, Grosfeld JL. Surgical repair of tracheoesophageal fistula and esophageal atresia. In: Fischer JE, Bland KI, et al., eds. *Mastery of Surgery*, 5th ed. Philadelphia, PA: Lippincott Williams & Wilkins; 2007, with permission.)

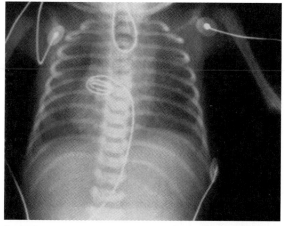

Radiograph of an infant with a blind-ending proximal esophageal pouch containing a Replogle tube and a gasless abdomen, indicating an isolated (type A) esophageal atresia. (From Engum SA, Grosfeld JL. Surgical repair of tracheoesophageal fistula and esophageal atresia. In: Fischer JE, Bland KI, et al., eds. *Mastery of Surgery*, 5th ed. Philadelphia, PA: Lippincott Williams & Wilkins; 2007, with permission.)

- **VACTERL** = **v**ertebral, **a**norectal (imperforate anus), **c**ardiac, **TE** fistula, **r**adius/renal, and **l**imb anomalies
- Tx: **right extrapleural thoracotomy** for most; perform primary repair; and place G-tube
  - Azygos vein often needs to be divided
- **Infants that are premature, <2,500 g, or sick** → Replogle tube, treat respiratory symptoms; delay repair; and place G-tube
- **Complications of repair** – GERD, leak, empyema, stricture, and fistula
- Survival related to birth weight and associated anomalies

MALROTATION
- Sudden onset of bilious vomiting (Ladd's bands cause duodenal obstruction, coming out from the right retroperitoneum); near ligament of Treitz
- Volvulus associated with compromise of the SMA, leading to infarction of the intestine
- Failure of normal counterclockwise rotation (270 degrees)

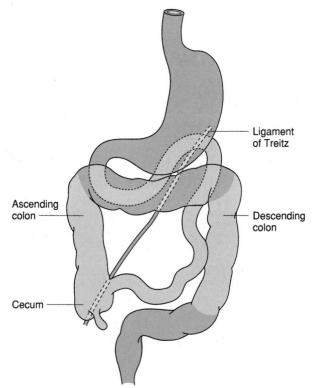

Normal oblique fixation of the midgut mesentery at the ligament of Treitz and in the right lower quadrant. The blue portions of the colon are extraperitoneal.

- 90% present by 1 year of age, 75% in the 1st month
- Any child with bilious vomiting needs a UGI to rule out malrotation
- Dx: UGI duodenum does not cross midline
- Tx: resect Ladd's bands, counterclockwise rotation (may require multiple turns), cecum in LLQ (cecopexy), duodenum in RUQ, and appendectomy

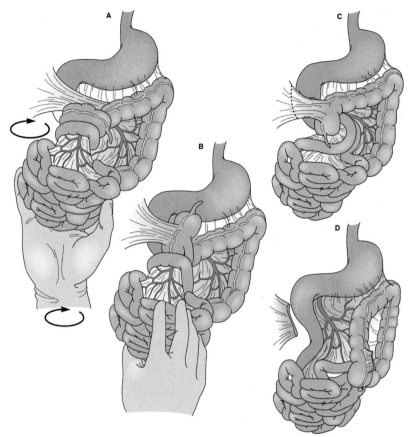

Correction of malrotation. (*A* and *B*) Detorsion of midgut. (*C* and *D*) Division of peritoneal attachments (Ladd's bands) of cecum to abdominal cavity.

MECONIUM ILEUS

- Causes **distal ileal obstruction**, abdominal distention, bilious vomiting, and distended loops of bowel
- Needs sweat chloride test or PCR for Cl channel defect
- Occurs in 10% of children with cystic fibrosis
- Abdominal x-ray: dilated loops of small bowel without air-fluid levels (because the meconium is too thick to separate from the bowel wall); can have ground glass or soap suds appearance
- Can cause perforation, leading to meconium pseudocyst or free perforation → requires laparotomy
- Tx: **Gastrografin enema** (effective in 80%); can also make the diagnosis and potentially treat the patient
- Can also use N-acetylcysteine enema
  - If surgery required, manual decompression and create a vent for **N-acetylcysteine antegrade enemas**

NECROTIZING ENTEROCOLITIS (NEC)
- Classically presents with bloody stools after 1st feeding in **premature infant (occurs in neonates)**
- Risk factors: prematurity, hypoxia, hypotension, anemia, polycythemia, and sepsis
- Symptoms: lethargy, respiratory decompensation, abdominal distention, vomiting, and blood per rectum
- Abdominal x-ray: may show pneumatosis intestinalis, free air, or portal vein air
- Needs serial lateral decubitus films to look for perforation
- Initial Tx: resuscitation, NPO, antibiotics, TPN, and orogastric tube
- Indications for operation: free air, peritonitis, clinical deterioration → resect dead bowel and bring up ostomies
- Needs barium contrast enema before taking down ostomies to rule out distal obstruction from stenosis
- Mortality 10%

CONGENITAL VASCULAR MALFORMATION
- Surgery for hemorrhage, ischemia, CHF, nonbleeding ulcers, functional impairment, and limb-length discrepancy
- Tx: embolization (may be sufficient on its own) and resection

IMPERFORATE ANUS
- More common in males
- Need to check for associated anomalies such as renal, cardiac, and vertebral (VACTERL)
- **High (above levators)** – meconium in **urine or vagina** (fistula to bladder/vagina/prostatic urethra)
  - **Tx**: colostomy, later anal reconstruction with posterior sagittal anoplasty
- **Low (below levators)** – perform **posterior sagittal anoplasty** (pull anus down into sphincter mechanism); **no colostomy needed**
- Need postop anal dilatation to avoid stricture; these patients are prone to constipation

Anatomic Classification of Anorectal Malformations	
Female	Male
HIGH	**HIGH**
Anorectal agenesis with rectovaginal fistula without fistula	Anorectal agenesis with rectoprostatic urethral fistula without fistula
Rectal atresia	Rectal atresia
INTERMEDIATE	
Rectovestibular fistula	Rectobulbar urethral fistula
Rectovaginal fistula	Anal agenesis without fistula
Anal agenesis without fistula	
LOW	
Anovestibular fistula[a]	Anocutaneous fistula[a]
Anocutaneous fistula[a,b]	Anal stenosis[a,c]
Anal stenosis[c]	Rare malformations
Cloacal malformations[d]	
Rare malformations	

[a]Relatively common lesion.
[b]Includes fistulas occurring at the posterior junction of the labia minora, often called *fourchette fistulas* or *vulvar fistulas*.
[c]Previously called *covered anus*.
[d]Previously called *rectocloacal fistulas*. Entry of the rectal fistula into the cloaca may be high or intermediate, depending on the length of the cloacal canal.

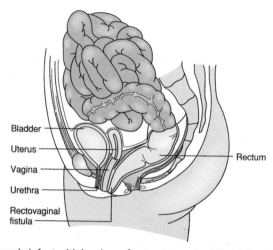

Bladder

Uterus

Vagina

Urethra

Rectovaginal
fistula

Rectum

Female infant with low imperforate anus and vestibular fistula.

GASTROSCHISIS

- **Intrauterine rupture of umbilical vein; does <u>not</u> have a peritoneal sac**
- ↓ congenital anomalies (only 10%) except malrotation
- To the right of midline, no peritoneal sac, stiff bowel from exposure to amniotic fluid
- Tx: initially place saline-soaked gauzes and resuscitate the patient; can lose a lot of fluid from the exposed bowel; TPN, NPO
  - Repair when patient is stable
  - At operation, try to place bowel back in abdomen, may need Vicryl mesh silo
  - Primary closure at a later date if mesh used

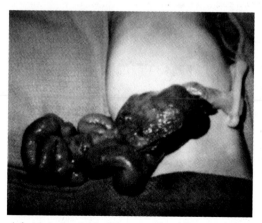

Gastroschisis. The defect is to the right of the normal umbilicus, and the bowel is thickened and inflamed.

OMPHALOCELE

- **Failure of embryonal development**; midline defect
- ↑ congenital anomalies (50%); has peritoneal sac with cord attached
- Sac can contain intra-abdominal structures other than bowel (liver, spleen, etc.)

- ■ **Cantrell pentalogy**
  - **Cardiac** defects
  - **Pericardium** defects (usually at diaphragmatic pericardium)
  - **Sternal** cleft or absence of lower sternum
  - **Diaphragmatic** septum transversum absence
  - **Omphalocele**
- ■ Tx: initially place saline-soaked gauzes and resuscitate the patient; can lose a lot of fluid from the exposed bowel; TPN, NPO
  - Repair when patient is stable
  - At operation, try to place bowel back in abdomen; may need Vicryl mesh silo
  - Primary closure at a later date of mesh used
- ■ Worse overall prognosis compared with gastroschisis secondary to congenital anomalies
- ■ **Malrotation** can occur with both gastroschisis and omphalocele

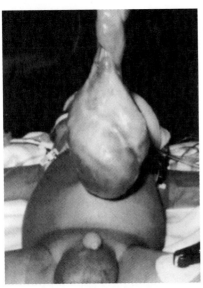

Omphalocele. The herniated intestines and liver are visible inside the sac. The umbilical cord attaches to the sac.

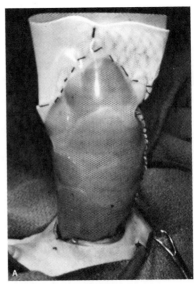

Silastic chimney or silo for temporary coverage of giant omphalocele.

Comparison of Gastroschisis and Omphalocele

Characteristic	Gastroschisis	Omphalocele
Defect size (diameter)	2–3 cm	2–15 cm
Sac	Never	Always, may be ruptured
Gestational age	Prematurity	Term common
Umbilical cord	Left of defect	Attached to sac
Herniated viscera	Small bowel, stomach, colon	Small bowel, stomach, colon, liver
Malrotation	Yes	Yes
Bowel character	Inflammatory, edematous	Normal
Enteral nutrition	Delayed	Normal
Associated anomalies	Uncommon (10% atresia)	Common (50%)

HIRSCHSPRUNG'S DISEASE
- #1 cause of colonic obstruction in infants; more common in males
- **Most common sign** → infants fail to pass meconium in 1st 24 hours
  - Can also present in older age groups as chronic constipation (age 2–3)
- Get distention, some get colitis
- Can get explosive release of watery stool with anorectal exam
- Barium enema can be normal, although often shows a spastic distal segment and dilated proximal segment
- Rectal biopsy diagnostic (**absence of ganglion cells in myenteric plexus**)
- Is due to failure of the neural crest cells (ganglion cells) to progress in craniocaudal direction
- Need to resect colon until proximal to where ganglion cells appear
- Tx: may need to bring up a colostomy initially, eventually connect the colon to the anus (Soave or Duhamel procedure); need colon resection to the point where ganglion cells appear
- Hirschsprung's colitis – may be rapidly progressive; manifested by abdominal distention and foul smelling diarrhea
  - Lethargy and signs of sepsis may be present
- Tx: rectal irrigation; may need emergency colectomy

HYDROCELE
- Most disappear by 1 year; noncommunicating will resolve; should transilluminate
- Tx: surgery at 1 year if not resolved or if thought to be communicating (waxing and waning size); resect hydrocele and ligate processus vaginalis

UMBILICAL HERNIA
- Failure of closure of linea alba; most close by age 3
- Increased in African-Americans and premature infants
- Tx: surgery if not closed by age 5 or incarceration or if patient has a VP shunt

INGUINAL HERNIA
- Due to persistent processus vaginalis; 3% of infants, M > F
- Right in 60%, left in 30%, bilateral in 10%
- Extension of the hernia into the internal ring differentiates hernia from hydrocele
- Tx: emergent operation if not able to reduce; otherwise elective repair with high ligation
- Explore the contralateral side if left sided, female, or child <1 year
- Need operation within next 2–3 days after reduction

CYSTIC DUPLICATION
- Most common in ileum; often on mesenteric border
- Tx: resect cyst

BILIARY ATRESIA
- Most common cause of neonatal jaundice requiring surgery
- Jaundice persisting >2 weeks after birth suggests atresia
- Can involve either the extrahepatic or intrahepatic biliary tree or both
- Progressive jaundice
- Dx: liver biopsy → periportal fibrosis, bile plugging, eventual cirrhosis
  - Ultrasound and cholangiography can reveal atretic biliary tree
- Get cholangitis, continued cirrhosis, and eventual hepatic failure
- Try Kasai procedure (hepaticoportojejunostomy) – ⅓ get better, ⅓ go on to liver transplant, and ⅓ die
  - Involves resecting the atretic extrahepatic bile duct segment

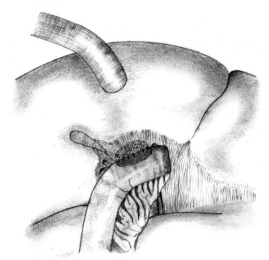

Anastomosis of Roux-en-Y hepatoportoenterostomy to liver. (From Qureshi FG, Ergun O, Ford HR. Biliary atresia. In: Fischer JE, Bland KI, et al., eds. *Mastery of Surgery*, 5th ed. Philadelphia, PA: Lippincott Williams & Wilkins; 2007, with permission.)

■ Need to perform Kasai procedure **before age 3 months**, o/w get irreversible liver damage

OSTEOSARCOMA
■ Can get pulmonary metastases
■ Tx: resection of primary and pulmonary metastases if isolated

TERATOMA
■ ↑ AFP and beta-HCG
■ Neonates – sacrococcygeal; adolescents – ovarian
■ Tx: excision
■ **Sacrococcygeal teratomas**
  • 90% benign at birth (almost all have exophytic component)
  • Great potential for malignancy
  • AFP – good marker
  • 2-month mark is a huge transition – <2 months → usually benign; >2 months → usually malignant
■ Tx: coccygectomy and long-term follow-up

UNDESCENDED TESTICLES
■ Wait until 2 years old to treat
■ Higher risk of testicular CA in these children
■ Cancer risk stays the same even if testicles brought into scrotum
■ Get **seminoma**
■ If undescended bilaterally, get chromosomal studies
■ If you cannot feel the testis in the inguinal canal, you need to get an MRI to confirm their presence
■ Tx: orchiopexy through inguinal incision; if not able to get testicles down → close and wait 6 months and try again; if will not come down, perform division of spermatic vessels

■ **Prune belly syndrome (rare)** – hypoplasia of the abdominal wall, urinary tract abnormalities with dilated urinary system, and bilateral cryptorchidism

LARYNGOMALACIA
- Most common cause of airway obstruction in infants
- Symptoms: intermittent respiratory distress and stridor exacerbation in the supine position
- Caused by immature epiglottis cartilage with intermittent collapse of the epiglottis airway
- Most children outgrow this by 12 months
- Surgical tracheostomy reserved for a small number of patients

CHOANAL ATRESIA
- Obstruction of choanal opening by either bone or mucus membrane, usually unilateral
- Symptoms: intermittent respiratory distress, poor suckling
- Tx: surgical correction

LARYNGEAL PAPILLOMATOSIS
- Most common tumor of the pediatric larynx
- Frequently involutes after puberty
- Can treat with endoscopic removal or laser but frequently comes back
- Thought to be caused from HPV in the mother during passage through the birth canal

CEREBRAL PALSY
- **Many develop GERD**

Neonatal Intestinal Obstruction

Diagnosis	History	Physical Examination	Diagnostic Studies
Intestinal atresia or stenosis	Bilious emesis	Abdominal distention	Plain abdominal film
Duodenal atresia or stenosis	Failure to pass meconium	Acholic meconium	Contrast enema
	Bilious emesis	Gastric distention	Plain abdominal film
		Trisomy 21	Upper GI contrast study
Imperforate anus	Failure to pass meconium	Absent anus or visible fistula	Plain chest, abdominal film
	Bilious emesis (late)	Abdominal distention	Ultrasound kidneys, sacrum, rectum
		VACTERL association	Echocardiogram
Necrotizing enterocolitis	High-risk, premature infant	Abdominal distention	Plain abdominal film
	Bilious emesis	Hematochezia, guaiac-positive stool	
Meconium ileus	Cystic fibrosis (10%)	Acholic meconium	Plain abdominal film
	Bilious emesis	Abdominal distention	Contrast enema
Malrotation	Bilious emesis	No abdominal distention	Plain abdominal film
	Term, healthy infant		Upper GI contrast study
Hirschsprung's disease	Delayed passage of meconium	Abdominal distention	Plain abdominal film
	Bilious emesis	Trisomy 21	Contrast enema
Uncommon causes of obstruction (intussusception, Meckel's diverticulum, duplication)		Abdominal mass, incarcerated hernia	Variable
Medical conditions associated with ileus	Bilious emesis	Sepsis, hypothyroidism, etc.	Plain abdominal film

GI, gastrointestinal; VACTERL, vertebral, anal, cardiac, tracheal, esophageal, renal, and limb anomalies.

4. STATISTICS

Ty... ejects null hypothesis incorrectly → falsely assumed there was a
difference when no difference exists
Type II error – accepts null hypothesis incorrectly because of **small sample size** → the
treatments are interpreted as equal when there is actually a difference
Null hypothesis – hypothesis that no difference exists between groups
    $p < 0.05$ rejects the null hypothesis
$p < 0.05$ = >95% likelihood that the difference between the populations is true
<5% likelihood that the difference is not true and occurred by chance
alone

Variance – spread of data around a mean
Parameter – population
Numeric terms – example: 2, 7, 7, 8, 9, 11, 15
    Mode – most frequently occurring value = 7
    Mean – average = 9
    Median – middle value of a set of data (50th percentile) = 8

TRIALS AND STUDIES
- **Randomized controlled trial** – prospective study with random assignment to
  treatment and nontreatment groups
  - **Avoids treatment biases**
- **Double-blind controlled trial** – prospective study in which patient and doctor are
  blind to the treatment
  - **Avoids observational biases**
- **Cohort study** – prospective study → compares disease rate between exposed and
  unexposed groups (nonrandom assignment)
- **Case–control study** – retrospective study in which those who have the disease are
  compared with a similar population who do not have the disease; the frequency of
  the suspected risk factor is then compared between the 2 groups
- **Meta-analysis** – combining data from <u>different studies</u>

QUANTITATIVE VARIABLES
- **Student's t test** – 2 independent groups and variable is **quantitative** → compares
  means (mean weight between 2 groups)
- **Paired t tests** – variable is **quantitative**; before and after studies (e.g., weight before
  and after, drug versus placebo)
- **ANOVA** – compares **quantitative** variables (means) for more than 2 groups

QUALITATIVE VARIABLES
- **Nonparametric statistics** – compare categorical (qualitative) variables **(race, sex,
  medical problems and diseases, medications)**
- **Chi-squared test** – compares 2 groups with **categorical (qualitative) variables** (number of obese patients with and without diabetes versus number of nonobese patients
  with and without diabetes)
- **Kaplan-Meyer** – small groups → estimates survival

Relative risk = incidence in exposed/incidence in unexposed
Power of test = probability of making the correct conclusion = 1 − probability of type II error
    Likelihood that the conclusion of the test is true
    Larger sample size increases power of a test

Prevalence – number of people with disease in a population (e.g., number of patients in US with colon CA)
    Long-standing disease increases prevalence
Incidence – number of new cases diagnosed over a certain time frame in a population (e.g., number of patients in US newly diagnosed with colon CA in 2003)
Sensitivity – ability to detect disease = true-positives/(true-positives + false-negatives)
    Indicates the number of people who have the disease who test positive
    With high sensitivity, a <u>negative test result means patient is very unlikely to have disease</u>

	Positive Test	**Negative Test**
Have disease	True-positive (TP)	False-negative (FN)
No disease	False-positive (FP)	True-negative (TN)

Specificity – ability to state no disease is present = true-negatives/(true-negatives + false-positives)
    Indicates the number of people who do not have the disease who test negative
    With high specificity, a <u>positive test result means patient is very likely to have disease</u>

Positive predictive value = true-positives/(true-positives + false-positives)
    Likelihood that with a positive result, the patient actually has the disease
Negative predictive value = true-negatives/(true-negatives + false-negatives)
    Likelihood that with a negative result the patient does not have the disease

Accuracy = true-positives + true-negatives/true-positives + true-negatives + false-positives + false-negatives

Predictive value - depends on disease prevalence
Sensitivity and specificity - independent of prevalence

↑	increased *or* high
↓	decreased *or* low
2,3-DPG	2,3-diphosphoglycerate
5FU	5-fluorouracil
AAA	abdominal aortic aneurysm
Ab	antibody
Abd	abdominal
abx	antibiotic
AC	doxorubicin (Adriamycin) and cyclophosphamide (Cytoxan)
ACE	angiotensin-converting enzyme
Ach	acetylcholine
ACT	activated clotting time
ACTH	adrenocorticotropic hormone
AD	autosomal dominant
ADH	antidiuretic hormone
ADL	activities of daily living
AFP	alpha-fetoprotein
Ag	antigen
AIDS	acquired immunodeficiency syndrome
AKA	above-knee amputation
ALL	acute lymphoblastic leukemia
ALND	axillary lymph node dissection
ALT	alanine aminotransferase
angio	angiography
ANOVA	analysis of variance
AP	aortopulmonary
APACHE	acute physiology and chronic health evaluation
APR	abdominoperineal resection
APUD	amine precursor uptake and decarboxylation
ARDS	acute/adult respiratory distress syndrome
ASA	acetylsalicylic acid
ASD	atrial septal defect
AST	aspartate aminotransferase
ATGAM	antithymocyte gamma globulin
AT-III	antithrombin III
ATN	acute tubular necrosis
ATP	adenosine triphosphate
ATPase	adenosine triphosphatase
A-V	arteriovenous
AV	atrioventricular
AVM	arteriovenous malformation
AVN	avascular necrosis
AXR	abdominal radiograph
BCG	bacille Calmette-Guérin
BKA	below-knee amputation
BM	bowel movement
BPH	benign prostatic hyperplasia
BSA	body surface area
BT shunt	Blalock-Taussig shunt
BUN	blood urea nitrogen
Bx	biopsy
Ca	calcium
CA	cancer, carcinoma
CABG	coronary artery bypass graft
cAMP	cyclic adenosine monophosphate
CaO_2	arterial oxygen content
CBD	common bile duct
CCK	cholecystokinin
cCMP	3_,5_-cyclic monophosphate (cytidine)
CD	cluster of differentiation (e.g., CD4, CD8)
CEA	carcinoembryonic antigen
CEA	carotid endarterectomy
cGMP	cyclic guanosine-3,5_-monophosphate
chemo	chemotherapy
CHF	chronic heart failure
CI	cardiac index
CLL	chronic lymphocytic leukemia
CMF	cyclophosphamide (Cytoxan), methotrexate, and 5-fluorouracil
CML	chronic myelogenous leukemia
CMV	cytomegalovirus
CN	cranial nerve
CNS	central nervous system
CO	cardiac output
COPD	chronic obstructive pulmonary disease
CPAP	continuous positive airway pressure
CPP	cerebral perfusion pressure
CPR	cardiopulmonary resuscitation
Cr	creatinine
CRH	corticotropin (ACTH)-releasing hormone
CSA	cyclosporin A
CSF	cerebrospinal fluid
CT	computed tomography
CVA	cerebrovascular accident (stroke)
CVHD	continuous venovenous hemodialysis

CvO$_2$	venous oxygen content	Fc	antibody fragment, crystallizable
CVP	central venous pressure		
Cx	complication	FEV$_1$	forced expiratory volume in 1 second
CXR	chest radiograph		
D/C	discontinue	FFP	fresh frozen plasma
DAG	diacylglycerol	FGF	fibroblast growth factor
DBP	diastolic blood pressure	FiO$_2$	fraction of inspired oxygen
DCIS	ductal carcinoma in situ	FNA	fine needle aspiration
DDAVP	desmopressin acetate, 1-desamino-8-d-arginine-vasopressin	FRC	functional residual capacity
		FSH	follicle-stimulating hormone
		FTSG	full-thickness skin graft
DES	diethylstilbestrol	FTT	failure to thrive
DIC	disseminated intravascular coagulation	Fx	fracture
		G6PD	glucose-6-phosphate dehydrogenase
DIT	diiodotyrosine		
DKA	diabetic ketoacidosis	GCS	Glasgow Coma Scale
DLCO	diffusing capacity of the lung for carbon monoxide	GCSF	granulocyte colony–stimulating factor
DM	diabetes mellitus	GDA	gastroduodenal artery
DPL	diagnostic peritoneal lavage	GERD	gastroesophageal reflux disease
DVT	deep venous thrombosis		
Dx	diagnosis	GFR	glomerular filtration rate
DZ	disease	GH	growth hormone
EBV	Epstein-Barr virus	GHRH	growth hormone–releasing hormone
ECA	external carotid artery		
ECHO	echocardiogram	GI	gastrointestinal
ECMO	extracorporeal membrane oxygenation	GIP	gastric inhibitory peptide
		GIST	gastrointestinal stromal tumors
EDRF	endothelium-derived relaxing factor		
		GNR	gram-negative rods
EDV	end diastolic volume	GnRH	gonadotropin-releasing hormone
EEG	electroencephalogram		
EF	ejection fraction	GPC	gram-positive cocci
EGD	esophagogastroduodenoscopy	GPR	gram-positive rod
EGF	epidermal growth factor	GRP	gastrin-releasing peptide
EKG	electrocardiogram	GSH	glutathione
ELAM	endothelial leukocyte adhesion molecule	GU	genitourinary
		H and P	history and physical
EPI	epinephrine	HA	headache
ER	emergency room or endoplasmic reticulum	HBIG	hepatitis B immunoglobulin
		HBV	hepatitis B virus
ERCP	endoscopic retrograde cholangiopancreatography	HCG	human chorionic gonadotropin
		HCl	hydrochloric acid; hydrochloride
ERV	expiratory reserve volume		
ESR	erythrocyte sedimentation rate	Hct	hematocrit
ESWL	extracorporeal shock wave lithotripsy	HCT	hematocrit
		HCV	hepatitis C virus
ET	endotracheal	HETE	hydroxyeicosatetraenoic acid
ETCO$_2$	end-tidal CO$_2$	HGB/Hgb	hemoglobin
ETOH	ethanol, alcohol	HIDA	hepatic iminodiacetic acid
F/U	follow-up	HIT	heparin-induced thrombocytopenia
FAP	familial adenomatous polyposis		
		HIV	human immunodeficiency virus
FAST	focused abdominal sonography for trauma		

HLA	human leukocyte antigen	LTA$_4$	leukotriene A$_4$
HMG CoA	_-hydroxy-_-methylglutaryl-CoA	LTB$_4$	leukotriene B$_4$
		LTC$_4$	leukotriene C$_4$
HMW	high molecular weight	LTD$_4$	leukotriene D$_4$
HPETE	hydroperoxyeicosatetraenoic acid	LTE$_4$	leukotriene E$_4$
		LV	left ventricle or left ventricular
HPF	high-power field		
HPV	human papillomavirus	LVEDV	left ventricular end-diastolic volume
HR	heart rate		
HSV	herpes simplex virus	LVEF	left ventricular ejection fraction
HTLV-1	human T-cell leukemia virus 1		
HTN	hypertension	LVESV	left ventricular end-systolic volume
HUS	hemolytic uremic syndrome		
HVA	homovanillic acid	LVOT	left ventricular outflow tract
IABP	intra-aortic balloon pump	MAC	minimum alveolar concentration
IBW	ideal body weight		
ICA	internal carotid artery	MALT	mucosal-associated lymphoproliferative tissue
ICAM	intracellular adhesion molecule		
ICP	intracranial pressure	MAO	monoamine oxidase
ICU	intensive care unit	MAOI	monoamine oxidase inhibitor
Ig	immunoglobulin	MAP	mean arterial pressure
IJ	internal jugular vein	MEN	multiple endocrine neoplasia
IL	interleukin	MHC	major histocompatibility complex
IMA	inferior mesenteric artery or internal mammary artery		
		MI	myocardial infarction
IMF	intermaxillary fixation	MIBG	radioactive iodine meta-idobenzoguanidine
IMV	inferior mesenteric vein		
INF	interferon	MIT	monoiodotyrosine
INH	isoniazid	MRA	magnetic resonance angiogram
INR	international normalized ratio		
ITP	idiopathic thrombocytopenic purpura	MRCP	magnetic resonance cholangiopancreatography
IV	intravenous	MRM	modified radical mastectomy
IVC	inferior vena cava	MRND	modified radical neck dissection
IVF	intravenous fluid		
IVP	intravenous pyelogram	MRSA	methicillin-resistant S. aureus
L	liter	MS	mental status
LA	left atrium	MSH	melanocyte-stimulating hormone
LAD	left anterior descending (coronary artery)		
		MTP	metatarsophalangeal
LAK	lymphokine-activated killer	MTX	methotrexate
LATS	long-acting thyroid stimulator	N/V	nausea and vomiting
LAR	low anterior resection	NADH	nicotinamide adenine dinucleotide
LCIS	lobular carcinoma in situ		
LD$_{50}$	dose that will kill 50% of test subjects	NADPH	nicotinamide adenine dinucleotide phosphate
LDH	lactate dehydrogenase	NAPA	n-acetylprocainamide
LES	lower esophageal sphincter	NE	norepinephrine
LFT	liver function test	NEC	necrotizing enterocolitis
LH	luteotropic hormone	NGT	nasogastric tube
LHRH	luteinizing hormone–releasing hormone	NHL	non-Hodgkin's lymphoma
		NIF	negative inspiratory force
LLQ	left lower quadrant	NO	nitric oxide
LR	lactated ringers	NPO	nil per os (nothing by mouth)
LS ratio	lecithin:sphingomyelin ratio	NS	normal saline (solution)

NSAID	nonsteroidal anti-inflammatory drug		PTCA	percutaneous transluminal coronary angioplasty
NSE	neuron-specific enolase		PTFE	polytetrafluoroethylene
NTG	nitroglycerine		PTH	parathyroid hormone
OCP	oral contraceptive pills		PTHrP	parathyroid hormone-related peptide
OKT3	murine monoclonal anti-CD3 antibody therapy		PTT	partial thromboplastin time
Op-DDD	2,4_-dichlorodiphenyl-dichloroethane (mitotane)		PTU	propylthiouracil
			PTX	pneumothorax
OR	operating room		PUD	peptic ulcer disease
ORIF	open reduction and internal fixation		PVC	premature ventricular contraction
PA	pulmonary artery		PVR	pulmonary vascular resistance
PABA	p-aminobenzoic acid		Qp/Qs	pulmonary-to-systemic flow ratio
PADP	pulmonary artery diastolic pressure		R/O	rule out
PAF	platelet-activating factor		RA	right atrium
PAS	periodic acid–Schiff stain		RBC	red blood cell
PCN	penicillin		RLL	right lower lobe
PCR	polymerase chain		RLN	recurrent laryngeal nerve
PDA	patent ductus arteriosus		RND	radical neck dissection
PDGF	platelet-derived growth factor		ROM	range of motion
			RPR	rapid plasma reagin
PE	pulmonary embolism		RQ	respiratory quotient
PECAM	platelet/endothelial cell adhesion molecule		RR	respiratory rate
			RUG	retrograde urethrogram
PEEP	positive end-expiratory pressure		RUL	right upper lobe
			RUQ	right upper quadrant
PEG	percutaneous endoscopic gastrostomy		RV	residual volume
			RV	right ventricle
PGD_2	prostaglandin D_2		S/E	side effect
PGE_1	prostaglandin E_1		S–B	Sengstaken–Blakemore (tube)
PGE_2	prostaglandin E_2		SBFT	small bowel follow-through
PGF_2	prostaglandin F_2		SBO	small bowel obstruction
PGG_2	prostaglandin G_2		SBP	spontaneous bacterial peritonitis
PGH_2	prostaglandin H_2			
PGI_2	prostaglandin I_2 (prostacyclin)		SBP	systolic blood pressure
PMHx	past medical history		SCC	squamous cell carcinoma
PMN	polymorphonuclear leukocytes		SCD	sequential compression device
PNMT	phenylethanolamine-N-methyl-transferase		SCM	sternocleidomastoid
			SCV	subclavian
POD	postoperative day		SFA	superficial femoral artery
PNA	pneumonia		SIRS	systemic inflammatory response syndrome
PPN	peripheral line parenteral nutrition		SLE	systemic lupus erythematosus
PRBC	packed red blood cells		SMA	superior mesenteric artery
PSA	prostate-specific antigen		SMV	superior mesenteric vein
PSSS	postsplenectomy sepsis syndrome		SOB	shortness of breath
			STSG	split-thickness skin graft
PT	prothrombin time		SVC	superior vena cava
PTA	percutaneous transluminal angioplasty		SvO_2	mixed venous oxygen saturation
PTC	percutaneous transhepatic cholangiography		SVR	systemic vascular resistance

SVRI	systemic vascular resistance index	TV	tidal volume
SVT	supraventricular tachycardia	Tx	treatment
Sx	symptom	TXA$_2$	thromboxane A$_2$
T bili	total bilirubin	TXP	transplant
TAG	triacylglyceride	U/S	ultrasound
TAH	total abdominal hysterectomy	UC	ulcerative colitis
		UDCA	ursodeoxycholic acid
TB	tuberculosis	UES	upper esophageal sphincter
TBG	thyroid-binding globulin	UGI	upper gastrointestinal
TCOM	transcutaneous oxygen measurement	URI	upper respiratory tract infection
TCR	T-cell receptor	UTI	urinary tract infection
TE	tracheoesophageal	UV	ultraviolet
TEN	toxic epidermal necrolysis	V/Q	ventilation/perfusion
TFT	thyroid function test	VC	vital capacity
TGF-β	transforming growth factor-beta	VCAM	vascular cell adhesion molecule
TIA	transient ischemic attack	V-fib	ventricular fibrillation
TIPS	transjugular intrahepatic portosystemic shunt	VIP	vasoactive intestinal peptide
TLC	total lung capacity	VIPoma	vasoactive intestinal peptide–producing tumor
TMJ	temporomandibular joint	VLDL	very-low-density lipids
TNF	tumor necrosis factor	VMA	vanillylmandelic acid
TOS	thoracic outlet syndrome	VO$_2$	oxygen consumption
tPA	tissue plasminogen activator	VP-16	etoposide
TPN	total parenteral nutrition	VRE	vancomycin-resistant *Enterococcus*
TRALI	transfusion-related acute lung injury	VSD	ventricular septal defect
TRAM	transverse rectus abdominis myocutaneous	V-tach	ventricular tachycardia
		vWD	von Willebrand's disease
TRH	thyrotropin-releasing hormone	vWF	von Willebrand factor
		W/U	workup
TSH	thyroid-stimulating hormone	WBC	white blood cell
TSI	thyroid-stimulating immunoglobulin	WDHA	watery diarrhea, hypokalemia, achlorhydria
TTP	thrombotic thrombocytopenic purpura	wedge	pulmonary artery wedge pressure
TURP	transurethral resection of the prostate; transurethral prostatectomy	WLE	wide local excision
		XRT	radiation therapy
		Z–E/ZES	Zollinger–Ellison syndrome

INDEX

Note: Page numbers in *italics* denote figures; those followed by a t denote tables

A